Hormone
Replacement
Therapy

Hormone Replacement Therapy

Edited by

Donald P. Swartz, M.D.
Professor and Head
Division of General Gynecology
Albany Medical College
Albany, New York

WILLIAMS & WILKINS
BALTIMORE • HONG KONG • LONDON • MUNICH
PHILADELPHIA • SYDNEY • TOKYO

Editor: Charles W. Mitchell
Managing Editor: Victoria M. Vaughn
Copy Editor: Thomas Lehr
Designer: Karen Klinedinst
Illustration Planner: Ray Lowman
Production Coordinator: Kathleen C. Millet
Cover Designer: Dan Pfisterer

Accurate indications, adverse reactions, and dosage schedules for drugs are provided in this book, but it is possible that they may change. The reader is urged to review the package information data of the manufacturers of the medications mentioned.

Printed in the United States of America

Library of Congress Cataloging-in-Publication Data

Hormone replacement therapy / edited by Donald P. Swartz.
p. cm.
Includes bibliographical references and index.
ISBN 0-683-08035-0
1. Menopause—Hormone therapy. 2. Osteoporosis—Hormone therapy. 3. Estrogen—Therapeutic use. I. Swartz, Donald P.
[DNLM: 1. Cardiovascular System—drug effects. 2. Estrogen Replacement Therapy. 3. Menopause—drug effects. 4. Osteoporosis—drug therapy. WP 580 H812]
RG186.H67 1992
618.1'75061—dc20
DNLM/DLC
for Library of Congress 91–40213
CIP

92 93 94 95 96
1 2 3 4 5 6 7 8 9 10

This book is dedicated to Dr. Georgeanna S. Jones, who did so much to strengthen my very early interest in reproductive endocrinology. As a result I am deeply indebted to her for opening many doors along my career path.

Preface

The study and practice of replacing the ovarian sex hormones in the woman who has reduced production of those hormones either through aberrant development, physiologic senescence, or surgical removal of ovaries is an area of exciting and rapidly advancing new knowledge. The philosophy followed for the first three or four decades after the identification of the ovarian sex steroid hormones—that their prescription should be for the briefest possible time required to alleviate specific acute vasomotor symptoms—is changing rapidly in response to a wealth of new information. The very diverse physiologic role of these hormones and the growing evidence for the pathology that results from their long-term deficiency are combining in a powerful way to change long-held beliefs.

The new knowledge is evolving at a time when all of the more advanced countries of the world are realizing that older women and specifically postmenopausal women are constituting as much as one-third of the female population, and also that those women are expected to survive another one-third of their lives in that state. Thus, the prospect that the new research may provide clear evidence for preventive health measures that can have a very substantive impact on even the two major areas of osteoporosis and cardiovascular disease has become a powerful stimulus to further investigation. Numerous investigators are exploring questions such as which patients can benefit the most from hormone administration on a longer-term basis; which patients should be excluded from such administration; how long should hormone therapy be continued; how late in life is commencement of hormone administration useful; can other therapeutic modalities substitute for hormone administration; what adjunctive measures can be employed along with hormone administration to obtain maximum preventive health benefit; and what safety parameters are involved in the administration of preventive hormonal therapy to a very large population of apparently healthy but generally elderly women? All of these questions are prompting a rapid expansion of research in this area.

It has been both a challenge and a privilege to have the opportunity to gather an international group of experts in this field to author the chapters of this publication. All are too scholarly to pretend that the answers to the listed questions can be found within these pages. However, a very serious effort has been made to bring the reader up to date across the spectrum of knowledge in the field at present and to point the reader in the directions toward which our knowledge seems to be moving at this time.

I am deeply indebted to all of the chapter contributors: Dr. Peter Horvath, Dr. Robert Lindsay, Dr. Charles Chesnut, Dr. Bruce Ettinger, Dr. Barbara A. Drinkwater, Dr. Graham A. Colditz, Dr. Malcolm I. Whitehead, Dr. David Crook, Mr. J. C. Stevenson, Dr. Paul Stumpf, Dr. Morrie M. Gelfand, and Dr. William T. Creasman. All are active researchers and recognized authorities in the areas that they have discussed.

I know that each contributor shares a common hope that this work will provide a broad overview of the rapidly advancing knowledge concerning ovarian sex steroid hormone replacement for the ovarian deficient woman and that it will encourage the reader to incorporate current knowledge into clinical practice and to consider further investigation in the field.

Donald P. Swartz, M.D.

Acknowledgments

First I want to acknowledge the support of my wife, Liz, who accepts so gracefully my busy life which is accentuated by these undertakings.

And without the skills and efforts of Laura Olf, my Divisional Secretary, I would neither have commenced nor finished the project.

Charles Mitchell of Williams & Wilkins deserves special credit for seeing the book through the processes of the merger of two publishers and for all of his assistance along the way.

Finally as editor, I wish to express my very deep personal appreciation to all of the chapter contributors who have given so generously of their time and expertise to this effort.

Contributors

Charles H. Chesnut III, M.D.
Department of Radiology
University of Washington School of Medicine
Seattle, Washington

Graham A. Colditz, M.D.
Associate Professor of Medicine
Harvard Medical School
Epidemiologist
Brigham and Women's Hospital
Boston, Massachusetts

Felicia Cosman, M.D.
Helen Hayes Hospital
Regional Bone Center
West Haverstraw, New York
Assistant Professor of Clinical Medicine
Columbia University
College of Physicians and Surgeons
New York, New York

William T. Creasman, M.D.
Sims-Hester Professor and Chairman
Department of Obstetrics and Gynecology
Medical University of South Carolina
Charleston, South Carolina

David Crook, Ph.D.
Laboratory Director
Wynn Institute for Metabolic Research
London, England

Barbara L. Drinkwater, Ph.D.
Department of Medicine
Pacific Medical Center
Seattle, Washington

Bruce Ettinger, M.D.
Division of Research
Kaiser Permanente Medical Care Program
Oakland, California

R. Don Gambrell Jr., M.D.
Clinical Professor of Endocrinology and Obstetrics and Gynecology
Department of Physiology and Endocrinology
Medical College of Georgia
Augusta, Georgia

Morrie M. Gelfand, M.D.
Professor
Department of Obstetrics and Gynecology
McGill University
Montreal, Quebec, Canada

Peter M. Horvath, M.D.
Assistant Professor
Division of Reproductive Endocrinology
Department of Obstetrics and Gynecology
Albany Medical College
Albany, New York

Robert Lindsay, M.D.
Chief, Internal Medicine
Helen Hayes Hospital
Regional Bone Center
West Haverstraw, New York
Professor of Clinical Medicine
Columbia University
College of Physicians and Surgeons
New York, New York

Meir J. Stampfer, M.D., Dr. P.H.
Assistant Professor of Medicine
Harvard Medical School
Associate Professor of Epidemiology
Harvard School of Public Health
Physician
Brigham and Women's Hospital
Boston, Massachusetts

John C. Stevenson, M.B., M.R.C.P.
Consultant Endocrinologist
Wynn Institute for Metabolic Research
London, England

Paul G. Stumpf, M.D.
Clinical Associate Professor of Obstetrics and Gynecology
University of Medicine and Dentistry of New Jersey
Robert Wood Johnson Medical School
New Brunswick, New Jersey
Program Director of Obstetrics and Gynecology
Director of Reproductive Endocrinology
Jersey Shore Medical Center
Neptune, New Jersey

Donald P. Swartz, M.D.
Professor
Department of Obstetrics and Gynecology
Albany Medical College
Albany, New York

Malcolm I. Whitehead, M.B., F.R.C.O.G.
Senior Lecturer/Consultant Gynaecologist
King's College School of Medicine and Dentistry
London, England

Introduction

It is usually estimated that in the 1990s there will be 50 million or more women in the United States who have become deficient in the production of the two main sex steroid hormones, estrogen and progesterone. Those who do not have ovarian tissue will also be relatively more deficient in testosterone. By far the greatest number of these women will have experienced a physiologic menopause, while an unknown smaller number of younger women will be deficient in one or more of the sex steroid hormones for other reasons:

Genetic (e.g., 45 × 0 karyotype and other variants)
Polycystic ovarian syndrome
Premature menopause
Resistant ovary syndrome
Surgical removal
Radiation therapy

In the United States, the average life expectancy of a woman who becomes deficient in ovarian hormones at the time of her menopause is approximately another 30 years. For the other causes of deficiency of ovarian hormone production listed above and occurring in much younger women, the expected life span in that deficiency state can be much longer.

The concept and philosophy of replacing one or more of the sex steroid hormones in the ovarian deficient woman have undergone classic pendulum-like vacillations typical of almost every medical discovery. Despite tremendous advances in knowledge in this area in the recent 15 years, there are many areas of incomplete scientific information, and this fact helps to perpetuate longstanding and strongly held views and practices not based on scientific evidence. Throughout the medical community, an entire spectrum of practices can still be found, such as "If you don't need hormones, don't take them"; "If you are really having trouble, take the hormone(s) for the shortest possible time and then stop." Prior to the 1975 publicity regarding an increased risk of

endometrial cancer in estrogen replacement users there was a rather strong medical and lay advocacy that hormone replacement therapy was a panacea to prevent aging, and that view was popularized by the expression "feminine forever." Following the 1975 publication of a study finding increased cancer risk in women using estrogen, many physicians adopted a completely negative view and announced to women patients, including those with marked estrogen deficiency symptoms, that they would not prescribe hormones.

The growth of scientific information since 1975 in the field has been rapid and voluminous. It is the purpose of this text to bring together a body of knowledge that can serve as a practical guide to any physician or other health provider who cares for women. The text is intended to be a summation of knowledge that specifically points toward the place of sex hormone replacement in medical practice. It would appear that new knowledge has moved practice in this area away from some of the empiric views mentioned above and toward a philosophy much closer to that of physiologic hormonal replacement practiced in all the other areas of hormonal deficiency. Perhaps one of the reasons for the slow evolution of a replacement philosophy with respect to sex steroid hormones compared, for example, to thyroid or pancreatic hormonal replacement may be the difference in the timing of the hormonal deficiency syndromes that result. In the case of thyroxin or insulin deficiency, the results are noted immediately in the form of well-known and relatively easily recognized derangements of physiology that are labeled as disease states.

The concept of sex hormonal replacement, on the other hand, except for the treatment of vaginal atrophy or the vasomotor symptoms of acute estrogen withdrawal, has required the much slower evolution of the concept of preventive health maintenance—maintenance of the potential for a better quality of life. This approach to the practice of sex hormone replacement has gained most of its impetus from two large, recent areas of study and emphasis: the role of the sex steroid hormones in the maintenance of bone mineral content with the resultant delay in the development or actual prevention of osteoporosis, and the many studies that point to a beneficial lipid and/or cardiovascular effect that may be a factor in reducing morbidity and mortality from cardiovascular disease. As in every medical intervention, therapeutic or preventive, there is a balance of risk and benefit. Medical practice has traditionally and properly practiced more critical and longer-delayed endorsement of preventive health measures than of life-saving and disease-treating therapeutic measures.

In the area of sex hormone replacement, the risks that have been most

Contents

1

Sex Steroids: Physiology and Metabolism

Peter M. Horvath

This is a book about hormonal replacement therapy in the ovarian deficient patient. While the emphasis of the book is clearly clinical, a basic scientific understanding of the physiology and metabolism of hormones is a necessary prerequisite to their judicious and safe use. In this context, it is the purpose of this chapter to provide a scientific framework that reviews basic concepts of steroid hormone synthesis, metabolism, and mechanism of action, upon which the clinician can build clinical decision making in utilizing these agents for exogenous replacement.

STEROIDOGENESIS

Steroidogenesis is the complex array of reactions that lead to the production of biologically active steroids. These reactions are primarily localized in two glands in the woman of reproductive age: the ovary and the adrenal cortex. (During pregnancy, the placenta is an additional organ that is capable of steroidogenesis, but this is another topic.) Even within these organs, steroid synthesis takes place only in certain specialized cells that contain the necessary substrates and enzymes, and the reactions occur only when appropriately stimulated.

The basic steroid skeleton is the cholestane ring (Fig. 1.1). There are four internal rings and 27 carbon atoms in the skeleton. Virtually all important naturally occurring steroids have this basic structure. The numbering system, which initially seems confusing, is actually straightforward. Further, it is important to understand, because the basic type of steroid (estrogen, progestin, androgen, or corticoid) can often be discerned simply by counting the number of carbon atoms present in the molecule. From cholesterol and its 21-carbon derivative pregnenolone (Fig. 1.2) are derived all classes of steroids: progestins (C_{21}), mineralocorticoids and glucocorticoids (C_{21}), androgens (C_{19}), and estrogens (C_{18}). For the purposes of this chapter we will concentrate only on the major sex steroids. Many enzymes are involved in

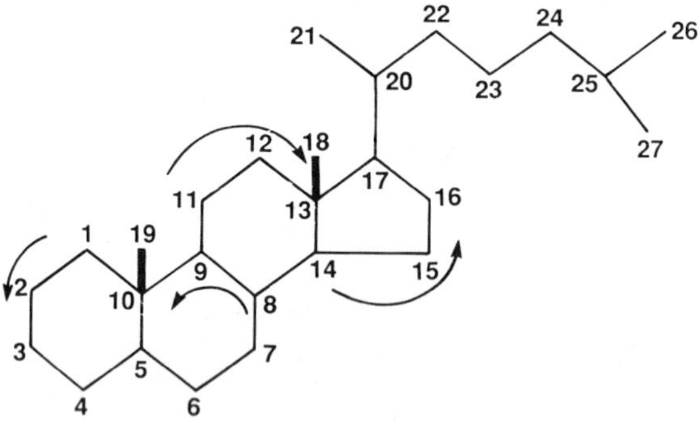

Figure 1.1. Cholestane ring.

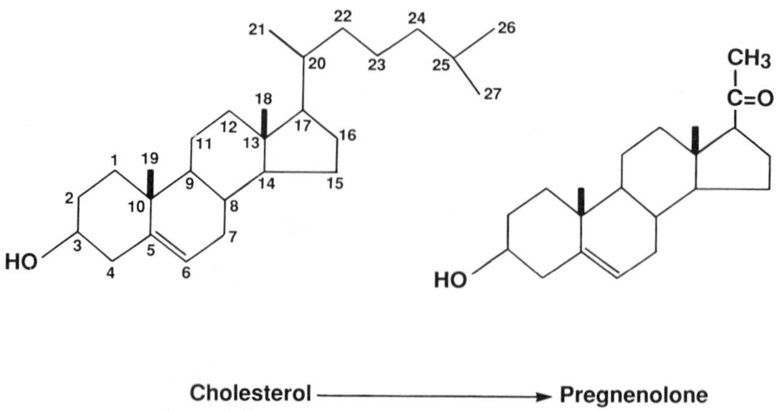

Figure 1.2. Cholesterol and pregnenolone.

these transformations from cholesterol. Some of the more important enzymes and their actions are listed in Table 1.1. The major interactions of these enzymes are schematically outlined in Figure 1.3.

Cholesterol can be synthesized de novo from acetate (except in the placenta) or can be ingested in the diet. Numerous studies have shown that ingested cholesterol, rather than de novo synthesized cholesterol, is the preferred substrate for subsequent synthesis to pregnenolone. Plasma cholesterol is carried in large molecules called lipoproteins.

There are five classes of lipoproteins, which are derived from each other in the following order of decreasing size and increasing density: chylomicrons, very low-density lipoproteins (VLDLs), intermediate-density lipoproteins (IDLs), low-density lipoproteins (LDLs), and high-density lipoproteins

Table 1.1.
Major Enzymes and Reactions of Steroidogenesis

Enzyme	Action	Location
17-hydroxylase/ 17-20 lyase	Hydroxylation of C-21 steroids at 17-position and conversion of C-21 steroids to C-19 steroids	Microsomal
3-B-ol dehydrogenase Δ^4-5-isomerase	Conversion of the 3-hydroxyl group to a ketone, and transfer of the double bond from the 5-6 to the 4-5 position	Microsomal
21-hydroxylase	Hydroxylation of C-21 steroids at 21-position	Microsomal
11-hydroxylase	Hydroxylation of C-21 steroids at 11-position	Mitochondrial
17-hydroxysteroid dehydrogenase	Reversible: interconversion of hydroxyl and ketone group at 17-position	Cytosol
Aromatase	Conversion of C-19 steroids to phenolic C-18 steroids	Microsomal

(HDLs). The primary carrier for cholesterol is LDL, and specific high-affinity receptors for LDL have been isolated in steroid-synthesizing cells.

The specific type of steroid synthesized and subsequently secreted by a given organ depends on the particular complement of enzymes that organ contains. For example, the ovary lacks significant 21-hydroxylase and 11-hydroxylase activity; the ovarian steroidogenic pathway, therefore, is shunted toward the production of sex steroids (Fig. 1.3). The zona glomerulosa of the adrenal gland, on the other hand, lacks 17-hydroxylase activity; its secretory products are therefore limited to the mineralocorticoids, particularly aldosterone.

One point of nomenclature should be mentioned because it is occasionally used when abbreviating and referring to certain steroids. Figure 1.3 shows that pregnenolone conversion may proceed along one of two pathways. The first is the so-called Δ^4-3-ketone pathway toward progesterone; the second, the Δ^5-3-β-hydroxysteroid pathway to 17-hydroxy-progesterone. An example of this nomenclature is the abbreviation for androstenedione, often referred to as Δ^4A.

Ovarian Steroidogenesis

Ovarian steroidogenesis occurs in different cells or compartments within the ovary and to a large extent is dependent on pituitary hormone stimulation.

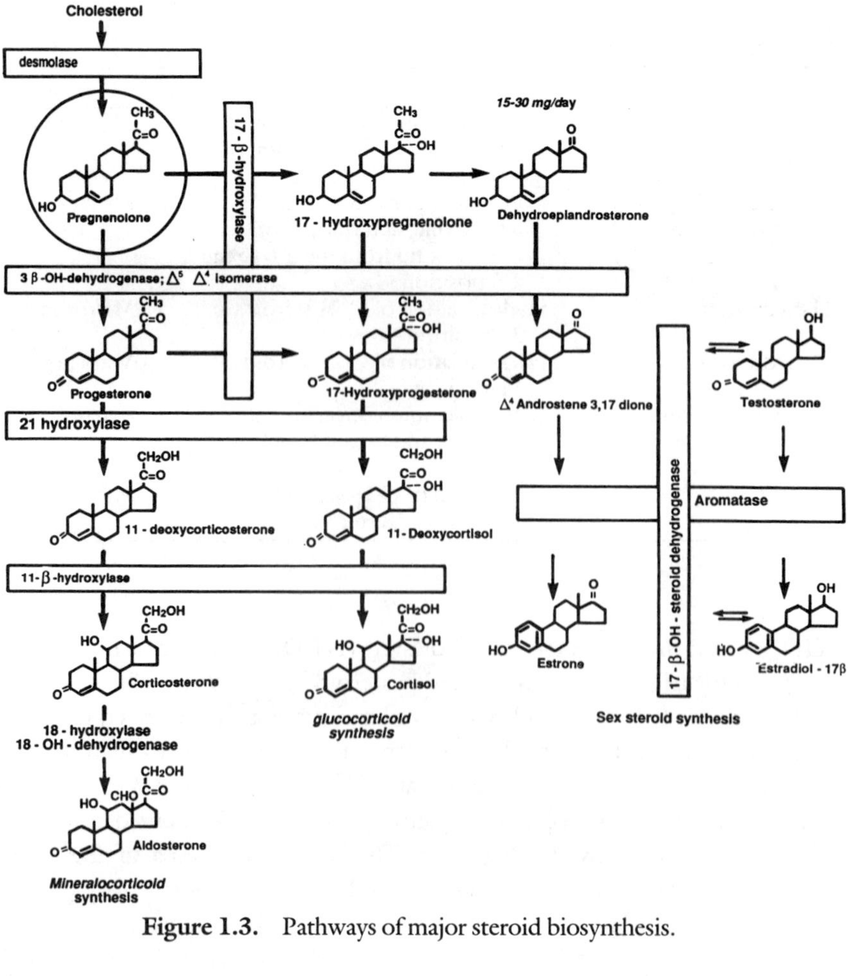

Figure 1.3. Pathways of major steroid biosynthesis.

The ovarian steroidogenic activity in these compartments is responsible for the coordination of the normal menstrual cycle and for the cyclic occurrence of ovulation in the woman of reproductive age. The first compartment is the ovarian stroma, which is composed of tissue originally derived from the thecal layer of developing ovarian follicles. These stromal (thecal) cells respond to pituitary gonadotropins, notably luteinizing hormone (LH), by producing androgens. The most important are Δ^4A and testosterone (T). These androgens are important because they serve as precursors for estrogen formation in a second compartment, the ovarian granulosa. Another androgen, dehydroepiandrosterone (DHEA), is also produced in the ovary; however, the majority (90%) is produced in the adrenal cortex (see below).

Once produced in the theca, androgens diffuse into the granulosa layer, where they are converted by aromatization into estrogens, especially estradiol (E_2). Pituitary follicle-stimulating hormone (FSH) stimulates this aromatase activity and thus enhances E_2 formation. Estradiol in turn enhances FSH activity in the granulosa. Under the influence of pituitary gonadotropins, the ovarian theca and the granulosa work together to coordinate ovarian steroidogenic activity so as to induce progressive follicular growth and development, and ultimately cyclic ovulation.

Parenthetically it should be noted that the normal follicular selection mechanisms and ovulatory processes are much more wondrous and complex than just outlined. (More complete discussions of the subject can be found in the books by Yen and Jaffe, Speroff et al., and Richardson (1–3). In addition to pituitary gonadotropins and ovarian steroids, many other substances affect these processes both directly and indirectly. One of the more important substances in this group is a dimeric peptide called inhibin (or folliculostatin). Inhibin is synthesized by the granulosa (or, in men, Sertoli) cells in response to FSH stimulation and is secreted into the follicular fluid and the ovarian venous effluent. The primary regulatory effect of inhibin is to inhibit FSH secretion by the pituitary. This negative feedback effect of inhibin is important in facilitating the emergence of the dominant follicle during the early to mid-follicular phase of the ovarian cycle. As inhibin levels rise in parallel with E_2, FSH support is withdrawn from the total cohort of recruited follicles. Only the single (dominant) follicle that is most sensitive to FSH continues to grow despite waning FSH levels; the lesser follicles become atretic and resorb.

Postmenopausally, ovarian granulosa function diminishes. In an attempt to stimulate ovarian activity—and E_2 production—pituitary gonadotropin levels increase. Loss of inhibin from aging granulosa may explain why FSH levels rise prior to LH levels during the early climacteric. Additionally, lack of inhibin may explain the inability of exogenous replacement therapy to fully suppress FSH to premenopausal levels. Despite high gonadotropin levels, the failing ovary cannot respond, and E_2 levels fall. The ovarian stroma is somewhat more resilient than the granulosa. Ovarian Δ^4A and T production therefore increases in response to elevated gonadotropins during the first few postmenopausal years. Thereafter, the stroma becomes atrophic as well, and levels of ovarian androgens fall in the older postmenopausal woman.

Adrenal Steroidogenesis

The zona reticularis of the adrenal cortex is the primary adrenal production site of sex steroids, particularly androgens. This zone is absent in young children, develops gradually beginning at about 6 years of age, and has a rapid period of growth and differentiation during puberty. The major androgens secreted by the adult adrenal cortex are DHEA, its sulfate (DHEAS), and Δ^4A.

Quantitatively, DHEA and DHEAS are the most abundantly produced adrenal androgens; however, they are the least potent biologically. Despite their abundance, the physiologic role of these Δ^5 steroids is unclear. Extraglandular conversion into the Δ^4 steroids (androstenedione and testosterone) or extraglandular aromatization to estrogens (see below) occurs in insignificant amounts only. As mentioned, the rise in DHEAS levels begins with the onset of puberty. Levels peak during the twenties and gradually decline thereafter. DHEAS levels can thus be utilized as a general hormonal marker of aging. This has led some to speculate that these steroids may be somehow important in certain biological events associated with the aging process.

Androstenedione is produced in significant amounts in both the adrenal gland and the ovary. Adrenal production varies with adrenocorticotropic hormone (ACTH) stimulation and thus has a circadian (diurnal) variation, with peak output occurring in the morning hours. Ovarian production is dependent on gonadotropin stimulation and thus varies with the time in the menstrual cycle. From a metabolic perspective, Δ^4A is an important androgen, in that it has a dual potential for conversion into more potent androgens or into estrogens. For example, peripheral conversion of Δ^4A to T (see below) accounts for approximately 50% of the total daily production of T in normal women. Additionally, Δ^4A can be aromatized, both peripherally and in the ovarian follicle, into estrone (E_1), a weak estrogen that can be further processed to the potent estrogen E_2.

Peripheral Tissue Metabolism

Glandular (ovarian and adrenal) production of sex steroids does not account for the total amount of these steroids present in the body. Significant peripheral metabolism occurs in extraglandular sites. This metabolism includes conversion of weak androgens into the more potent androgens, conversion of androgens into estrogens, and catabolism (breakdown and excretion) of steroids.

Liver, blood, skin, fat, and skeletal muscle possess 17-hydroxysteroid dehydrogenase activity, which is responsible for the conversion of Δ^4A to T. As much as 30% of this conversion takes place in the liver. DHEA is not converted to T in significant amounts in the normal woman.

In addition to serving as a precursor for conversion into T, Δ^4A also serves as a substrate for conversion into the weak estrogen E_1. This conversion (aromatization) occurs largely in muscle and in adipose tissue, although other sites (such as skin) also possess aromatizing activity. Of the 3 mg of Δ^4A produced per day, approximately 1% is peripherally converted to E_1; this accounts for nearly one-third of the daily E_1 production.

Extraglandular production of estrogens may be excessive in numerous pathophysiologic states, including polycystic ovarian syndrome (PCOS), obesity, Cushing's syndrome, and thyroid disease. Aromatase activity in adipose tissue also increases with aging, and this accounts for the large (two- to fourfold) increase in peripheral E_1 production in the elderly. Over a period of time, increased peripheral conversion of androgens into estrogens results in an (acyclic) hyperestrogenic state. This may cause serious clinical pathology such as endometrial hyperplasia, with its attendant risks of hemorrhage and neoplastic change. Intermittent exposure to progestins is necessary to avoid the risks of long-term unopposed estrogen.

Steroid excretion is largely via the biliary and urinary systems and is accomplished by hepatic conjugation of steroids with various acids (such as glucuronic and sulfuric acid). Conjugation diminishes or inactivates the biological potency of most steroids, and serves as an essential step in deactivation preliminary to excretion. Estrogens, androgens and progestins are all excreted via similar mechanisms.

STEROID TRANSPORT

The major sex steroids circulate in the bloodstream bound to carrier proteins. Sex hormone binding globulin (SHBG), a β-globulin with a molecular weight of about 80,000 to 90,000, is the primary carrier for E_2 and T. SHBG binds T very avidly; E_2 is also strongly bound, but only about one-third as strongly as T. Cortisol, many other corticoids, and progesterone (P) are carried primarily by another hepatically synthesized protein, corticosteroid-binding globulin (CBG, or transcortin). Additionally, most major hormones are bound loosely by albumin. Current evidence indicates that hormone-carrier protein complexes may have some functional role in target cell uptake or other cellular processes; however, it is generally felt that effective biological action of the major steroids is restricted to the free, unbound fraction of hormone. In other words, free hormone is biologically active; bound hormone is not. This is important, because the majority of hormone exists in its bound state (Table 1.2), and routine clinical laboratory assessments of hormone levels measure total hormone (bound plus free), not the biologically active fraction. Thus, only a small percentage of hormone circulates in its free, biologically active form in the bloodstream.

Numerous factors affect SHBG levels (Table 1.3). Due to the positive influence of estrogens on SHBG production by the liver, adult women have about twice as much circulating SHBG as adult men. Because SHBG levels are highly sensitive to the estrogen and androgen milieu (estrogen stimulatory/androgen inhibitory), the amount of circulating SHBG is of primary importance in controlling the balance between biologically active estrogens and androgens. When SHBG levels are altered, therefore, clinically important changes can occur in the action of the major sex steroids.

One clinical example of how alterations in SHBG can have significant clinical effects is in women with PCOS. The pathophysiology of PCOS is certainly complex; indeed, women with PCOS represent a very heterogeneous group. Nevertheless, the "classical" patient with PCOS—the patient with so-called Stein-Levinthal syndrome—is worth discussing briefly. A historical perspective and thorough pathophysiologic discussion of PCOS can be found in Futterweit's text (4).

Table 1.2.
Binding of Major Sex Hormones to Plasma Carrier Proteins

Hormone	Percent Bound		Percent Free
	SHBG	Albumin	
Estradiol	40	59	1
Testosterone	60	38	2
Dihydrotestosterone	80	18	2

Table 1.3.
Factors Affecting Sex Hormone Binding Globulin Levels

Hormone Class	Effect
Estrogens	Increase
Thyroid hormones	Increase
Androgens	Decrease
Progestins[a]	Decrease
Glucocorticoids	Decrease

[a]Particularly 19-nor progestins.

The typical Stein-Levinthal patient is one who is obese, oligo- or anovulatory, and hirsute. Patients with PCOS have inappropriately elevated LH release and low or low-normal FSH secretion. Persistently elevated LH stimulates the ovarian theca and causes a state of hyperandrogenemia, which causes hirsutism. Elevated androgen precursors are in turn available for extraglandular conversion to estrogens (particularly in muscle and fat), and a chronic acyclic hyperestrogenic state results. Such chronically elevated estrogen suppresses FSH and causes a failure in the recycling mechanism. Oligoovulation, or complete failure of ovulation, results. As already mentioned, if left untreated, chronic unopposed estrogen stimulation of the endometrium will cause hyperplasia, hemorrhage, and potential neoplastic change. Progestational therapy must be utilized intermittently or continuously (such as in the oral contraceptive pill) to avoid these risks.

Key Points

- Steroidogenesis occurs primarily in the ovary and in the adrenal glands in women of reproductive age.
- Dietary cholesterol is the primary substrate for steroidogenesis.
- Ovarian steroidogenesis is compartmentalized: the granulosa cells synthesize estrogens and progestins; the stromal (thecal) cells synthesize androgens.
- Ovarian steroid production is stimulated by pituitary gonadotropins: follicle stimulating hormone (FSH) and luteinizing hormone (LH).
- Gonadotropins and sex steroids have an intricate feedback mechanism, which is responsible for cyclic ovarian function in the woman of reproductive age; this cyclic function is further modulated by many non-steroidal substances such as the peptide inhibin.
- Dehydroepiandrosterone (DHEA) and its sulfate (DHEAS) are the most abundant adrenal androgens. DHEAS can be utilized as a marker for adrenal function and aging.
- Significant metabolism of steroids occurs in peripheral tissues, notably aromatization of androgens into estrogens, which occurs primarily in muscle and fat.
- Steroids circulate bound to carrier proteins. Sex hormone binding globulin (SHBG) is the primary carrier for estradiol and testosterone. Bound

hormone is biologically inactive; only free, unbound hormone exerts biological effects.

- The steroid milieu affects SHBG levels (estrogen stimulates SHBG production; androgen inhibits it). Alterations in SHBG levels may consequently affect the availability of biologically active steroids.

References

1. Yen SSC, Jaffe RB. Reproductive endocrinology. Philadelphia: WB Saunders Company, 1986.
2. Speroff L, Glass RH, Kase NG. Clinical gynecologic endocrinology and infertility. 4th ed. Baltimore: Williams & Wilkins, 1989.
3. Richardson GS. Steroidogenesis. In: Sciarra JJ, ed. Gynecology and obstetrics. 11th ed. New York: Harper and Row, 1987; 5.
4. Futterweit W. Polycystic ovarian disease. New York: Springer-Verlag, 1984.

2

The Perimenopause

Donald P. Swartz

Menopause is usually accepted to have occurred when no menses have taken place for 12 months, providing the woman is not pregnant. Some define the menopause as occurring when the interval from the last menstrual flow has persisted for 6 months. The perimenopause cannot be defined so precisely. The semantic precision might be improved by discarding the term perimenopause and using the term premenopause to designate the time in a woman's life during which some symptoms or signs of approaching menopause begin to appear; then, when her duration of amenorrhea fits the definition of menopause, the term menopause could be employed. Climacteric, although synonymous with menopause, is sometimes used as a comprehensive term encompassing the period of time that includes the premenopausal era when some signs or symptoms of approaching menopause begin to appear, the period of acute menopausal symptoms, and a period of years following the menopause when some menopausal symptoms may persist and, in addition, the late changes of estrogen deficiency begin to appear.

The spontaneous cessation of menses occurs between the approximate ages of 40 to 60 years. If it occurs earlier than age 40, it is called premature menopause. The cessation of menses is presumed to occur because of the exhaustion of ovarian follicles. The fetal supply of follicles numbering 7 million is reduced at birth to 2 million and by puberty to 300,000. Throughout the remainder of the woman's premenopausal years this number is eventually completely depleted. In the immediate premenopausal phase, it is believed that there are a smaller number of primordial follicles remaining to be stimulated by follicle-stimulating hormone (FSH) in the normal cyclic fashion. Thus, quantitatively it is felt that total estrogen production in a given cycle becomes somewhat less than it was in the normal cycles throughout the regularly ovulating years. The diminution in the estrogen negative feedback to the pituitary allows FSH in particular to rise. During this premenopausal era, rather wide fluctuations in FSH can be noted.

There is evidence that, during these early premenopausal changes, there can be some beginning acceleration of loss of bone mineral content from the bony skeleton as well as some reduction in HDL cholesterol and elevation in LDL cholesterol.

These reported changes provide a rationale for an alternative therapeutic approach to the patient who presents with some or all of the above premenopausal changes. Some practitioners recommend and practice the prompt commencement of full sequential estrogen progestin replacement therapy.

It is not the purpose of this discussion to present a review or analysis of the extensive psychiatric writings concerning the perimenopausal and postmenopausal years. However, a number of observations deserve emphasis here.

The physician whose practice requires the discussion of menopause, either surgically induced or physiologically impending, with any relatively large number of women is painfully aware that some past teachings and beliefs have persisted quite stubbornly. The following quotation from *100 Years of Gynecology—1800 to 1900* was apparently written in 1850 (1):

> Compelled to yield to the power of time, women now cease to exist as for the species, and henceforward live only for themselves. Their features are stamped with the impress of age, and their genital organs are ceiled with the signet of sterility . . . It is the dictate of prudence of all such circumstances as might tend to awaken any erotic thoughts in the mind and reanimate a sentiment that ought rather to become extinct . . . In fine, everything calculated to cause regrets for charms, that are lost, and enjoyments that are ended forever.

Although knowledge of sexual activity and satisfaction among women long beyond the menopause is much more widespread today than even 2 or 3 decades ago, fear of loss of libido in herself or apprehension regarding her ability to be a satisfactory sexual partner to her mate after cessation of the menstrual function continue to cause great apprehension among large numbers of women. Such apprehension is noted particularly when a medical need for premenopausal hysterectomy develops.

A publication from 1857 brings out two additional aspects (2):

> A large class of women are thoroughly unhinged by the change of life being left to take its course: eccentricity embitters their existence and the lives of those around them . . . I cannot repeat too often that this crisis, like puberty weighs upon the subsequent life time of women and the nervous symptoms of the change of life assume vast importance.

The very term "change of life" conveys to women some foreboding course of events beyond their control; and past medical writings such as these quotations and woman-to-woman personally embellished accounts might seem to justify their worst fears.

Sometimes an ancient quotation seems strikingly current in its implication for the practitioner of medicine (2):

> It is not unusual with women to refer all their extraordinary sensations to the change of life, and to consider that when they have thus accounted for their diseases they have at the same time cured them; and in this, most medical men, judging at least from their practice, seem to be of the same option.

This warning of Sir C. M. Clarke, quoted by Pilt in 1857, thus reminds all current practitioners that the only characteristic identifiable symptom of the menopause is the vasomotor response that we commonly call the hot flush or flash. It is essential that as practitioners we do not follow the tendency of many women to do as Clarke described, namely, to ascribe every symptom that occurs in this perimenopausal era to "The Change." It is important that each physician follow the standard recognized diagnostic algorithm for significant symptoms other than hot flushes in this age group in the same way that such symptoms would be investigated if presented by a patient who is not having menopausal signs and symptoms.

On occasion, when symptoms presented by the patient along with symptoms of acute estrogen withdrawal seem somewhat obscure and nondescript, it may be entirely appropriate to initiate hormonal replacement therapy and to review the patient's total status in 2 to 4 weeks. Symptoms related to the patient's estrogen deficiency, including many miscellaneous complaints that may be related to sleep deprivation, should be absent or markedly alleviated within that time span if the patient complies with the prescribed hormonal replacement. It may then be possible to delineate much more clearly if there are additional symptoms requiring investigation.

Ditkoff and colleagues have undertaken comprehensive double-blind placebo controlled psychologic testing of post menopausal women to whom they administered placebo or one of two doses of conjugated estrogen. The women had serum estradiol levels below 20 pg/ml but were asymptomatic. The major finding was a "significant improvement in the income management scales of the Profile of Adaptation to Life and in depression scores of the Beck Depression Inventory." Another conclusion was the suggestion that "estrogen may have the ability to improve quality of life even in asymptomatic women" (3).

If the patient benefits by having a diminished tendency toward depression and improved mood and feeling of well-being, other presenting complaints for which no pathological process can be found may be ameliorated.

Studies of the menstrual patterns of large numbers of women as they approach their last menstrual flow indicate that the most common signal of impending cessation is a shortened cycle (4). Further study shows that it is the follicular phase that begins to decrease in length.

The shortening cycle length brings some women to their physician. Many other variations of prior menstrual pattern may occur. Menses may cease abruptly; one or more menses may be skipped and then normal menstrual flow may occur again. If ovulation occurs sufficiently frequently, even though not monthly in this phase, endometrial hyperplasia and its resultant dysfunctional bleeding will probably not occur. If, however, the patient continues to produce a level of estrogen (ovarian or extragonadal) that stimulates endometrial proliferation and if there is no postovulatory counterbalancing progesterone, endometrial hyperplasia and abnormal uterine bleeding will probably follow in a relatively short time.

During this premenopause (or perimenopause), some women begin to experience some symptoms that they themselves describe as a "change" and may inquire if they are beginning to experience the "change of life." Symptoms are generally reported as milder early in the process and may not be volunteered. The woman who presents with the early changes in menstrual pattern may reveal other symptoms only on direct inquiry. These may include sleeplessness, irritability, increased tendency to weep, loss of concentration, mild depression, increased avoidance of social contact, and some vaginal dryness.

If the pattern of intermittent bleeding (skipped menses, shortened cycle length, etc.) indicates sufficient estrogen production to produce endometrial proliferation, it seems most rational to prescribe cyclic progestin to assist in restoring a more customary menstrual pattern. Medroxyprogesterone acetate 10 mg daily for 10 to 14 days monthly has proven very satisfactory for this purpose. Some women may continue to produce endogenous estrogens at a level that will stimulate endometrial growth and regular cyclic shedding within 24 to 72 hours of the last medroxyprogesterone acetate tablet for many months. And most women will report a return to normal well-being and the disappearance of the previously mentioned symptoms.

Since endometrial adenocarcinoma begins to make a significant appearance in these pre- and perimenopausal years, the physician must be alert to the occurrence of intermenstrual bleeding or menorrhagia, which demand histologic testing by endometrial biopsy or curettage. The Pipelle[a] has proven to be

[a]Unimar Inc., Wilton, CT.

an innovation that, in most women in these circumstances, allows for easy and relatively painless endometrial sampling. Oral administration of any of the anti-prostaglandin synthetase inhibitors 30 minutes prior to the procedure further decreases procedural discomfort.

While it would be admirable if women would maintain a menstrual calendar throughout their postpubertal years, the premenopausal era is a time when a written record of the menstrual cycles permits the physician to assess the menstrual history more accurately and promptly. Thus the woman who is more than 40 years of age should be encouraged to do so. An incentive in this direction is to provide her with one of the convenient small cards printed for this purpose.

In addition, as women enter the decade of their 40s, it is extremely helpful for the physician to provide an authoritative educational booklet or other educational materials to acquaint the patient with current knowledge in this field. Accurate information can dispel much of the mystery and fear, can counteract much inaccurate older-to-younger woman information, and can encourage the patient to bring her questions and concerns for clarification.

Key Points

- Total estrogen production may decline in some women as they approach menopause and may account for the onset of symptoms of irritability, sleep disturbance, and some vasomotor symptoms, even though relatively regular menses are still occurring.
- Irregularity of the menstrual interval may accompany this premenopausal period.
- Cyclic oral progestin can restore menstrual regularity and relieve symptoms in many of these women.
- Full sequential estrogen/progestin replacement is also effective.
- The only absolutely characteristic symptom of the menopause is the vasomotor response called "hot flush" or "hot flash."
- Health care providers must avoid the pitfall of attributing other symptoms to the menopause and failing to initiate appropriate diagnostic procedures because the woman is coincidentally experiencing menopausal symptoms.
- When the menstrual pattern departs from its normal regularity (and especially if intermenstrual bleeding occurs but also if significant menor-rhagia occurs), if conventional D&C is not performed, or felt to be

indicated, endometrial sampling by means of one of the many small devices now available must be employed to avoid failure to diagnose early adenocarcinoma of the endometrium in its most curable stage. Hysteroscopy is also proving to be a useful adjunct.

- The use of a menstrual calendar card can aid in the practitioner's rapid and accurate assessment of the woman's changing menstrual pattern.

References

1. L'Iserem C, trans. Meigs CD. 100 years of gynecology—1800 to 1900. Philadelphia: Blakiston, 1850:532.
2. Pilt EF. The change of life in health and disease. London: John Churchill, 1857.
3. Ditkoff EC et al. Estrogen improves psychological function in asymptomatic postmenopausal women. Obstet Gynecol 1991;78:991.
4. Sherman BM, Karenman SG. Hormonal characteristics of the human menstrual cycle throughout reproductive life. J Clin Invest 1975;55:669.

3

Osteoporosis: The Estrogen Relationship[a]

Robert Lindsay and Felicia Cosman

It is only since the original and compelling clinical studies of Fuller Albright that the role of the menopause in the pathogenesis of osteoporosis has been recognized (1, 2). In fact, the majority of information about the epidemiology (3, 4) and pathophysiology of this disorder has been generated only in the past 20 years or so, stimulated, in part at least, by the development of precise tools for noninvasive measurement of bone mass (5). Consequently, there has been some change in our thinking about the disorder. The original designation of osteoporosis as a variety of fracture syndromes has become surpassed by a definition that emphasizes reduction in bone mass and the consequent alteration in architecture increase the risk of fracture. The relationship between bone mass, osteoporosis, and fracture syndromes is similar to that between blood pressure, hypertension, and vascular catastrophes. Blood pressure, like bone mass, is a variable that changes with age, albeit in the opposite direction. At some arbitrary point in this change, which may be exaggerated in susceptible individuals, there is a sufficient increase in the risk of a catastrophic outcome that intervention is warranted to reduce the risk. In both circumstances, therapeutic interventions (as well as other lifestyle alterations) can be shown to reduce risk. Thus, early identification of the individuals at greatest risk of osteoporosis is as important as it is for those with even mildly elevated blood pressure, since the greatest therapeutic benefits can be achieved at this stage. Treatment after the clinical catastrophe has occurred is less than satisfactory.

Bone loss with age occurs throughout the skeleton and thus increases the risk of fracture for all bones. The most common fractures are those of vertebrae, hip, and wrist (Colles' fracture), which together account for some 70% of all osteoporotic fractures (3, 4). The incidence of these fractures increases with age, preceded by a long period of asymptomatic bone loss. Thus, examination of fractures among the elderly population requires analyses

[a]Work for this chapter was supported in part by PHS Grant AR 39191.

of the factors that predispose to bone loss and subsequently low bone mass, which in turn increases the risk of fracture.

EPIDEMIOLOGY OF BONE LOSS

Bone loss appears to be an inevitable age-related process that occurs in all populations studied thus far (5). Therefore it is fair to say that all individuals, should they live long enough, will eventually become osteoporotic. Not all osteoporotic individuals will experience fractures, just as not all hypertensive individuals will develop strokes. Indeed, the converse is also true in both circumstances. Fractures obviously can and do happen in the absence of osteoporosis. Thus, while osteoporosis is a major risk factor for fracture, it is only one of several.

Factors Determining Bone Mass

Some of the factors thought to alter bone mass are listed in Table 3.1. Each may operate throughout life or only at specific time periods (Fig. 3.1). Genetic factors are probably most important in determining peak bone mass (6), that is, the amount of bone present in the skeleton in early adult life (ages 20 to 40 years). As demonstrated by the fact that concordance in bone mass between twins declines with age, genetic factors appear to be less important in later years. Caucasian women have low peak mass in comparison to black women or to men of any race (7). The presence of relatively sudden and ubiquitous gonadal failure (at menopause), and the consequent acceleration of bone mass that results, places women at further risk (8). Additionally, pathologic cessation of gonadal function prior to menopause in women or at

Table 3.1.
Possible Risk Factors for Osteoporosis

Genetic	Race
	Sex
	Familial prevalence
Nutritional	Low calcium intake
	High alcohol intake
	High caffeine intake
	High sodium intake
	High animal protein intake
Lifestyle	Cigarette use
	Low physical activity
Endocrine	Menopausal age (oophorectomy)
	Low body weight
	Glucocorticoid excess
	Thyroid hormone excess

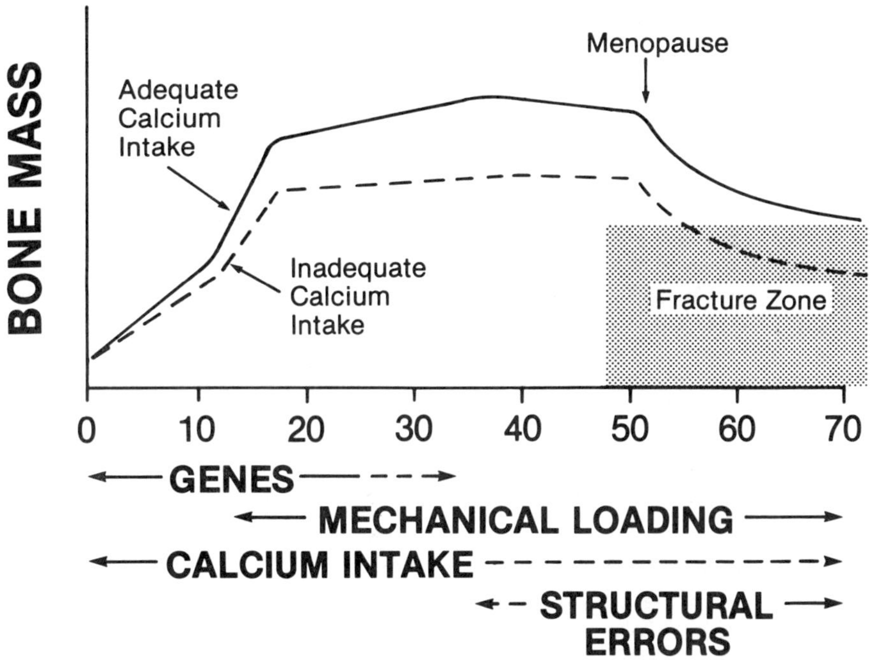

Figure 3.1. A hypothetical schema illustrating the changes in bone mass in women throughout life together with the proposed factors of greatest importance that impact upon skeletal mass (Courtesy of R.P. Heaney, with permission).

any age in men also contributes to bone loss. True age-related bone loss begins later in life and affects both sexes (9). Extremes of physical activity—from disuse (bed rest, space flight) to indulgence in athletic pursuits at a competitive level—clearly influence the skeleton, resulting in significant loss of skeletal tissue during disuse (10–15) and increase in tissue with high levels of activity (16, 17). Whether or not normal everyday activity is sufficient to maintain the skeleton is less certain (3, 18), but it is nonetheless attractive to assume that modest stress is important for mineral homeostasis. This is supported by significant ex vivo data (19, 20). It is also thought that long-term inadequacies in nutritional status can negatively affect the skeleton (21). However, data on this point are conflicting (22–24). Even in the case of calcium, of which 99% of the body's load is contained in the skeleton, it has been remarkably difficult until recently to produce convincing human data that a significant deficiency in dietary calcium can result in the mobilization of skeletal calcium. Calcium deprivation clearly produces osteoporosis in animals, however, and can probably do so in humans also (24a). Alcohol consumption and cigarette smoking both appear to be directly injurious to the skeleton (25–28), and there are various drugs—of which glucocorticoid and thyroxine are the most common—that can influence skeletal metabolism (29).

Role of Ovarian Failure

Considering the wide range of factors influencing the skeleton, it is perhaps not surprising that it has taken great effort to determine the role of even the most important factor. However, it now seems clear that loss of gonadal function is an important, if not the major, determinant of skeletal status in adults (8). Among older women, the number of years with a deficiency in sex hormones (i.e., postmenopausal years) is a more important indicator of skeletal status than age (30, 31). Albright originally drew attention to this issue (1, 2), but it was not until the development of noninvasive techniques for the measurement of bone mass that it became possible to investigate this in detail. In our early studies (30) we were able to demonstrate that oophorectomy, when performed prior to menopause, resulted in significant reduction in bone mass. Most cross-sectional studies have confirmed that bone mass in women is stable until the onset of ovarian failure and that there is an acceleration of bone loss as ovarian function declines (32–47). The studies that have been unable to demonstrate such an increase in the rate of bone loss after menopause are few (48–51) and are beset by a variety of problems including, for example, sample size in the appropriate groups (principally the premenopausal). Almost all data show increased bone loss from the radius after menopause, and indeed bone loss from other sites of principally cortical bone occurs in a similar pattern. This has led to the suggestion that there are different patterns of loss from different skeletal sites, especially cancellous bone of the spine, with perhaps different factors operative at these different sites (50). However, data obtained using computerized axial tomography suggest that the changes in purely cancellous bone of the spine are qualitatively similar to those that occur at cortical sites, although quantitatively greater (33, 41). Cross-sectional data from our laboratory (Fig. 3.2) summarize the lumbar spine findings in 400 Caucasian women who fit pre-established normal criteria. Loss of bone in the femoral neck is similar, but with a somewhat greater premenopausal loss than is seen in the spine. There is still a clear postmenopausal acceleration, however.

As indicated above, using oophorectomy as a model for postmenopausal bone loss, our group began to investigate this issue some 20 years ago (30). We were able to demonstrate that oophorectomized individuals within the first 3 years after surgery had significantly lower cortical bone mass in

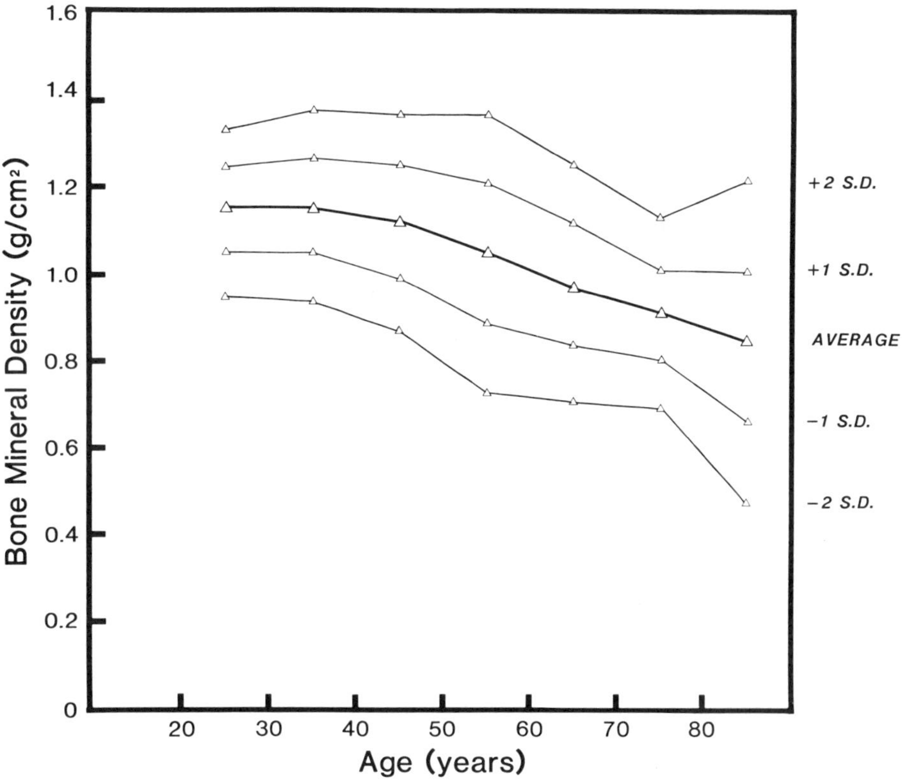

Figure 3.2. Distribution of bone mass with age in the lumbar vertebrae in normal women by dual photon absorptiometry.

peripheral bone than women who had hysterectomy with ovarian conservation, despite being of identical age (Fig. 3.3) (30). More recently, the Mayo Clinic group repeated this experiment in a somewhat different fashion. Comparing 50-year-old women who had been oophorectomized at age 30 years, they were able to demonstrate that reductions in bone mass in spine, hip, and wrist were similar to those of 70-year-old women who had undergone a natural menopause (31).

Prospective data in which changes in bone mass have been associated with ovarian function are few. In our original study (52, 53) we demonstrated that bone turnover measured biochemically and cortical bone loss estimated prospectively were significantly related to the supply of endogenous estrogen in postmenopausal women when this was carefully estimated throughout the study period. Similar data have been published by other groups (53–55). These results have been remarkably consistent, suggesting that relatively low

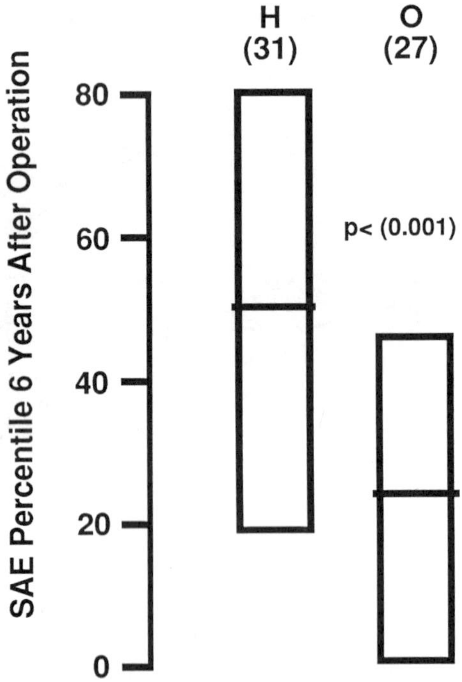

Figure 3.3. Bone mass by radiographic absorptiometry in two groups of women 3 years after either hysterectomy (*H*) or hysterectomy plus bilateral oophorectomy (*O*). Results are mean ± SD. The average age of each group was 46 years at time of measurement.

levels of circulating estradiol (within early to mid-follicular range) can positively affect skeletal remodeling and bone loss. If this is true, it suggests that modest circulating levels of estrogen need to be achieved when estrogens are given exogenously to postmenopausal women for prevention of bone loss.

Among younger women, oligomenorrhea and amenorrhea resulting from primary or secondary ovarian insufficiency cause low bone mass (56). Excessive physical activity (which can produce secondary failure of the hypothalamic-pituitary-ovarian axis) fails to mask this effect (56–63). Hyperprolactinemia only results in low bone mass when secondary ovarian failure results (64). In anorexia nervosa the reduction in bone may be exacerbated by the abnormal diet (65). Administration of gonadotropin superagonists or antagonists may also result in premature accelerated rates of bone loss (66–69). It has been suggested that temporary creation of a state of estrogen deficiency using a gonadotropin-releasing hormone antagonist may allow prediction of those particularly at risk of osteoporosis (70), although this thesis requires confirmation.

In males hypogonadism also results in bone loss, irrespective of its cause (71–73), and testicular failure appears to contribute significantly to the risk of osteoporosis among the aging male population (74, 75), although in general osteoporosis among males has been inadequately studied.

Mechanism of Estrogen Action

The mechanism of the effect of ovarian insufficiency on the skeleton has been difficult to unravel, perhaps not surprisingly. The elegant studies of Heaney first demonstrated that menopause caused increased skeletal turnover with greater movement of calcium into and out of the skeleton (76–78). However, the gap between influx and efflux widens and bone loss ensues. The latter has been amply demonstrated in the wide variety of studies using noninvasive techniques for bone mass measurement (32–50). The principal mechanism within the skeleton by which this occurs appears to be increased activation of skeletal remodeling cycles, but it is likely that there must also be a change in the relative performance of teams of osteoclasts and the osteoblasts that follow them (79). The preponderance of evidence suggests that in the absence of sex steroids, osteoclast teams work harder, excavating more bone, while osteoblast teams fail to repair the damage. The result, in cancellous bone, is a gradual thinning of trabeculae, with trabecular perforation and eventual removal. In cortical bone, inadequate filling of resorption cavities leaves spaces, a process often referred to as trabecularization of the cortex. Once complete trabeculae have been removed, no mechanisms exist to reconstitute the structure (Fig. 3.4).

The metabolic control of these alterations in skeletal metabolism is not well understood. The original data from Heaney suggested an accompanying decline in the efficiency of calcium absorption across the intestine, as well as relatively increased loss of calcium in urine (76, 77). Both of these, or a change intrinsic to the skeleton, could account for bone loss, but only an intrinsic change in skeletal metabolism explains both of the other events (Fig. 3.5). Recent descriptions of putative estrogen receptors in osteoblasts maintained in cell culture and osteoblast-like cells lend weight to the concept of direct control of skeletal homeostasis by estrogen (80, 81). However, the changes that occur when estrogen deficiency appears are principally in the recruitment or activity of osteoclasts. These cells have yet to be shown to respond directly to estrogens in physiologic concentrations (82), although recent preliminary data suggest that osteoclasts may also have functional estrogen receptors (82a). This lack of direct effect on osteoclasts by estrogen, though, is similar to most other skeletal hormones, including parathyroid hormone (PTH). Since osteoblasts are potent synthesizers of a variety of peptides, it is tempting to

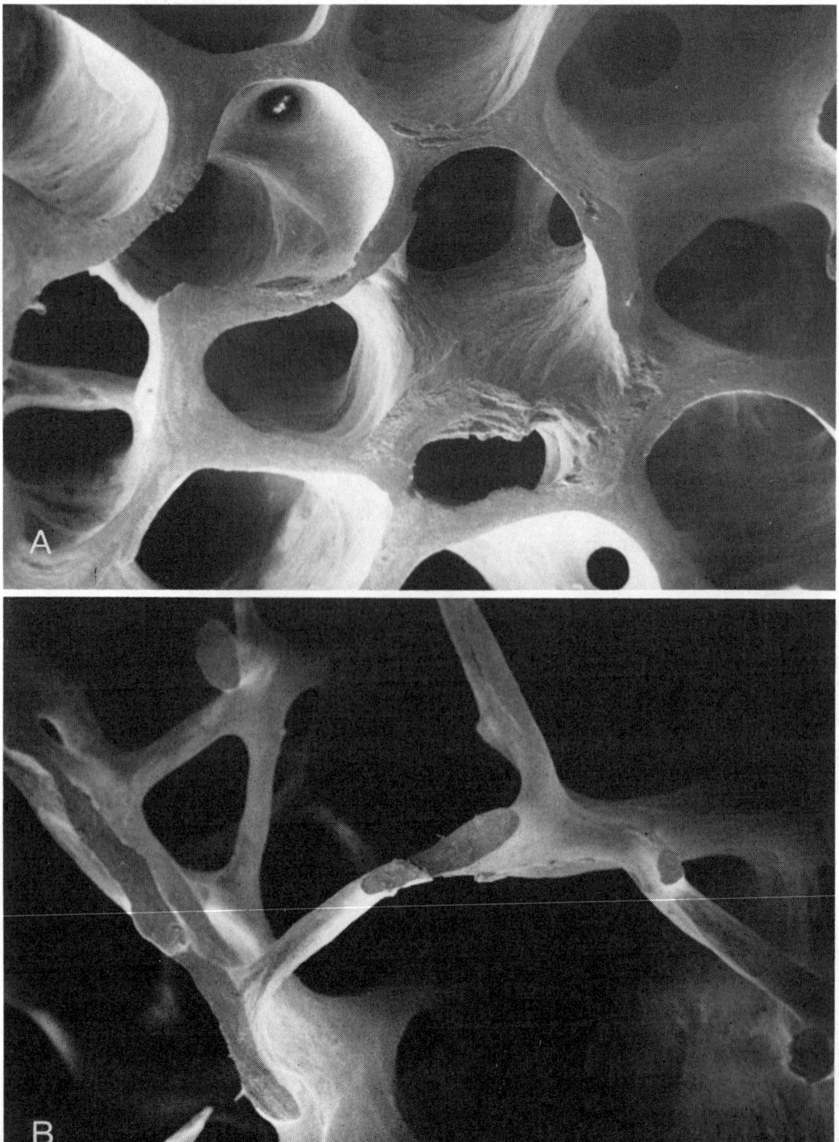

Figure 3.4. Scanning electron micrographs of normal and osteoporotic cancellous bone. Normal cancellous bone has trabecular plates interconnecting with small regular marrow spaces (**A**). As bone is lost the trabeculae are penetrated, become rod-like, and eventually are completely resorbed (**B**). All stages of this process can be observed. (From Dempster DW et al. J Bone Min Res 1986;1:15.)

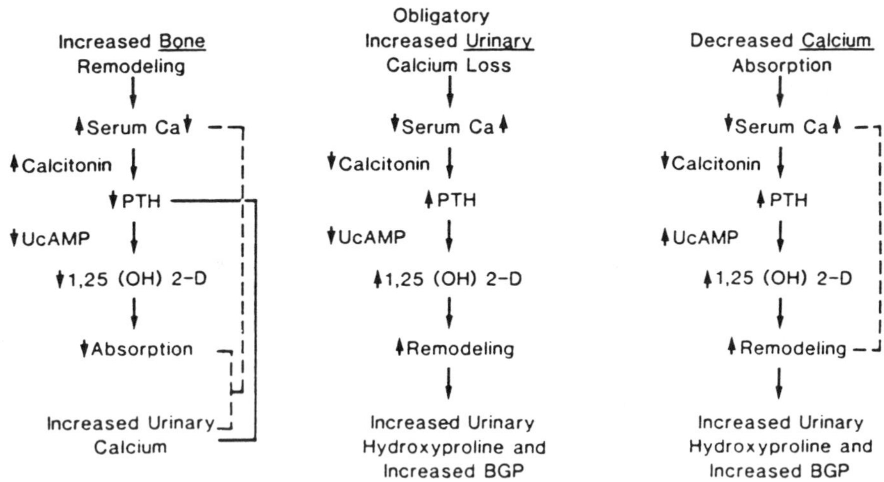

Figure 3.5. Postulated impairments in hormonal control of calcium metabolism that might occur after menopause and account for the observed changes in mineral and skeletal status.

speculate on the existence of a second messenger secreted by osteoblasts, controlled by estrogen status, that modulates osteoclasts (83–85). Potential mediators include TGF-β, interleukins, insulin-like growth factors, or perhaps even osteocalcin, the most common noncollagenous protein in bone, secreted by osteoblasts with an as yet unknown function (86).

The rate of bone loss after ovarian failure declines exponentially with the duration of the postmenopausal period. Bone loss continues, at least on a population basis, until old age at a somewhat slower rate than occurs early after ovarian failure. Whether the patients who are likely to develop osteoporotic fractures are those who lose bone at the greatest rate or those who enter their menopausal years with the lowest values for bone mass, or both, is still not entirely clear. Nevertheless, it is clearly important, since it has a great impact on the capacity to identify those most at risk at the time of menopause, when prevention is likely to be the most effective.

Age-related Bone Loss

Since bone loss occurs universally in both sexes, and men are not universally affected by testicular failure with age, it seems probable that there is some contribution of age itself that predisposes to the loss of bone tissue (74, 75). The Mayo Clinic group has hypothesized that this age-related bone loss affects sites with a greater proportion of cortical bone (29, 87, 88). In addition, although other osteoporotic fractures occur more frequently after the initial fracture, they are still somewhat less common than would be hypothesized if all osteoporotic fractures were consequent upon the same etiologic event (4).

One mechanism suggested for bone loss of this type involves the age-related decline in calcium absorption across the intestine that has been observed to occur in both sexes (89, 90). It can be argued that this will increase the calcium requirement of the organism at a time when calcium intake is declining (91). Consequently, more calcium must be mobilized from the skeleton (see Fig. 3.5). In an attempt to mobilize calcium and to improve intestinal calcium absorption, the secretion of parathyroid hormone increases, as has been shown to occur with increasing age (92). There appears also to be an age-related decline in the responsiveness of the renal 1-α-hydroxylase to parathyroid hormone (93, 94) and of the intestinal calcium absorption process to $1{,}25(OH)_2D$. Therefore, improvement in calcium absorption is less than expected. However appealing this hypothesis, it has yet to be causally linked to bone loss. It is entirely possible that the variabilities in fracture recurrence are related to the different rates in expression of extraskeletal factors.

EPIDEMIOLOGY OF FRACTURES

In addition to the presence of osteoporosis, contributions to fracture risk result from a variety of other sources. In general, these are factors that increase the frequency of falls. The relative importance of trauma and falling varies according to fracture site, but is clearly of major importance in two of the three main osteoporotic fractures, the hip and distal radius (3). Since less than 2% of falls result in fracture, however, other contributing factors are clearly important (95). Among elderly individuals who fall once, 50% will fall repeatedly (96, 97). Women fall more frequently than men, at least up to the age of 75 years, after which the incidence appears to be similar in both sexes. The incidence of falls is higher among the institutionalized elderly, who in general are more debilitated than those living at home (98). Thus, not surprisingly, most falls among the elderly result from the cumulative effects of several intrinsic factors, coupled often with extrinsic factors that increase the risk of injury (Table 3.2 and 3.3).

The risk factors for fracture among the elderly, therefore, include both those of low bone mass (Table 3.1) and those affecting the risk of injury (99).

Throughout life, patterns of fracture frequency and location change (Fig. 3.6). Fracture occurrence in general tends to be high at the extremes of life, with a secondary peak in young adults (3, 4). Each peak is associated with different fractures, and those most common among the aged are thought to be consequent upon osteoporosis. In the United States, approximately 1.5 million osteoporotic fractures are thought to occur each year (4). Of these there are approximately 500,000 vertebral fractures (although precise data on the incidence of vertebral fractures do not exist), 250,000 fractures of the hip, and 150,000 Colles' fractures. The remainder include proximal humerus, pelvis, and other limb fractures, for which osteoporosis accounts for at least one-half of the total fracture incidence among the elderly in the United States. Nonvertebral fracture incidence at any age is dependent on both trauma and the capacity of the body and skeleton to resist the injury.

Vertebral fractures probably occur mostly because of low bone mass (4), and sufficient force to fracture the vertebrae is generated during the normal activities of life. Finally, qualitative changes in the skeleton that accompany reduced mass also contribute to the likelihood of fracture, but their contribution in quantitative terms is difficult to evaluate.

The natural history of osteoporotic fractures is not well understood. While clinically it is generally assumed that patients who have one fracture will be more likely to sustain other fractures, data to substantiate that statement are

Table 3.2.
Intrinsic Factors Increasing the Risk of Falling among the Elderly[a]

- Long term
  - Neurologic disease
    - e.g., Parkinson's disease
    - Hemiparesis
    - Alzheimer type dementia
  - Cognitive disorders
    - Vision
    - Hearing
    - Vestibular function
    - Proprioception
  - Musculoskeletal disorders
    - Muscle weakness
    - Slow gait (senile gait)
  - Medications
    - Sedatives, tranquilizers
    - Hypotensive agents
    - Diuretics
    - Anticonvulsants
    - Alcohol
- Short term
  - Acute illness (or acute exacerbation of chronic illness)
  - Postural hypotension
  - Medications

[a]Adapted from Lindsay R. Osteoporosis, and its relationship to estrogen. Contemp Obstet Gynecol 1984;63:201–224.

Table 3.3.
Extrinsic Factors Increasing the Risk of Falling among the Elderly[a]

Lighting
Glare
Excessive shadows
Floors
Rug
Trailing cords
Small objects (litter)
Waxed surfaces
Stairs
Inadequate lighting
Absence of rails
Noncontrasting steps
Inadequate repair
Kitchen
Cupboards not within reach, etc.
Bathroom
Absence of grab bars in showers, toilets, baths
Absence of non-skid floor in shower
No shower chair
Footwear
Non-form-fitting shoes
Soles not non-skid
Outdoors
Ice, snow
Uneven terrain
Tools, etc.
Inadequate lighting

[a]Adapted from Lindsay R. Osteoporosis, and its relationship to estrogen. Contemp Obstet Gynecol 1984;63:201–224.

difficult to find. Prior fractures of the proximal humerus are twice as common among patients with hip fracture, and vertebral fractures may be 2 to 10 times more common in this population (4). The converse is also true, that is, there is some increase in the risk of hip fracture in patients with either radius or vertebral fracture (4). Melton has suggested that the relationship between fractures is not as strong as expected, and, as previously noted, this forms part of the basis for the hypothesis that there are two forms of osteoporosis, accounting for the difference in fracture relationships (4). Nonetheless, the occurrence of one fracture is clearly a risk factor for subsequent fractures.

Fractures of the Proximal Femur

The age-specific increase in hip fracture is exponential in both sexes (3, 100–102) but begins at a much later age among men (Fig. 3.5). The incidence increases from negligible to more than 3% per year for the very old (more than

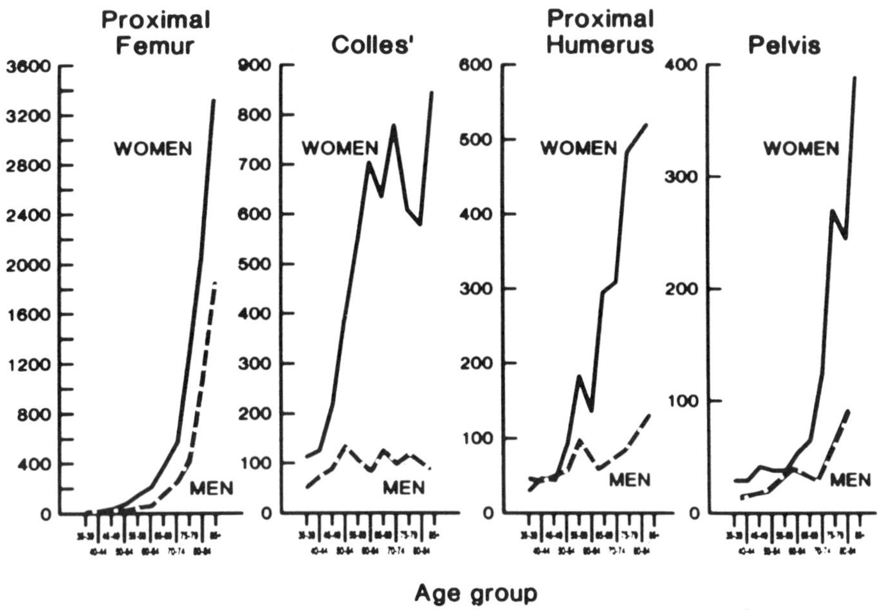

Figure 3.6. Distribution of all fractures as a function of age in males and females.

85 years). Eighty percent of all hip fractures occur among women (3, 4). Part of this female predominance is due to a greater proportion of females than males entering the at-risk age group, but the risk of an elderly female suffering hip fracture remains at least twice the risk for an elderly male. This underscores the importance of the menopause in the pathogenesis of hip fracture and the importance of estrogen treatment in reducing the risk of fracture. The lifetime risk of hip fracture is 15% for the average perimenopausal woman and probably significantly greater for the women (about 30 to 40%) who enter menopause with low bone mass.

Fractures of the hip occur in two types: across the femoral neck itself or between the trochanters (intertrochanteric). Both increase in a similar fashion with age, although there appears to be a greater increase in intertrochanteric fractures among the very old. The latter type also appears to have a closer relationship to previous vertebral fracture. When a fracture of one type has occurred there is a significantly greater chance of recurrence of the same type of hip fracture on the opposite side.

Although hip fractures are generally associated with trauma superimposed on osteoporosis, some may be spontaneous and others may be associated with other underlying pathology, such as malignancy or Paget's disease. Most fractures of the hip require moderate trauma such as occurs in a fall from standing height (95, 99). The frequency of falls increases with age (95, 96), and one fall increases the risk of future falls. Women may have a greater risk of falling than men at least until age 70 years (97). It has been suggested that an increased risk of fracturing after falls in the elderly is due to a slower gait and an increased tendency to land on the side or back, directly on the hip. The direction of the fall is important in that falls directly on the hip generate enough force to fracture the bone at all levels of bone mass in humans (103). Thus, protective factors including muscle activity, fat, and reflex responses are required to prevent serious injury. The increased frequency of hip fracture among the elderly, therefore, depends on low bone mass, falls, and reduced capacity to protect the bone from the trauma (104–106).

Hip fractures are more common in all white populations studied, with lower incidence in black populations in Africa and America (107, 108), as well as among Maoris (109). Low fracture incidence in Asian populations may be due in part to under-reporting, and good epidemiologic data are still lacking for a major portion of the world (110).

Since the actual number of individuals over the age of 65 years is increasing in most Western countries, it is perhaps not surprising that the frequency of fractures of the femoral neck is also increasing (106, 111). Solely on the basis of the changes in the elderly population, the total number of hip fractures in the United States would be expected to double in the next 50 years (3). In addition, a number of studies, mostly from Europe, suggest that there is also an increase in the age-specific incidence of the disorder. Secular changes in hip fracture have been observed in several Scandinavian countries, United Kingdom, Belgium, Finland, and Canada, and is suggested by some data from the United States, although other data suggest that the rise has leveled off in the United States (106, 111–117). The reasons for those increases in age-specific incidence are not at all clear. It may be that privation in early life is the cause and that we are now seeing a cohort of these individuals reaching the age at risk of hip fracture. This might be conjectured from the Yugoslav data, which suggested that lower peak bone mass from early calcium deprivation resulted in increased hip fracture frequency among the elderly (22). However, considerably more data are required before this can be proved.

Even if the secular increase in hip fracture frequency has ceased in the United States, the financial burden from these fractures continues to increase and the financial cost is enormous. About 35% of patients with limb fractures require inpatient care, including all patients with hip fracture, who may require up to 33 days in an acute care setting. It is thought that osteoporotic fractures result in 750,000 million visits to physicians annually in the United States (118). In 1984 dollars, the cost was estimated to be $18 billion for all fractures and $7 billion for hip fractures (Table 3.4). These costs can only be expected to increase as the number of elderly persons in the population continues to grow. By the year 2050 the elderly will constitute 22% of the entire population and those over 85 years, 5%. A recent estimate of the costs of hip fracture, based on conservative estimates of inflation, calculated that by 2040, hip fracture costs would exceed $16 billion (119).

the global costs of hip fracture are now estimated to be significantly greater than those that accrue to the United States alone. From current international incidence rates of hip fracture and secular changes in the demography of third-world countries, it has been suggested that the largest increments in hip fracture will occur in the Asian continent. Currently Asia contributes only about 31% to the estimated 1,660,297 fractures occurring each year. By the year 2050 it is estimated that the global number of hip fractures will increase to 6,262,100, of which some 51% will occur in Asia (119a).

Hip fracture is associated with significant morbidity and mortality (Fig. 3.7) (120). Estimates of post–hip fracture mortality vary, but generally it is accepted that these fractures are associated with a 5 to 20% excess mortality

Table 3.4.
Annual Cost of Fractures in the United States

	All Fractures	Hip Fractures Only
Direct costs		
Hospital inpatient services	$4,467,440,000	$1,136,030,000
Outpatient and emergency room institutional services	88,410,000	2,530,000
Outpatient diagnostic and therapeutic services	3,200,400,000	24,650,000
Patient inpatient services	1,570,340,000	739,310,000
Physician office, outpatient and emergency room services	356,850,000	10,220,000
Other practitioner services	211,990,000	82,450,000
Drugs	120,020,000	3,440,000
Nursing home services	4,534,520,000	4,001,930,000
Prepayments and administration	654,750,000	27,030,000
Non–health sector goods and services	2,182,500,000	900,080,000
Total direct costs	$17,387,220,000	$7,170,670,000
Indirect costs		
Lost earnings: wage earners	425,960,000	9,240,000
Lost earnings: homemakers	330,870,000	83,400,000
Total indirect costs	$756,830,000	$92,640,000
Total costs	$18,144,050,000	$7,263,340,000

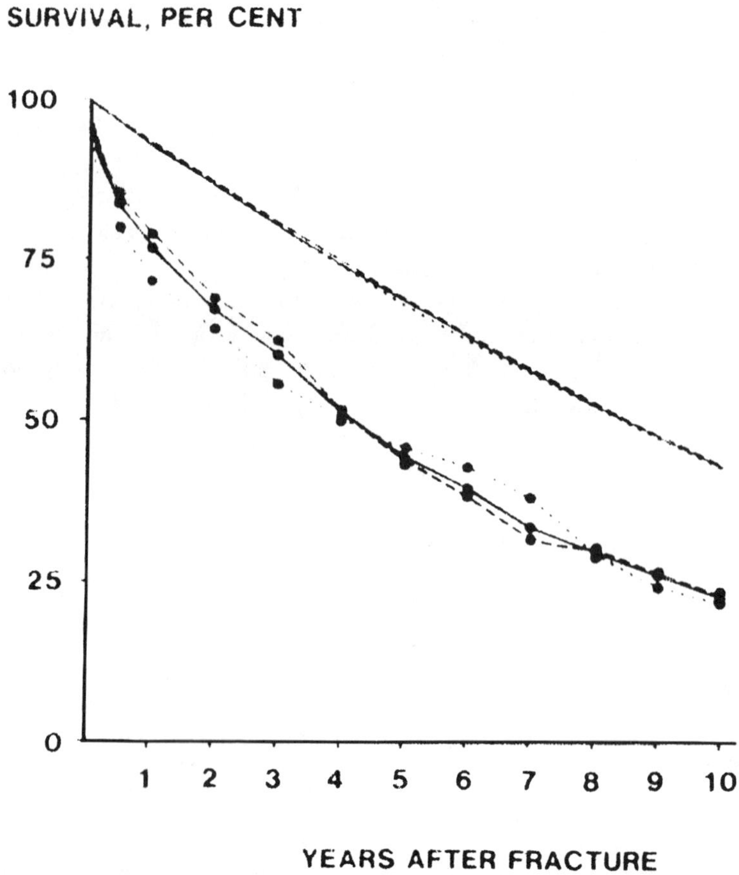

Figure 3.7. Survival of all 288 patients, 207 women and 81 men, after hip fracture. Survival of the age-matched population is shown: all (———), females (-----), and males (·····) as well as survival of the fracture patients: all (○———○), females (○-----○) and males (○·····○). (Reprinted with permission from reference 122.)

(i.e., above that expected for age and sex) that occurs within the first 6 to 12 months following the fracture (121, 122). Mortality varies with age and sex, with survival being higher among women and somewhat lower for the very old, although not dramatically so. Institutionalized patients are especially at risk, as are those with concomitant disease. The complications of the often-required emergency surgery account for some of the mortality in this population, and this is exacerbated by the increased later risk of later thromboembolic disease. Hip fracture is thought to account for about 30,000 deaths each year in the United States (118).

Chronic complications of the fracture and hospitalization also take a significant toll. Of those surviving a hip fracture, one-half will be unable to walk independently afterward and will experience reduced social activity. For almost one-third of patients, hip fracture precipitates entry to nursing home care, such that almost 10% of nursing home patients have experienced a hip fracture. Hip fractures lead to over 7 million days of restricted activity, while vertebral fractures and Colles' fractures are estimated to result in 5 and 6 million restricted days, respectively (118).

Most troublesome in terms of the capacity to treat and rehabilitate patients with hip fracture is the recent suggestion that the institution of the prospective payment system in the United States increases the morbidity following hip fracture (122a). In that study which documented the shorter duration of hospital stay in the acute care setting for patients with hip fracture, the proportion of patients requiring long-term nursing care appeared to have increased since the institution of the system that imposes set length of stays on individual diagnoses, independent of the needs of individual patients. This phenomenon requires a more intensive evaluation, but perhaps stresses the importance of rehabilitation following surgical repair of the fracture.

Vertebral Fractures

The prevalence of vertebral fractures among the aging population is extremely high and may exceed 75% for older women if wedging is included (123–127). Vertebral fractures may be painless and gradual, or acute and accompanied by severe back pain. Asymptomatic fractures are detected on radiographs with increasing frequency as age increases. The suggested higher incidence of acute episodes among younger individuals may be an anomaly caused by the higher activity patterns in that population. True incidence rates have been difficult to determine because of the insidious appearance of these fractures. Nontraumatic fractures probably affect about one-third of women by age 65 years, or 5 million women in the United States currently. Estimates of incidence based on the available prevalence data show that incidence begins to increase around the time of the menopause and continues to rise throughout life (123). Based on these estimates, patients with vertebral fractures are three times more common than those affected by hip fracture, while the number of vertebral fracture incidents exceeds hip fractures by a considerably greater amount.

Little reliable information is available on the distribution of vertebral fractures in different countries. Most estimates are similar to the data for the United States, but the difficulty in determining population-based prevalence probably accounts for some data that suggest lower prevalence in some countries. The influence of race is also poorly documented, although clinical experience and one study suggests that black women have vertebral fractures only rarely. Vertebral fracture prevalence among men is probably 8 to 12 times lower than among women.

The problem in acquiring reliable data about the incidence of vertebral fracture is also related to the difficulty in deciding on a specific definition of fracture. Vertebral deformities are extremely common among the elderly and are usually recognized on routine radiographs. One general classification of these as fractures requires reduction of anterior, central, or posterior vertebral height by 25% visualized on lateral radiographs. Each measurement has to be vertebra specific, since vertebral shape changes according to position with some degree of anterior wedging normal in the mid-thoracic spine. This definition results in the inclusion of many relatively asymptomatic individuals. Recently it has been suggested that a change in shape of more than four standard deviations from normal is required before symptoms result (127a), and this may be a more valid although stringent definition. This issue currently remains unresolved.

Colles' Fractures

The incidence of Colles' fracture increases among women after menopause but then plateaus, unlike fractures of vertebrae or hip (100). The explanation for this phenomenon is unknown. It seems likely that the phenomenon of increased bone loss after menopause accounts for the postmenopausal rise, but the mechanism of the plateau effect remains obscure. Explanations based on gradual changes in falling patterns with age seem unsatisfactory, although they undoubtedly occur. In older women the incidence of Colles' fracture is around 600 per 100,000 person-years, but only 80 per 100,000 person-years among men. In general, Colles' fractures tend to have a seasonal variation, with increased incidence during the winter, presumably related to the increased risk of falling (102).

There is little information on the geographic variation in Colles' fracture, although in general regional differences are somewhat similar to those recorded for hip fracture. This was not found to be the case in certain areas of Yugoslavia associated with a relatively high calcium intake, where hip fracture incidence was lower (compared to incidence in a region with low calcium intake), but Colles' fractures remained relatively frequent (22). The same problem exists for epidemiologic studies of Colles' fractures as for vertebral crush fractures. The majority of cases do not require hospital admission, and therefore accurate data are difficult to obtain.

Other Fractures

Since bone loss after menopause affects all bones to a variable degree, fracture of any bone can occur as part of the osteoporotic syndrome. After the most common fractures, described above, the most frequent fractures encountered are of the proximal humerus, pelvis, and proximal tibia (128). The age-specific incidence of these fractures follows closely that seen for fractures of the hip. Incidence rates rise with age to a greater extent among women than men, and the rate continues to increase with age.

IDENTIFYING THE "AT-RISK" POPULATION

For a woman entering menopause the lifetime risk of suffering a hip fracture is on the order of 15%, which is equal to the combined risk of breast, uterine, and ovarian cancer (129). Applied across the entire population, however, this figure is insufficient to allow recommending preventive therapy for all individuals as they pass menopause. Nonetheless, menopause is probably a useful time at which to evaluate women for their risk of osteoporosis and to target those thought to be at increased risk for treatment.

As bone mineral density accounts for 75 to 80% of the strength of bone, as bone density falls with age so does the strength of bone. The likelihood that a fracture will be sustained following an incident of trauma is determined by bone strength. Recent studies have demonstrated this increased risk of fracture as bone density falls for hip, vertebral, Colles', and other limb fractures.

Estimates of bone density can predict the future risk of fracture because bone density at one age is fairly predictive of bone density in that individual in later years (130, 131). Thus, a bone density measurement made at the time of menopause gives a reasonable idea of what will happen to that woman's skeleton as she ages. A recent model based on these assumptions estimated that the lifetime risk of hip fracture is negligible if a woman has a femoral neck bone density above 1.3 g/cm^2 at age 40 years, and the risk increases to more than 25% for both intertrochanteric and femoral neck fractures if the bone mass is less than 0.6 g/cm^2 (130). Thus, bone density at menopause is a useful method of triaging patients for treatment to prevent osteoporosis.

Bone mass measurements in women with fractures overlap the normal population (132). Bone mass cannot and should not be used to diagnose fracture, but can be used to stratify patients into groups of varying risk. This is analogous to the use of cholesterol for coronary artery disease, or even blood pressure for cerebrovascular disease risk. Recent data have confirmed the feasibility of this use of bone mass measurements. Measurement of bone mass in the radius or os calcis predicts the risk of fracture (131). Women with the lowest bone mass (in the bottom quintile) had four times the risk of subsequent fracture when compared with women in the topmost quintile (Fig. 3.8). Bone mass at one site can predict fracture risk at another. Measurement of bone mass at the os calcis, for example, predicted vertebral fracture risk, as well as the risk of radius and os calcis fractures. Measurement in the radius predicts hip fractures. In one study the risk of subsequent fracture was shown to increase with declining bone mass at all ages (Fig. 3.9). It seems intrinsically reasonable that one mass measured at one specific site (e.g., the femoral neck) will be more highly predictive of fractures at that site. One recent large study has shown that the gradient of risk is indeed greater for fractures at the site of measurement (132a).

Clinical data are often used to identify individuals at risk of osteoporosis. Indeed, most clinicians have a set of favored risk factors that are used clinically. However, there are no data that confirm that clinical observations can be used in this way. Risk factors do not allow estimation of bone mass, and patients cannot be stratified into high and low risk using any grouping of clinical facts with the data currently available. Risk factor analysis does have some more

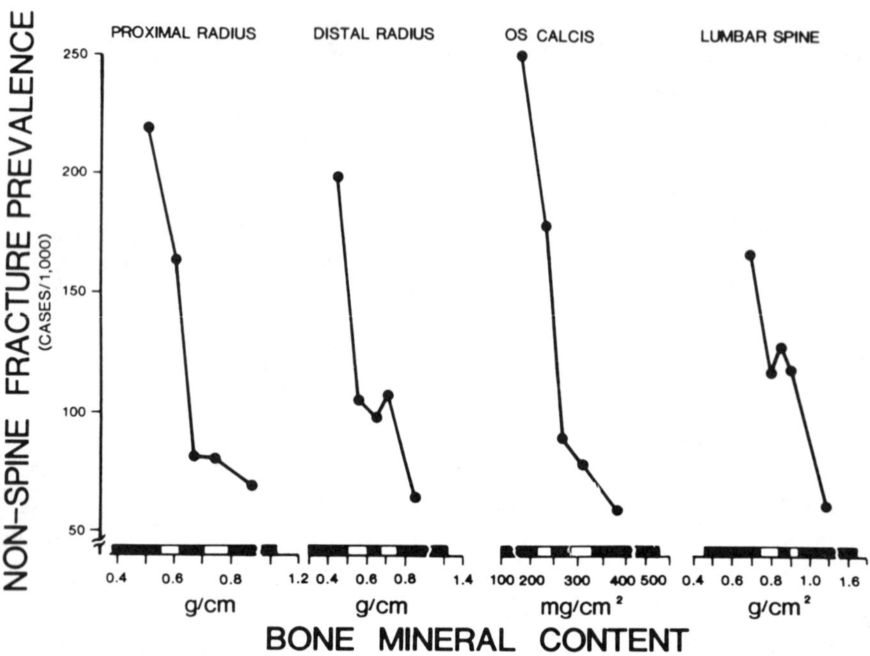

Figure 3.8. Risk of nonspinal fractures as a function of initial bone mass at four different sites. All sites predict fracture risk. (Reprinted with permission from Reference 131.)

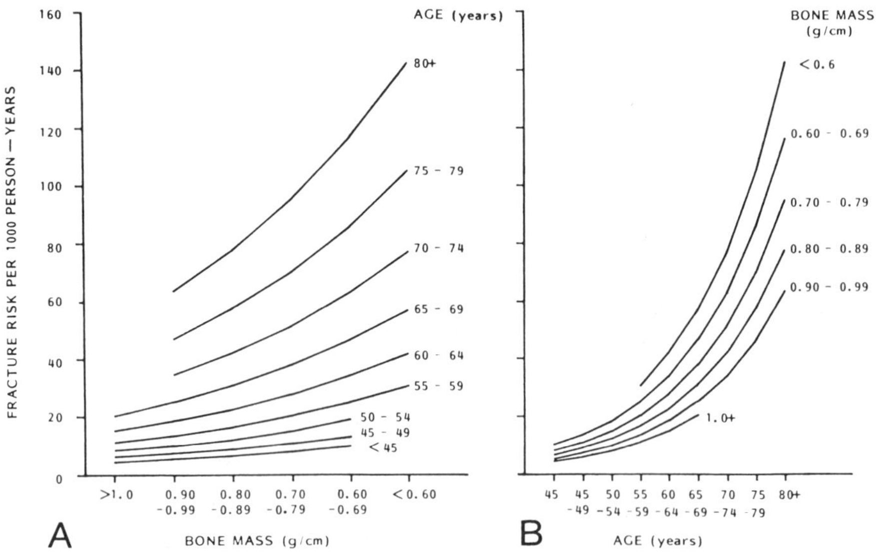

Figure 3.9. **A,** Fracture risk plotted as a function of initial bone mass (SPA-radius) plotted at different ages. Fracture risk increases as bone mass declines at all ages. **B,** Fracture risk as a function of age plotted at different values of radial bone mass. Risk increases with age at all levels of bone mass. (Reprinted with permission from Reference 132b.)

general use, since many of the factors that putatively increase risk for osteoporosis have also been implicated in other disorders of aging. Evaluation of these factors with the patient is a useful way of motivating better general health, but to determine the risk of future fracture, a bone mass measurement is necessary (130). Certain biochemical markers of bone turnover might help identify those patients likely to lose bone faster (133) and suffer greater risk of future fracture, but as yet these markers have not been standardized well enough with the rate of bone loss to be clinically useful.

PREVENTION

With the interrelationship between bone loss and the decline in ovarian function, it is not surprising that the introduction of estrogen therapy reduces the rate of bone loss in hypogonadal women. To investigate this we began a series of studies more than 20 years ago in which we evaluated the effects of estrogen therapy in women after oophorectomy (134–138). These originally double-blind controlled studies allowed us to determine that introduction of estrogen reduced the rate of cortical bone loss in comparison to a placebo (Fig. 3.10). Bone mass measured by single-photon absorptiometry remained

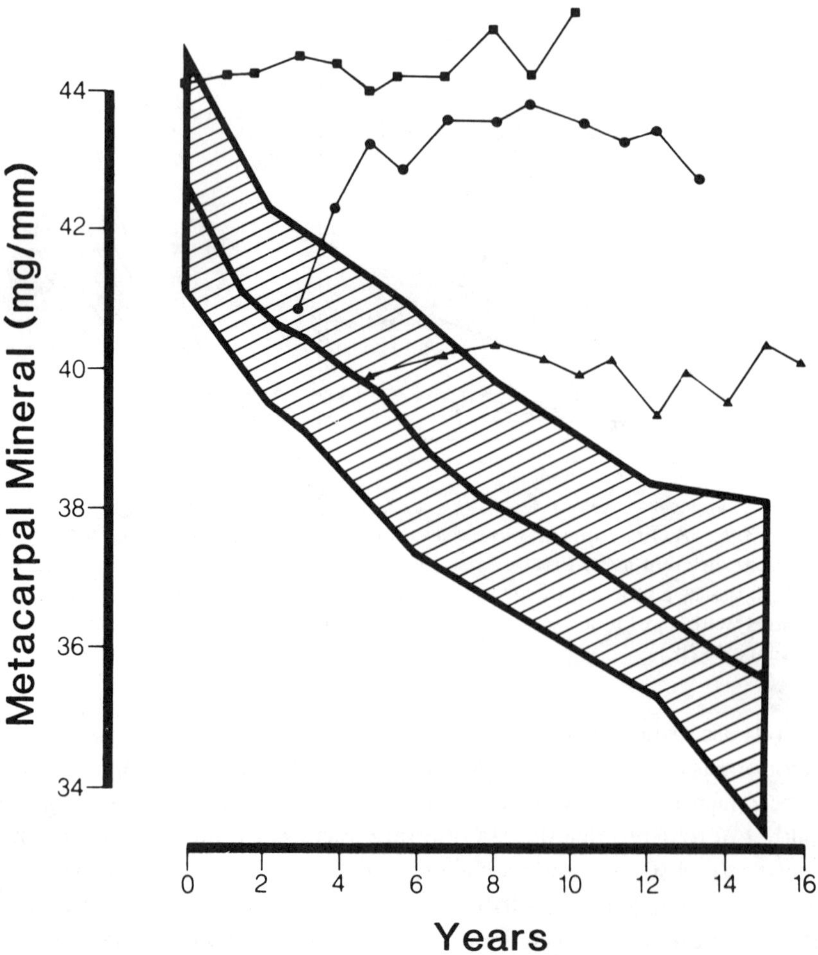

Figure 3.10. Long-term prevention of bone loss by estrogen. The hatched area represents the placebo-using group (mean ± SD) from a prospective controlled study in oophorectomized women. The three lines show the mean values only for three estrogen-treated groups; treatment initiated at the time of oophorectomy (squares), 3 years after oophorectomy (circles), and 6 years after oophorectomy (triangles). Bone loss is prevented in all three situations. However, the earlier treatment is begun, the better the outcome, in terms of bone mass after 10 years of therapy. (From Lindsay R, Hart DM, Abdalla H, Al-Azzawi F. Interrelationship of bone loss and its prevention and fracture expression. In: Christiansen C, Johnson JS, Riis BJ, eds. Osteoporosis. Copenhagen: Osteopres, 1988;2:508–512, with permission).

stable in estrogen-treated patients for at least 10 years, while bone mass declined continuously in the placebo-treated groups (139). Estrogens were effective independently of the duration of time from oophorectomy that had preceded the introduction of treatment. In those studies therapy was introduced as long as 6 years after surgery and bone loss was subsequently prevented. Since bone loss had occurred prior to the initiation of therapy, however, the group in which therapy was not started until 6 years after surgery had lower bone mass after 10 years of active treatment than either the group in which treatment was initiated immediately after surgery or the third group, in which treatment was begun 3 years after ovarian removal (Fig. 3.10). Thus, treatment effects were independent of the point at which intervention was begun. More recently we have examined an older population and demonstrated that these effects can be seen at least up to and probably beyond the age of 70 years (140).

Curiously, if estrogens are initiated during relatively rapid bone loss a small but significant increase in bone mass is almost always evident. It has been hypothesized that this occurs because of the differential immediate effects of estrogen on bone resorption and formation (79, 141). During the phenomenon of accelerated bone loss that occurs after menopause, there is increased activation of bone remodeling units and in addition an increase in the deficit between resorbed bone and newly formed bone. In other words, the osteoblast team will form less bone than has previously been removed by the osteoclast population. This phenomenon creates the irreversibility of bone loss, since once the remodeling cycle is complete there is no mechanism for synthesizing more bone at that site until a new remodeling cycle is activated. In addition, the increase in the frequency of activation of new remodeling sites creates a larger than normal temporary deficit in skeletal tissue, since more osteoclast teams are working at the same time resorbing bone.

In vivo, estrogens primarily reverse the effects that occur across the menopause, thereby reducing remodeling activation and inhibiting osteoclast activity or recruitment. There is a time, therefore, during which those remodeling units that are in the stage of synthesizing new bone when treatment is initiated complete their cycle, while bone resorption at other sites is slowed by the inhibitory effects of estrogen on activation and osteoclasts. Thus, there is a transient period after the introduction of estrogen therapy during which net bone formation will be proceeding faster than net bone resorption, and this will result in a temporary increase in bone mass as assessed by noninvasive techniques for bone mass measurement. This temporary state of positive bone balance can continue only until the remodeling units active when estrogens are initiated have completed their formative process; that is, when all active remodeling sites have been initiated after the introduction of estrogen. Thus within 1 to 2 years the increase in bone mass ceases. At that point, if estrogen affected only activation frequency, bone loss should begin again but at a slower rate. In our studies, however, we failed to detect a significant reduction in bone mass even when patients were observed for 10 years, implying that estrogens must also affect the balance between resorption and formation within each remodeling unit.

Many other studies of a variety of designs have demonstrated that estrogens reduce the acceleration of bone loss after menopause (35, 142–159). In fact, remarkably few negative studies have been published. In a study to examine the effects of estriol on bone loss we were unable to detect effects at least up to 12 mg/day, although our data suggested that higher doses might be effective (160). Estriol binds weakly to the estradiol receptor, and the pharmacokinetics of the compound require that it be given in multiple doses throughout the day. Thus, estriol would appear to have no place in the prevention of osteoporosis, a conclusion also reached by other investigators (161).

The skeleton appears to be extremely sensitive to estrogen. In a study designed to evaluate the minimum effect dose that would reduce bone loss, we demonstrated that 0.625 mg/day of conjugated equine estrogen (Premarin) is required (Fig. 3.11) (151). The dose response appears to be very steep, with only modest effects being seen at 0.3 mg/day and yet 100% efficacy at double

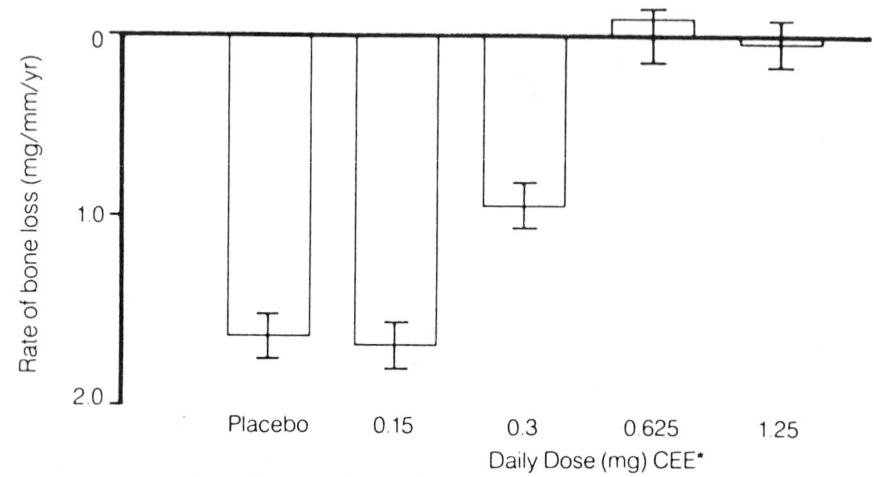

Figure 3.11. Effect of varying doses of conjugated equine estrogens (CEE) on bone loss. Five groups of patients were treated randomly with either placebo or one of four different daily doses of equine estrogen. (Reprinted with permission from Reference 151.)

this dose. Because of the reported variability in both tablet concentration of estrogen and bioavailability in generic sources of conjugated estrogen, we do not regard these sources as appropriate alternatives for use in prevention of osteoporosis (162, 163). The sensitivity of the skeleton to estrogen has been demonstrated by the decline in bone mass that precedes the overt menopause, occurring during the gradual decrease in ovarian function before menstrual periods cease entirely (55). From these data it can be suggested that circulating levels of estradiol adequate to prevent bone loss must be within the mid-follicular range, perhaps 60 to 120 pg/ml. There is much inter-individual variation, however, and achievement of these levels in one patient may not be predictive of an effect on the skeleton in that patient.

Given that circulating estrogen levels are important, it appears that the method by which these levels are achieved is irrelevant. Thus, different routes of administration can be used. Therapeutic effects have been demonstrated after oral (142–159), percutaneous (164), subcutaneous (159), and transdermal (165) administration of estrogen.

The effects of estrogen can be seen at every skeletal site that is amenable to measurement. Although we could measure bone only at a peripheral site by single-photon absorptiometry when our long-term studies began, we undertook a cross-sectional evaluation of these patients to determine if similar effects were seen in spine and hip, the sites of the most important osteoporotic fractures (166). After 10 years of therapy bone mass was 29% greater in the lumbar spine and 12% higher in the femoral neck in the estrogen-treated group in comparison with the placebo-treated individuals (Fig. 3.12) (166). These results are compatible with the virtual elimination of bone loss in the spine but a somewhat lesser effect in the hip. The reasons for this are not clear. However, there also appears to be more bone loss in the hip prior to menopause than in the spine (167), and perhaps this site is more dependent than the spine on other factors such as the stress from physical activity and thus is less dependent on endocrine status. This will require evaluation in prospective studies, something that has yet to be achieved in this young population. In our prospective study of older individuals we demonstrated a more marked increase in bone mass in the spine after the introduction of estrogen than we could see in the femoral neck, perhaps confirming that hypothesis (140).

If estrogen treatment is discontinued, bone loss begins again (168–170). The rate of bone loss appears to approximate the rate that occurs after oophorectomy. In other words, the sudden cessation of an exogenous estrogen supply is similar to the cessation of ovarian function induced by surgery. At least two studies have been able to demonstrate the recurrence of

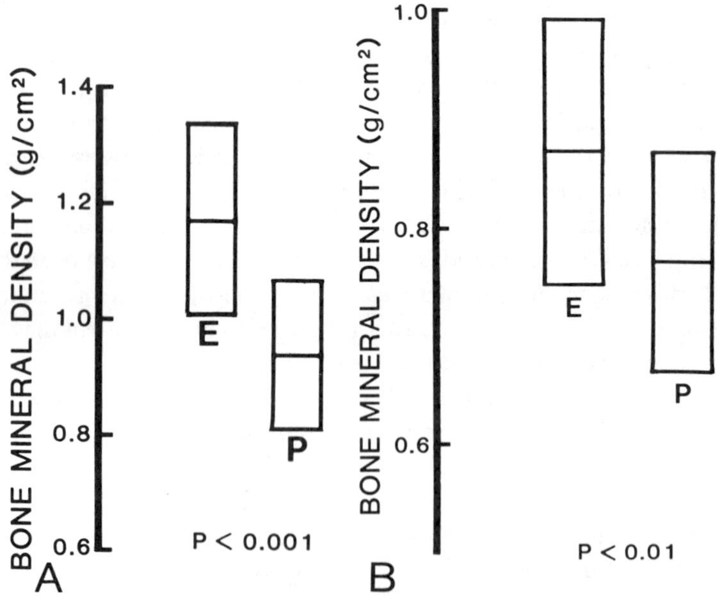

Figure 3.12. A, Bone mineral density in the lumbar spine, determined by dual-photon absorptiometry (DPA), after 10 years of treatment with estrogen (E) or placebo (P). Results are mean ± SD. **B,** Bone mineral density in the femoral neck, determined by DPA, after 10 years of treatment with estrogen (E) or placebo (P). Results are mean ± SD. (Reprinted with permission from Reference 166.)

bone loss after estrogen withdrawal, and these two, although of different design, resulted in very similar conclusions.

Estrogens cause very specific alterations in mineral homeostasis that are reflected in changes in serum and urine biochemistry (Table 3.5) (150). In most studies serum calcium tends to fall within the normal range. Serum phosphate also declines, as does alkaline phosphatase. Excretion of calcium and hydroxyproline also fall, indicative of the decline in bone resorption. The tubular maximum for phosphate resorption declines, suggestive of increased parathyroid hormone bioactivity at the level of the kidney. We have also seen increased secretion of cAMP in estrogen-treated patients (171), again suggestive of increased PTH activity. In contrast to these findings is the hypothesis originally proposed by Heaney that estrogens increase the resistance of the skeleton to PTH (172). In a series of studies designed to evaluate that issue we demonstrated that the increase in biochemical indicators of bone resorption seen after infusion of (1-34)hPTH was significantly reduced among estrogen-treated women (173). Thus, there appears to be skeletal

Table 3.5.
Effect of Oral Estrogen on the Biochemistry of Mineral Homeostasis

	SERUM			
	Calcium	PO_4	Alk. Phos.	
Placebo	9.76 ± 0.08	3.32 ± 0.03	87.8 ± 5.3	
Estrogen	9.52 ± 0.04	2.94 ± 0.09	70.0 ± 3.1	
	p<0.01	p<0.01	p<0.01	
	URINE			
	Ca/Cr	OHp/Cr	$TmPO_4$	Cyclic AMP μmol/g Creatinine
Placebo	9.76 ± 0.08	0.02 ± 0.01	3.38 ± 0.1	3.56 ± 0.4
Estrogen	0.082 ± 0.01	0.013 ± 0.01	2.87 ± 0.1	4.90 ± 0.36
	p<0.01	p<0.01	p<0.01	p<0.01

resistance, at least to the bone-resorbing effects of PTH without evidence of resistance to its renal actions.

These effects of estrogen on the skeleton translate into reduction in the risk of fracture for the postmenopausal female population. Several epidemiological studies have evaluated the magnitude of the effect, mostly for fractures of the hip, but also for Colles' fractures (143, 146, 147, 174–178). General conclusions from these studies are that estrogen use early in the postmenopausal period for a duration of at least 6 years will reduce hip fracture risk by 60% and Colles' fracture risk by a similar percentage. These effects are remarkably consistent among the studies that have been performed and are not confounded by other factors likely to alter risk (e.g., Tables 3.1, 3.2, and 3.3). Because of the effect of estrogen withdrawal and the consequent resumption of bone loss, it is not surprising that long-term treatment is required to reduce risk. It is also not surprising that the effects appear most marked if estrogen therapy is introduced soon after ovarian failure is manifested. If the 12% increment in bone mass at the hip seen after 10 years of therapy were maintained until the age of highest risk for hip fracture, this could account for the difference in hip fracture risk. In addition, if bone loss begins after estrogen therapy is stopped, one could argue that 5 to 6 years of therapy would be sufficient to produce a protective effect against fractures, especially of the femoral neck (179). The argument is as follows: Bone loss begins around the time of menopause, 50 years of age on average. Hip fracture risk begins to rise most steeply at age 75 years. Life expectancy is on average around 80 years for women at the present time. Thus, delaying bone loss by 5 years, to age 55, might be expected to delay the rise in fracture risk by the same amount, i.e., to age 80, when it would be an irrelevant issue for the majority of the population. It is entirely possible that the maximal beneficial effects of estrogen on fractures are seen only in those who currently remain on long-term therapy (178).

Significantly fewer data are available about the effects of estrogen on vertebral fractures, which are feared by women as much as if not more than hip fracture because of the accompanying changes in body configuration that result. Cross-sectional evaluation of chest radiographs from an HMO setting suggested that exposure to estrogen even for periods as short as 1 year resulted in a reduction in vertebral fracture prevalence of about 50%. Radiographs of the dorsolumbar spine (151) from women participating in our long-term study at the end of 10 years of therapy were evaluated and suggested a decline of some 75 to 90% in the occurrence of vertebral deformity with long-term estrogen use.

Some studies have tried to investigate interactions between estrogens and other modalities for the prevention of bone loss. In one study, the authors concluded that if calcium intake were increased to 1500 mg/day the minimum dose of estrogen required to prevent bone loss could be reduced to 0.3 mg/day (157) (as conjugated equine estrogen, Premarin). Since this was not a randomized study, the data require confirmation. In another study, patients were randomly assigned to estrogen with or without the addition of an exercise program (180). In this setting the group using estrogen and participating in the activity program had a greater increment in lumbar spine bone mass than the control group using estrogen alone. Although clearly more data are required to evaluate the interactions of estrogen with lifestyle factors, it is reasonable to try to improve nutrition and physical activity when intervening to prevent osteoporotic fracture. Increasing calcium intake to 1000 to 1500 mg/day is not difficult, even when calcium supplements are utilized, and is generally considered to be without risk for most individuals (care should be taken to obtain a history of renal stones before advice about calcium is given). Increasing activity has such general beneficial effects that neglecting this recommendation is probably a mistake. For those undertaking an exercise program for the first time a cardiologic evaluation, including a stress test, should be performed prior to initiation of the program. We insist that the activity be fun, to improve compliance, and do not usually give specific advice about the type of activity.

The effects of estrogen on the skeleton are not unique to estrogens alone. There is evidence that some progestogens can also reduce the rate of bone loss when given to postmenopausal women (159, 181–183). Androgenic steroids (those derived from 19-nortestosterone) appear to be somewhat more effective than pure C-21 progestogens. Norethindrone inhibits bone loss at a daily dose of 5 mg, a dose often used clinically, while at least 20 mg/day of medroxyprogesterone acetate is required to produce similar effects. It seems unlikely that these agents can or should be used as alternatives to estrogen for long-term prevention of bone loss, since they have negative effects on the plasma lipid profile, tending to lower HDL and raise LDL in a fashion similar to androgens (184, 185). Perhaps more importantly these agents, commonly used with estrogens to reduce the risk of endometrial carcinoma (186, 187), do not interfere with the dominant effects of estrogen. Some data suggest that the effects of estrogen on bone may be enhanced when a progestogen is added (188). Further evaluation of this is required. Anabolic agents also reduce the rate of bone loss (147, 156, 189, 190), and such agents were originally suggested by Albright (2) as being potentially useful in the treatment of osteoporosis. Asymptomatic female patients do not in general tolerate these agents well because of masculinizing side effects, and they are not approved for use in the United States. Some in vitro data suggest that anabolic agents, and thus perhaps the progestogens derived from androgens, can stimulate bone formation (191).

Estrogen therapy can also be used in established osteoporosis to prevent further loss of bone in patients with an already compromised skeleton (140, 192–194). Indeed, estrogens appear to be capable of reducing bone loss in all estrogen-deficient women, irrespective of age, at least up to the eighth decade (140, 158). Recent data suggest that estrogens, in addition to their effects on bone mass, also reduce fracture recurrence in the osteoporotic population (194a). Clinical impressions as well as uncontrolled data (192) certainly suggest this is so, and the trend in our data supports the conclusion.

Alternatives to estrogen include calcitonin and perhaps also the bisphosphonates (195–208). Neither has the global effects of estrogen and should be used only for the prevention or treatment of osteoporosis in estrogen-deficient women when there is a specific contraindication to the use of estrogen, or when the patient refuses such treatment and can be shown to be at high risk of osteoporosis (or has osteoporotic fractures). Calcitonin may become available in an intranasal spray form, which will be advantageous for those who do not wish to use an injectable agent (201, 202). Further studies on this route of administration are required to establish the exact dose required to prevent spinal bone loss, especially in the established disorder. Bisphophonates are oral alternatives to calcitonin. Etidronate is currently the only available agent in the United States, but it is not approved for use in osteoporosis. These agents act like osteoclast poisons and have a long skeletal half-life. Preliminary data suggest that very low doses can reduce bone loss in patients with osteoporosis but appear to have little effect on future recurrence

(206–208). Long-term data are required before these agents can be considered for more general use in patients with a high risk of fracture. Excess doses may inhibit bone remodeling so powerfully that the normal repair processes cease and the mean age of the tissue increases. If this occurs, fracture risk might potentially increase (209). Bisphosphonates remain experimental agents.

The exact mechanism of estrogen action in reducing bone remodeling is not well understood. In his original observations Albright noted the biochemical accompaniments of estrogen therapy, particularly the marked reduction in urinary calcium (2) and the improvement in calcium balance. Similar data have been reported by others (8, 76–78). The data suggest improved efficiency in the use of available dietary calcium, elegantly demonstrated by the work of Heaney (76–78). Thus calcium absorption across the intestine, which declines after menopause, improves with estrogen therapy. Reductions in 1,25-dihydroxyvitamin D receptor number have been shown in rats after oophorectomy, providing a mechanism for the effects on intestinal calcium absorption (210, 211). The improved calcium absorption coupled with reduced renal loss can reduce calcium mobilization from the skeleton, again demonstrated by Heaney using kinetic data (76–78). The prime event has been the source of discussion for many years, but assessment of the available data leads to the conclusion that the main effect of estrogen must be at the skeletal level and that other effects are consequent upon this (see Fig. 3.5).

Heaney first hypothesized that estrogen increased the resistance of the skeleton to the effects of PTH (172) and, as we have noted, without causing similar effects in the kidney (171, 173). Some data suggest that this effect is mediated by increased endogenous calcitonin secretion (212–216). In vitro data suggest that physiologic concentrations of estrogen increase the release of calcitonin from C-cells in culture (213). However, not all data agree with the concept that estrogen can lead to increased circulating concentrations of calcitonin (217, 218). In part this results from the difficulty in performing the immunoassay of calcitonin in interpreting the results (205, 219). Increments in calcitonin have been demonstrated by some, but not all. In the latter case, when calcitonin monomer is measured after separation of the dimer and other immunoreactants, no changes in monomeric calcitonin can be observed. It is not clear if this is biologically relevant or if the results are induced by the purification technique. Other circumstantial evidence supports the calcitonin hypothesis for estrogen action. Increased calcitonin levels during pregnancy, particularly in the third trimester, have been suggested to be a mechanism for protection of the maternal skeleton from the demands of the fetus for calcium (215). In addition, higher levels of calcitonin in men and blacks has been suggested to be a mechanism for higher peak bone mass in these populations, and may be one mechanism for reduced incidence of osteoporotic fractures (220–223).

In addition, as we have noted above, a fall in serum phosphorus and reduced $TmPO_4$ are consistent with increased PTH activity, which has been difficult to demonstrate by immunoassay (224). An alternative explanation for the changes in phosphate homeostasis would be a decrease in the effect of growth hormone or insulin-like growth factors (225). These biochemical effects of estrogen continue for as long as estrogens are prescribed, at least up to 10 years. Thus the conclusion might be that estrogen effects a relative resistance to PTH in bone, confirmed by our recent data during infusion of (1-34)hPTH, with increased sensitivity to PTH at the level of the kidney. The alternative is to require a separate effect mediated by alterations in growth hormone secretion. However, growth hormone product is stimulated by estrogen (225, 226).

These results and the difficulty in explaining the effects of estrogen stimulated a search for estrogen receptors in bone cells, which until recently was largely unsuccessful (227). In 1988 two groups separately identified high-affinity estradiol receptor in osteoblasts or osteoblast-like cells in culture (80, 81). Estrogens stimulate replication and collagen gene expression in the primary calvarial cells of rats (83, 84, 228). In osteosarcoma cells estradiol reduces cAMP production (229). In addition, estradiol is mitogenic in both primary cultures of calvarial cells and in immortalized cell lines (83). In the same cells estradiol increases IGF-1 mRNA and reduces the response of the cells to PTH. These data suggest the interaction of estradiol with osteoblasts. PTH acts primarily on osteoblasts, and it has been proposed that these cells control bone resorption either by providing the stimulus for activation or by assisting in the recruitment of osteoclasts to the bone resorption site (230). Thus, affecting bone resorption through osteoblasts would be a potential mechanism of action for estrogens. Other potential mechanisms of action exist. Following ovarian failure there is increased production of interleukin-1 by circulating monocytes. It has been suggested that this is suppressed by estrogen, although not all data agree (231–233). Interleukin-1 is a potent stimulator of bone resorption synergistically with PTH (234). Prostaglandins, which increase both formation and resorption, increase after oophorectomy in rats and are reduced in vivo but not in vitro by estrogens (235). Prostaglandins also appear to work synergistically with PTH (236). In terms of the effects of PTH on resorption, the cellular effects of estrogen would appear to be appropriate for decreased responsivity to PTH. As noted above, there are recent reports that osteoclasts may also have estrogen receptors (81a). However, it has proved difficult to demonstrate convincingly the effects of estrogen on osteoclast function in vitro except at toxic concentrations (82), and therefore the functional significance of these putative receptors remains unclear.

Although they are difficult to define, the effects of estrogen are clinically clear and evident. The almost universal finding of reduced bone remodeling and the decreased loss of skeletal tissue that follows the introduction of estrogen to estrogen-deficient women highlights the importance of the menopause in the pathogenesis of osteoporosis. The judicious use of bone mass measurements allows us to target specific groups for preventive therapy against osteoporosis. Other effects of estrogen will of course influence the individual's decision whether or not to use the therapy.

TREATMENT

The treatment of patients who present with clinical fracture syndromes is difficult. Initially, for patients presenting with an acute fracture syndrome, the approach to the patient is surgical (for hip and Colles' fracture) or rehabilitative for patients presenting with acute symptoms of vertebral fracture. It is the therapeutic approaches to skeletal status that are more controversial. The preferred approach would be to increase skeletal mass and restore architecture to eliminate the possibility of further atraumatic fracture. At the present such approaches are not feasible. The therapeutic agents currently available are those likely to be more effective in the prevention of the disorder. These include estrogen, calcitonin, and possibly the bisphosphonates, all of which are essentially antiresorptive agents. Each has some advantages over the others, and all have certain disadvantages. Thus the physician must discuss the benefits and risks of each therapy with each patient.

Estrogen

The effects of estrogen are best documented for prevention. However, several recent studies have evaluated the effects of estrogen intervention both in older women and in women with established osteoporosis (140, 192–194). These studies are consistent in their conclusions and can be summarized easily. All data published thus far indicate that estrogen intervention when provided to estrogen-deficient women reduces the rate of bone loss. In studies of women with established osteoporosis there is a small but significant increase in bone mass, especially in the spine (Fig. 3.13). In our controlled study in which we compared estrogen therapy plus calcium supplementation to calcium alone, we demonstrated that estrogen treatment prevented bone loss at least up to age 75 years, while bone loss continued in patients given only calcium

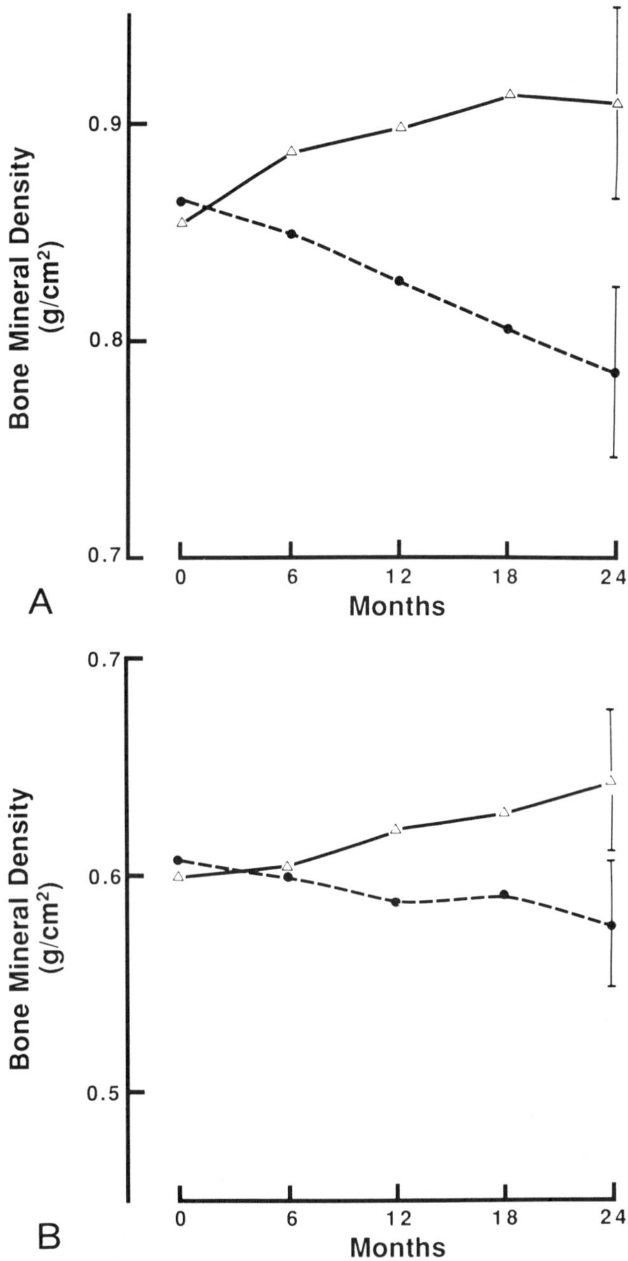

Figure 3.13. Mean changes in bone mineral density of the lumbar spine (**A**) and the femoral neck (**B**) during 2 years' therapy with estrogen and calcium (triangles) or calcium (circles). At the end of 2 years, the mean bone mineral density of the lumbar spine was significantly greater in the calcium and estrogen–treated group than at the initiation of the study ($p<0.01$) and than the final mean for the calcium-treated group ($p<0.01$). (Reproduced with permission from Reference 140.)

supplements (140). The effects were more obvious in the lumbar vertebrae than in the femoral neck, since bone loss in the hip appeared to be slower than in the spine in the calcium-treated group. Other studies have confirmed these data (192–194). As with younger patients, a progestin must be added to the regimen to protect the uterus. We have had somewhat more success with a combined continuous regimen in this older group of patients.

Calcitonin

Calcitonin in controlled studies produces essentially the same effects as estrogen (195–199). There is preservation of bone mass with doses of salmon calcitonin of 50 to 100 units daily or on alternate days. A clear dose-response relationship has been described over this limited range. Recently, one study divided patients biochemically into those with "high" turnover and "low" turnover and demonstrated a more pronounced therapeutic effect in those with increased skeletal remodeling. The effects of calcitonin on bone mass may be only one reason to use calcitonin immediately following fractures such as vertebral fracture whose main symptom is pain. Several reports, including controlled experiments in animals, indicate that calcitonin in certain circumstances is an effective analgesic agent (205). Thus, immediately following vertebral fracture, if pain is a major symptom calcitonin may speed the recovery of the patient, reducing the requirement for narcotic analgesia and perhaps shortening the period of bed rest required. The main disadvantage to the use of calcitonin in the United States at present is the necessity for parenteral administration. Recent studies in which preparations of calcitonin have been administered in an intranasal spray have demonstrated that the drug effectively reduces bone loss by this route. Calcitonin is relatively devoid of serious side effects. Flushing, nausea, and abdominal fullness are the most frequent. These are usually transient, and if they are problematic the dose should be reduced. Initiation of treatment at a low dose and gradually increasing the dose every 2 to 3 days until the therapeutic dose is reached is the most effective method of reducing the likelihood of side effects. In addition, since calcitonin is a potent inhibitor of gastric acid secretion it should be administered several hours after food. We generally administer calcitonin in the evening prior to retiring to minimize the side effects. An antiemetic may be given 30 minutes beforehand if nausea is a problem.

Bisphosphonates

The effects of bisphosphonates have recently been tested in several studies (206–208). Preservation of bone mass is somewhat similar to that found in other studies of antiresorptive agents. In two studies that evaluated the effects of etidronate, reductions in fracture frequency were reported (206–208). Therefore, bisphosphonates will be alternatives to other therapies if approved by the FDA. Etidronate, the only bisphosphonate currently available in the United States, is given in daily doses of 400 mg for 2 weeks each 3 months, and the dose must be given at least 2 to 3 hours before or after food. In addition, calcium supplements should not be taken at the same time as the daily dose of bisphosphonates. This so-called intermittent approach to treatment is probably a misnomer because of the long half-life of the compound in the skeleton. Bisphosphonates are potent inhibitors of osteoclasts. Bisphosphonates bind to calcium in bone, and in the process of bone resorption osteoclasts are subjected to high concentrations of the drug, which acts as a cell poison. The long-term effects of these agents in patients with osteoporosis have yet to be examined, and they remain experimental at present.

Other Alternatives

A variety of other potentially useful agents are currently being evaluated for the treatment of osteoporosis. Anabolic agents also stabilize bone mass and small but significant increases in total body calcium have been demonstrated (147, 156, 189, 190). Their androgenicity limits their use among postmenopausal women. Thiazides have been shown to be associated with decreased bone loss and a reduced risk of hip fracture (237). Limited formal controlled studies are available, and the overall benefit-to-risk ratio still requires evaluation before these agents can be advocated for use in osteoporosis. Fluoride is the one agent that increases bone mass, especially in the vertebrae. As such it has long been considered to be a potentially useful therapeutic approach to patients with crush fracture syndrome. However, recent controlled studies could not demonstrate a significant reduction in fracture recurrence despite dramatic increments in bone mass (238, 239). In addition, there was an apparent increase in peripheral fractures, perhaps confirming the uncontrolled studies that had previously suggested that fluoride use is associated with an increased risk of hip fracture. Curiously, antiestrogens may also protect against bone loss. Tamoxifen, in doses usually used in the prevention of secondary breast cancer, appears to reduce the rate of bone loss and reduces the risk of osteoporosis among women with breast cancer (240).

It is therefore possible to develop a rational approach to osteoporosis prevention and treatment. While primary prevention is most likely to be achieved by maximizing peak bone mass, this will remain difficult to achieve until public attitudes are changed toward nutrition and exercise during growth. It is at the time of ovarian failure, through the judicious use of bone mass measurements, that those most at risk can be identified and targeted for treatment. Estrogens remain the principal therapeutic approach to both prevention and treatment of established osteoporosis. The goal in general is to achieve physiologic levels of circulating 17β-estradiol. Alternatives to estrogen are available for patients who cannot or will not participate in hormone replacement therapy. These agents, however, target only the skeleton, and therefore patients will accrue none of the other benefits of estrogen therapy.

Key Points

- Osteoporosis is a disorder in which bone mass is reduced sufficiently to significantly increase the risk of fracture.
- Osteoporosis is a major public health problem in the United States and other developed countries.
- Approximately 1.5 million new fractures each year are caused by osteoporosis in the United States.
- The most common fractures are those of hip, spine (vertebral crush fractures), and wrist (Colles' fracture), but fracture of any bone can occur.
- Hip fracture is the most serious fracture, occurring in 0.25 million individuals each year and resulting in 5 to 20% excess mortality, with 30 to 50% of individuals becoming dependent after their fracture.
- The frequency of osteoporotic fracture is increasing, in part because the population over age 65 is increasing.
- There may also be an age-specific increase in the incidence of osteoporosis, the causes of which are not known.
- Ovarian failure, whatever its cause, is a major etiologic factor in the development of osteoporosis.
- Osteoporosis therefore occurs more commonly in postmenopausal women; the female:male ratios are 10:1 for vertebral fracture and 2:1 for hip fracture.
- Other factors are superimposed upon menopause to alter the individual's risk of osteoporosis. These include hereditary factors, diet (low calcium intake, high alcohol and caffeine intake), lifestyle (cigarette smoking, inactivity), and secondary factors (endogenous or exogenous excess of glucocorticoid and thyroid hormone).

- A measurement of bone mass by a noninvasive technique at menopause is a useful indicator of risk for future fracture. The lower bone mass is, the greater the risk of fracture.
- Bone mass can therefore be used as an indicator for intervention.
- Estrogen intervention reduces bone loss and reduces the risk of fracture. In general, the earlier treatment is initiated, the greater the response is likely to be. At least 5 to 10 years of therapy may be required.
- The minimum effective dose of estrogen is 0.625 mg conjugated equine estrogen or its equivalent. The route of administration does not appear to be important.
- The addition of a progestogen does not alter the skeletal response to estrogen.
- Estrogen therapy is also useful for the treatment of patients who present with osteoporotic fractures, since estrogen will reduce further loss of bone at least up to age 70 years.
- Calcitonin and perhaps also the bisphosphonates, progestogens, or tamoxifen are alternatives to estrogen for patients who cannot or should not take estrogen.

References

1. Albright F, Bloomberg F, Smith PH. Postmenopausal osteoporosis. Trans Assoc Am Phys 1940;55:298–305.
2. Albright F. The effect of hormones on osteogenesis in man. Recent Prog Horm Res 1947;1:293–353.
3. Cummings SR, Kelsey JL, Nevitt MC, O'Dowd KJ. Epidemiology of osteoporosis and osteoporotic fractures. Epidemiol Rev 1985;7:178–188.
4. Melton LJ III. Epidemiology of fractures. In: Riggs BL, Melton LJ III, eds. Osteoporosis: etiology, diagnosis and management. New York: Raven Press, 1988:133–154.
5. Johnston CC, Melton LJ. Bone density measurement and the mangement of osteoporosis. In: Favus MJ, ed. Primer on the metabolic bone diseases and disorders of mineral metabolism. Kelseyville, California: American Society for Bone and Mineral Research, 1990:93–100.
6. Smith DM, Nance WE, Kang K, et al. Genetic factors in determining bone mass. J Clin Invest 1973;52:2800–2811.
7. Garn SM, Nagy JM, Sandusky ST. Differential sexual dimorphism in bone parameters of subjects of European and African ancestry. Am J Phys Anthropol 1972;37:127–130.
8. Lindsay R. Sex steroids and osteoporosis. In: Riggs BL, Melton LJ III, eds. Osteoporosis: etiology, diagnosis and management. New York: Raven Press, 1988:333–358.
9. Albanese AA, Edelson AH, Lorenze EJ Jr, Woodhull ML, Wein EH. Problems of bone health in the elderly: ten year study. NY State J Med 1975;75:326–336.
10. Donaldson CL, Hulley SB, Vogel JM, Hattner RS, Bayers JH, McMillan DE. Effect of prolonged bed rest on bone mineral. Metabolism 1970;19:1071–1084.

11. Hansson TH, Roos BO, Nachemson A. Development of osteopenia in the fourth lumbar vertebrae during prolonged bed rest after operation for scoliosis. Acta Orthop Scand 1975;46:621–630.
12. Jenkens DB, Cochran TH. Osteoporosis: the dramatic effect of disuse of an extremity. Clin Orthop 1969;64:128–134.
13. Krolner B, Toft B. Vertebral bone loss: an unheeded side effect of therapeutic bed rest. Clin Sci 1973;64:537–540.
14. Mack PB, LaChance PA, Vose GP, Vogt FB. Bone demineralization of foot and head of Gemini-Titan IV, V and VII astronauts during orbital flight. Am J Roentgenol 1967;100:503–511.
15. Rambaut PC, Goode AW. Skeletal changes during space flight. Lancet 1985;2:1050–1052.
16. Margulies JY, Simkin A, Leichter I, Bivas A, Steinberg R, Giladi M, Stein M, Kashtan H, Milgrom C. Effect of intense physical activity on the bone mineral content in the lower limbs of young adults. J Bone Joint Surg 1986;68A:1090–1093.
17. Aloia JF, Cohn SH, Babu T, Abesamis C, Kalici N, Ellis K. Skeletal mass and body composition in marathon runners. Metabolism 1978;27:1793–1796.
18. Dalen N, Olsson KE. Bone mineral content and physical activity. Acta Orthop Scand 1974;45:170–174.
19. Lanyon LE. Bone remodeling, mechanical stress and osteoporosis. In: DeLuca HF, Frost HM, Jee WSS, Johnston CC Jr, Parfitt AM. Osteoporosis: recent advances in pathogenesis and treatment. Baltimore: University Park Press, 1980:129–138.
20. Lanyon LE. Functional strain as a determinant for bone remodeling. Calcif Tissue Int 1984;36(suppl):56–61.
21. Heaney RP. Nutritional factors in bone health. In: Riggs BL, Melton LJ III, eds. Osteoporosis: etiology, diagnosis and management. New York: Raven Press, 1988:359–372.
22. Matkovic V, Kostial K, Simonovic I, Buzina R, Brodarec A, Nordin BEC. Bone status and fracture rates in regions of Yugoslavia. Am J Clin Nutr 1979;32:540–549.
23. Nilas L, Christiansen C, Rodbro P. Calcium supplementation and postmenopausal bone loss. Br Med J 1984;289:1103–1106.
24. Riis B, Thomsen K, Christiansen C. Does calcium supplementation prevent postmenopausal bone loss? N Engl J Med 1987;316:173–177.
24a. Dawson-Hughes B, Dallal GE, Krall GE, et al. A controlled trial of the effect of calcium supplementation on bone density in postmenopausal women. N Engl J Med 1990;323: 878–883.
25. Bikle DD, Genant HK, Cann CE, Recker RR, Halloran BP, Strewler GJ. Bone disease in alcohol abuse. Ann Intern Med 1985;103:42–48.
26. Farley JR, Fitzsimmons R, Taylor AK, Jarch WM, Lau KHW. Direct effects of ethanol on bone resorption and formation in vitro. Arch Biochem Biophys 1985;238:305–314.
27. Daniell HW. Osteoporosis of the slender smoker: vertebral compression fractures and loss of metacarpal cortex in relation to postmenopausal cigarette smoking and lack of obesity. Arch Intern Med 1983;143:1678–1682.
28. Daniell HW. Postmenopausal tooth loss. Contributions to edentulism by osteoporosis and cigarette smoking. Arch Intern Med 1983;143:1678–1682.
29. Melton LJ III, Riggs BL. Clinical spectrum in osteoporosis. In: Riggs BL, Melton LJ III, eds. Osteoporosis: etiology, diagnosis and management. New York: Raven Press, 1988: 155–179.
30. Aitken JM, Hart DM, Anderson JB, Lindsay R, Smith DA. Osteoporosis after oophorectomy for non-malignant disease. Br Med J 1973;1:325–328.
31. Richelson LS, Wahner HW, Melton LJ III, Riggs BL. Relative contributions of aging and estrogen deficiency to postmenopausal bone loss. N Engl J Med 1984;311:1273–1275.

32. Bloom RA, Laws JW. Humeral cortical thickness as an index of osteoporosis in women. Br J Radiol 1970;43:522–527.
33. Cann CE, Genant HK, Kolb FO, Ettinger B. Quantitative computed tomography for prediction of vertebral fracture risk. Bone 1985;6:1–7.
34. Cohn SH, Aloia JF, Vaswani AN, Zanzi I, Vestsky D, Ellis KJ. Age and sex related changes in bone mass measured by neutron activation. In: Menzcel J, ed. Osteoporosis. Chichester: John Wiley & Sons, 1982:33–43.
35. Davis ME, Lanzl LH, Cox AB. Detection, prevention and retardation of postmenopausal osteoporosis. Obstet Gynecol 1970;36:187–198.
36. Garn SM, Nagy JM, Sandusky ST. Differential sexual dimorphism in bone parameters of subjects of European and African ancestry. Am J Phys Anthropol 1972;37:127–130.
37. Garn SM, Rohmann CG, Wagner B. Bone loss as a general phenomenon in man. Fed Proc 1977;26:1729–1736.
38. Jasani C, Nordin BEC, Smith DA, Swanson I. Spinal osteoporosis and the menopause. Proc R Soc Med 1965;58:441–444.
39. Krolner B, Nielsen SP. Bone mineral content of the lumbar spine in normal and osteoporotic women: cross sectional and longitudinal studies. Clin Sci 1982;62:329–336.
40. Lindsay R. Osteoporosis, and its relationship to estrogen. Contemp Obstet Gynecol 1984; 63:201–224.
41. Madsen M. Vertebral and peripheral bone mineral content by photon absorptiometry. Invest Radiol 1977;12:185–188.
42. Mazess RB. Advances in total body and regional bone mineral by dual-photon absorptiometry. In: Menczel J et al., eds. Osteoporosis. Chichester: John Wiley & Sons, 1982:80–86.
43. Maziere B, Kuntz D, Dughesnay M. In vivo analysis of bone calcium by local neutron activation of the hand in postmenopausal osteoporosis. In: Menczel J et al., eds. Osteoporosis. Chichester: John Wiley & Sons, 1982:117–125.
44. Meema HE. Cortical bone atrophy and osteoporosis as a manifestation of aging. Am J Roentgenol 1963;89:1287–1295.
45. Meema HE. Menopausal and aging changes in muscle mass and bone mineral content. J Bone Joint Surg 1966;48A:1138–1144.
46. Nordin BEC, MacGregor J, Smith DA. The incidence of osteoporosis in normal women: its relation to age and the menopause. Q J Med 1966;137:25–38.
47. Solomon L. Bone density of aging Caucasian and African populations. Lancet 1979; 1:1326–1330.
48. Arnold JS, Bartley MH, Tont SA, Jenkins DP. Skeletal changes in aging and disease. Clin Orthop Rel Res 1966;49:17–38.
49. Leichter I, Wermreb A, Hazan G, Loewinger E, Robin GC, Steinberg R, Mencyer J, Makin M. The effect of age and sex on bone density, bone mineral content and cortical index. Clin Orthop Rel Res 1981;156:232–239.
50. Riggs BL, Wahner HW, Dunn WL, Mazess RB, Offord KP, Melton LJ III. Differential changes in bone mineral density of the appendicular and axial skeleton with aging: relationship to spinal osteoporosis. J Clin Invest 1981;67:328–335.
51. Trotter M, Hixon BB. Sequential changes in weight, density and percentage weight of human skeletons from an early fetal period through old age. Anat Rec 1974;179:1–8.
52. Lindsay R, Hart DM, Sweeney A, Coutts JRT, Clark A. Endogenous estrogen and bone loss following oophorectomy. Calc Tissue Res 1977;22(suppl):213–216.
53. Lindsay R, Coutts JRT, Hart DM. The effect of endogenous oestrogen on plasma and urinary calcium and phosphate in oophorectomized women. Clin Endocrinol 1977;6:87–93.
54. Riis BJ, Christiansen C, Deftos LJ, Catherwood BD. The role of serum concentrations of estrogens in postmenopausal osteoporosis and bone turnover. In: Christiansen C et al., eds. Osteoporosis. Denmark: Aalborg Stiftsbogtrykkeri, 1984:333–336.

55. Slemenda C, Hui SL, Longcope C, Johnston CC. Sex steroids and bone mass: a study of changes about the time of menopause. J Clin Invest 1987;80:1261–1269.
56. Cann CE, Martin MC, Genant HK, Jaffe RB. Decreased spinal mineral content in amenorrheic women. JAMA 1984;251:626–629.
57. Crosby LO, Kaplan FS, Pertschuk MJ, Mullen JL. The effect of anorexia nervosa on bone morphometry in young women. Clin Orthop Rel Res 1985;201:271–277.
58. Drinkwater BL, Nilson K, Chestnut CH III, Bremner WJ, Shainholtz S, Southworth MB. Bone mineral content of amenorrheic and eumenorrheic athletes. N Engl J Med 1984; 311:277–281.
59. Fisher EC, Nelson ME, Frontera WR, Turksoy RN, Evans WJ. Bone mineral content and levels of gonadotropins and estrogens in amenorrheic running women. J Clin Endocrinol Metab 1986;62:1232–1236.
60. Gonzalez ER. Premature bone loss found in some nonmenstruating sportswomen. JAMA 1982;248:513–514.
61. Lindberg JS, Fears WB, Hunt MM. Exercised induced amenorrhea and bone density. Ann Intern Med 1984;101:647–649.
62. Linnel SL, Stager MM, Blue PW. Bone mineral content and menstrual regularity in female runners. Med Sci Sports Exec 1983;16:343–348.
63. Marcus R, Cann C, Madvig D. Menstrual function and bone mass in elite women distance runners. Ann Intern Med 1985;102:158–163.
64. Klibanski A, Neer RM, Beitins IZ, Ridgway C, Zervas NT, MacArthur J. Decreased bone density in hyperprolactenemic women. N Engl J Med 1980;303:1151–1514.
65. Rigotti NA, Nussbaum SR, Herzog DB, Neer RM. Osteoporosis in women with anorexia nervosa. N Engl J Med 1984;311:1601–1606.
66. Gudmundsson JA, Ljunghall S, Bergquist C, et al. Increased bone turnover during gonadotrophin releasing hormone superagonist-induced ovulation inhibition. J Clin Endocrinol Metab 1987;65:159–163.
67. Henzl MR, Corson Sl, Moghissi K, et al. Administration of nasal nafarelin as compared with oral danazol for endometriosis. A multicenter double-blind comparative clinical trial. N Engl J Med 1988;318:485–489.
68. Steingold K, DeZeigler D, Cedars M, et al. Clinical and hormonal effects of chronic gonadotropin-releasing hormone against treatment of polycystic ovarian disease. J Clin Endocrinol Metab 1987;65:773–777.
69. Frasen HM, Waxman J. Gonadotropin releasing hormone analogues for gynecological disorders and infertility. Br Med J 1989;298:475–476.
70. Abbasi R, Hodgen GD. Predicting the predisposition to osteoporosis. Gonadotropin-releasing hormone agonist for acute estrogen deficiency test. JAMA 1986;255:1600–1604.
71. Greenspan SL, Neer RM, Ridgway EC, Klibanski A. Osteoporosis in men with hyper-prolactinemic hypogonadism. Ann Intern Med 1986;104:777–782.
72. Jackson JA, Kleerekoper M, Parfitt AM. Symptomatic osteoporosis in a man with hyperprolactinemic hypogonadism. Ann Intern Med 1986;105:543–545.
73. Rigotti NA, Neer RM, Jameson L. Osteopenia and bone fractures in a man with anorexia nervosa and hypogonadism. JAMA 1986;256:385–388.
74. Seeman E, Melton LJ III, O'Fallon WM, Riggs BL. Risk factors for spinal osteoporosis in men. Am J Med 1983;75:977–983.
75. Meier DE, Orwoll ES, Jones EM. Marked disparity between trabecular and cortical bone loss with age in healthy men. Measured by vertebral computed tomography and radial photon absorptiometry. Ann Intern Med 1984;101:605–612.
76. Heaney RP, Recker RR, Saville PD. Calcium balance and calcium requirements in middle-aged women. Am J Clin Nutr 1978;30:1603–1611.

77. Heaney RP, Recker RR, Saville PD. Menopausal changes in calcium balance performance. J Lab Clin Med 1978;92:953–963.
78. Heaney RP, Recker RR, Saville PD. Menopausal changes in bone remodeling. J Lab Clin Med 1978;92:964–970.
79. Parfitt AM. The coupling of bone resorption to bone formation. A critical analysis of the concept and of its relevance in the pathogenesis of osteoporosis. Metab Bone Dis Rel Res 1982;4:1–6.
80. Komm BS, Terpening CM, Benz DJ, et al. Estrogen binding, receptor mRNA, and biologic response to osteoblast-like osteosarcoma cells. Science 1988;241:81–84.
81. Eriksen EF, Colvard DS, Berg NJ, et al. Evidence of estrogen receptors in normal human osteoblast-like cells. Science 1988;241:84–86.
82. Arnett TR, Dempster DW, Lindsay R. Effect of estrogen and anti-estrogens on osteoclast activity in vitro. J Bone Min Res 1986;1(suppl 1):99.
82a. Owsler M, Pyfferaen J, Osdoby P, et al. Osteoclasts express mRNA for estrogen receptor. J Bone Miner Res 1990;5:A517.
83. Ernst M, Schmid C, Frankenfoldt C, Fraesch ER. Estradiol stimulation of osteoblast proliferation in vitro: mediator roles for TGFβ, PGE_2, IGF-1. Calcif Tissue Res 1988; 42(suppl):A117.
84. Gray TK, Mohan S, Linkhart TA, Williams ME, Baylink DJ. Estrogen may mediate its effects on bone cells by signalling the observation of growth factors. J Bone Min Res 1988;3:A552.
85. Pacifici R, Rifas L, Vered I, et al. Interleukin secretion from human blood monocytes in normal and osteoporotic women effect of menopause and estrogen/progesterone treatment of bone. J Bone Min Res 1988;3:A541.
86. Price P. Osteocalcin. In: Peck WA, ed. Bone and mineral research. Amsterdam: Excerpta Medica. 1983:157–190.
87. Riggs BL, Melton LJ III. Evidence for two distinct syndromes of involutional osteoporosis. Am J Med 1983;75:899–901.
88. Riggs BL, Melton LJ III. Involutional osteoporosis. N Engl J Med 1986;314:1676–1686.
89. Alevizaki CC, Ikkos DG, Singhelakis P. Progressive decrease of true intestinal calcium absorption with age in normal man. J Nucl Med 1973;14:760–762.
90. Avioli LV, McDonald J, Lee SW. The influence of age on the intestinal absorption of Ca^{47} in women and its relation to Ca^{47} absorption in postmenopausal osteoporosis. J Clin Invest 1965;44:1960–1965.
91. Avioli LV. Calcium and osteoporosis. Am Rev Nutr 1984;4:471–491.
92. Endres DB, Morgan CH, Garry PJ, et al. Age-related changes in serum immunoreactive parathyroid hormone and its biological action in healthy men and women. J Clin Endocrinol Metab 1987;65:724–731.
93. Slovik DM, Adams JS, Neer RM, et al. Deficient production of 1,25 dihydroxyvitamin D in elderly osteoporotic patients. N Engl J Med 1981;305:372–374.
94. Tsai KS, Heath H, Kumar R, et al. Impaired vitamin D metabolism with aging in women. Possible role in pathogenesis of senile osteoporosis. J Clin Invest 1984;73:1668–1672.
95. Baker SP, Harvey AH. Fall injuries in the elderly. Symposium on falls in the elderly. Biological and behavioral aspects. Clin Geriatr Med 1985;1:501–508.
96. Gryfe CI, Amies A, Ashley MJ. A longitudinal study of falls in an elderly population: I. Incidence and morbidity. Age Ageing 1977;6:201–210.
97. Tinetti ME, Speechley M. Prevention of falls among the elderly. N Engl J Med 1989;320:1055–1059.
98. Campbell AJ, Renken J, Allen BC, Martinez GC. Falls in old age: a study of frequency and related clincial factors. Age Ageing 1981;10:264–270.

99. Melton LJ III, Riggs BL. Risk factors for injury after a fall. Clin Geriatr Med 1985;1:525–539.
100. Garraway WM, Stauffer RN, Kurland LT, O'Fallon WM. Limb fractures in a defined population. I. Frequency and distribution. Mayo Clin Proc 1979;54:701–707.
101. Gallagher JC, Melton LJ, Riggs BL, Bergstralh E. Epidemiology of fractures of the proximal femur in Rochester, Minnesota. Clin Orthop 1980;150:163–171.
102. Melton LJ, Riggs BL. Epidemiology of age-related fractures. In: Avioli LV, ed. The osteoporotic syndrome: detection, prevention, and treatment. New York: Grune & Stratton, 1983:45–72.
103. Hayes WC, Myers ER, Morris JN, Rejdc SA, Gerhart TN. Fall biomechanics as determinants of osteoporotic hip fracture risk. Proceedings of the Steenbock Symposium on Osteoporosis, Madison, Wisconsin, 1989;abstract 40.
104. Pogrund H, Makin M, Robin G, Menczel J, Steinberg R. Osteoporosis in patients with fractured femoral neck in Jerusalem. Clin Orthop 1977;124:165–172.
105. Gallagher JC, Melton LJ, Riggs BL. Examination of prevalence rates of possible risk factors in a population with a fracture of the proximal femur. Clin Orthop 1980;153:158–165.
106. Lindsay R, Dempster DW, Clemens T, et al. Incidence, cost, and risk factors of fracture of the proximal femur in the USA. In: Christiansen C, Arnaud C, Nordin BEC, Parfitt AM, Peck WA, Riggs BL, eds. Osteoporosis. Denmark: Aalborg Stiftsbogtrykkeri, 1984:311–315.
107. Solomon L. Osteoporosis and fracture of the femoral neck in the South African Bantu. J Bone Joint Surg 1968;50B:2–13.
108. Fesmer ME, White LR, Brody JA. Race and sex differences in hip fracture incidence. Am J Public Health 1984;44:1374–1380.
109. Stott S, Gray DH. The incidence of femoral neck fractures in New Zealand. N Z Med J 1980;91:6–9.
110. Consultation in Osteoporosis: Report of the World Health Organization. Geneva: World Health Organization, 1988.
111. Melton LJ, Ilstrup DM, Riggs BL, Beckenbaugh RD. Fifty-year trend in hip fracture incidence. Clin Orthop 1983;162:144–149.
112. Wong PCN. Femoral neck fractures among the major racial groups in Singapore. Incidence patterns compared with non-Asian communities. Singapore Med J 1964;5:150–157.
113. Hedlund R, Aulbom A, Lindgren U. Hip fracture incidence in Stockholm 1972–1981. Acta Orthop Scand 1964;57:30–34.
114. Elabdien BSZ, Olerud S, Karlstrom G, Smedley B. Rising incidence of hip fracture in Uppsala 1965–1980. Acta Orthop Scand 1984;55:284–289.
115. Finsen V, Benun P. Changing incidence of hip fractures in rural and urban areas of central Norway. Clin Orthop 1987;218:104–110.
116. Felch JA, Liebekk A, Slumbaard W. Epidemiology of hip fractures in Norway. Acta Orthop Scand 1985;56:12–16.
117. Martin AD, Silverthorn Houston CS. Age-specific increase in hip fractures in Canada. In: Christiansen C, Johansen JS, Riis BJ, eds. Osteoporosis. Copenhagen: Osteopres, 1987;111–112.
118. Holbrook TL, Grazier K, Kelsey JL, et al. The frequency of occurrence, impact, and cost of musculoskeletal conditions in the United States. Chicago: American Academy of Orthopedic Surgeons, 1985:163–166.
119. Cummings SR, Rudin SM, Black D. The future of hip fracture in the United States: numbers, costs and potential effects of postmenopausal estrogen. Clin Orthop Rel Res 1985;252:163–166.
119a. Cooper C, Campion G, Melton LJ III. Hip fractures in the elderly: a world-wide projection. Osteo Int 1992 (in press).

120. Lord SR, Sunnett PF. Femoral neck fractures: admissions, bed use, outcome and projections. Med J Aust 1986;145:493–496.
121. White BL, Fisher WD, Lauren CA. Rate of mortality for elderly patients after fracture of the hip in the 1980s. J Bone Joint Surg 1987;69A:1335–1340.
122. Fitzgerald JF, Moore PS, Dittus RS. The care of elderly patients with hip fracture: changes since implementation of the prospective payment system. N Engl J Med 1988;319:1392–1397.
123. Melton LJ III, Kan SH, Frye MA, et al. Epidemiology of vertebral fractures in women. Am J Epidemiol 1989;129:1000–1011.
124. Peacock M, Heyburn PJ, Aaron JE, et al. Osteomalacia treated with 1α-hydroxyvitamin or 1,25 dihydroxvitamin D. In: Norman AW, Schaefer K, Herrath DV, et al., eds. Vitamin D: basic research and its clinical applications. Berlin: Walter de Gruyter, 1979;1153–1162.
125. Papapoulos SE, Clemens TL, Fraher LJ, et al. Metabolites of vitamin D in human D deficiency: effect of vitamin D3 or 1,25-dihydroxycholecalciferol. Mineral Electrolyte Metab 1981;5:212–227.
126. Lund B, Charles P, Egmose C, et al. Changes in vitamin D metabolites and bone histology in rats during recovery from rickets. Calcif Tissue Int 1985;37:478–483.
127. Parfitt AM, Villaneuva AR. Hypophosphatemia and osteoblast function in human bone disease. In: Massry SG, Letteri JM, Ritz E, eds. Proceedings of the Fifth International Workshop on Phosphate and Other Minerals. Regulation of Phosphate and Mineral Metabolism. Adv Exp Med Biol 1982;151:209–216.
127a. Ettinger B, Black DM, Nevitt MC, et al. Contribution of vertebral deformities to chronic back pain and disability. J Bone Miner Res 1992;7:449–456.
128. Weinstein RS, Underwood JL, Hutson MS, DeLuca HF. Bone histomorphometry in vitamin D-deficient rats infused with calcium and phosphorus. Am J Physiol 1984;246:E499–E505.
129. Cummings SR. Osteoporotic fractures: the magnitude of the problem. In: Christiansen C, Johansen JS, Riis BJ, eds. Osteoporosis. Osteopres, Copenhagen, 1987;2:1193–1196.
130. Johnston CC Jr. Melton LJ III, Lindsay R, Eddy DM. Clinical indications for bone mass measurements. J Bone Min Res 1989;4(suppl):1–28.
131. Ross PD, Wasnich RD, Vogel JM. Detection of prefracture spinal osteoporosis using bone mineral absorptiometry. J Bone Min Res 1988;3:1–11.
132. Cummings SR. Are patients with hip fractures more osteoporotic? Review of the evidence. Am J Med 1985;78:487–494.
132a. Black DM, Cummings SR, Genant HK, et al. Axial bone mineral density predicts fractures in older women (abstract). J Bone Miner Res 1991;6:A862.
132b. Hui SL, Slemenda CW, Johnston CC Jr. Baseline measurement of bone mass predicts fracture in white women. Ann Intern Med 1989;111:355–361.
133. Christiansen C, Riis BJ, Rodbro P. Prediction of rapid bone loss in postmenopausal women. Lancet 1987;1:1105–1107.
134. Lindsay R, Aitken JM, Anderson JB, Hart DM, MacDonald EB, Clark AC. Long-term prevention of postmenopausal osteoporosis by oestrogen. Lancet 1976;1:1038–1041.
135. Lindsay R, Hart DM, MacLean A, Clark AC, Kraszewski A, Garwood J. Bone response to termination of oestrogen treatment. Lancet 1978;1:1325–1327.
136. Lindsay R, Coutts JRT, Hart DM. The effect of endogenous oestrogen on plasma and mineral calcium and phosphate in oophorectomized women. Clin Endocrinol 1977;6:87–93.
137. Lindsay R, Hart DM, Forrest C, Baird C. Prevention of spinal osteoporosis in oophorectomized women. Lancet 1980;2:1151–1154.
138. Lindsay R, Coutts JRT, Sweeney A, Hart DM. Endogenous oestrogen and bone loss following oophorectomy. Calcif Tissue Res 1977;22:213–216.
139. Lindsay R, Hart DM, Abdalla H, Al-Azzawi F. Interrelationship of bone loss and its

prevention and fracture expression. In: Christiansen C, Johnson JS, Riis BJ, eds., Osteoporosis. Copenhagen: Osteopres, 1987;2:508–512.

140. Lindsay R, Tohme JF. Estrogens in the prevention and treatment of osteoporosis. Obstet Gynecol 1990;76:290.
141. Parfitt AM. Bone remodeling: relationship to the amount and structure of bone, and the pathogenesis and prevention of fractures. In: Riggs BL, Melton LJ III, eds. Osteoporosis: Etiology, Diagnosis and Management. New York: Raven Press 1988:45–93.
142. Bogdonoff MD, Shock NW, Parsons J. The effects of stilbestrol on the retention of nitrogen, calcium, phosphorus and potassium in aged males with and without osteoporosis. J Gerontol 1954;9:262–275.
143. Burch JC, Byrd BF, Vaughn WK. The effects of long-term estrogen on hysterectomized women. Am J Obstet Gynecol 1974;118:778–782.
144. Christiansen C, Christiansen MS, McNair P. Prevention of early postmenopausal bone loss: conducted 2-year study in 315 normal females. Eur J Clin Invest 1980;10:273–279.
145. Christiansen C, Rodbro P. Does postmenopausal bone loss respond to estrogen replacement therapy independent of bone loss rate. Calcif Tissue Int 1983;35:720–722.
146. Ettinger B, Genant HK, Cann CE. Long-term estrogen therapy prevents bone loss and fracture. Ann Intern Med 1985;102:319–324.
147. Gordan GS, Picchi J, Roof BS. Antifracture efficacy of long-term estrogens for osteoporosis. Trans Assoc Am Phys 86:326–332.
148. Horsman A, Gallgher JC, Simpson M, Nordin BEC. Prospective trial of estrogen and calcium in postmenopausal women. Br Med J 1976;2:789–792.
149. Horsman A, James M, Francis R. The effect of estrogen dose on postmenopausal bone loss. N Engl J Med 309;1405–1407.
150. Lindsay R, Hart DM, Purdie P, Ferguson MM, Clark AC, Kraszewski A. Comparative effects of oestrogen and a progestogen on bone loss in postmenopausal women. Clin Sci Mol Med 1978;54:193–195.
151. Lindsay R, Hart DM, Clark DM. The minimum effective dose of estrogen for prevention of postmenopausal bone loss. Obstet Gynecol 1984;63:759–763.
152. Marshall H, Nordin BEC. The effect of 1-hydroxy-α-vitamin D3 with and without oestrogen on calcium balance in postmenopausal women. Clin Endocrinol 7:159s–168s.
153. Miller GJ, Miller ME. Plasma-high-density-lipoprotein concentration and development of ischemic heart disease. Lancet 1975;1:16–19.
154. Recker RR, Saville PD, Heaney RP. The effect of estrogens and calcium carbonate on bone loss in postmenopausal women. Ann Intern Med 1977;87:649–655.
155. Riggs BL, Jowsey J, Kelly PJ, Jones JD, Maher FT. Effect of sex hormones on bone in primary osteoporosis. J Clin Invest 48:1065–1072.
156. Riggs BL, Wahner HW, Dunn WL, Mazess RB, Offord KP, Melton LJ III. Differential changes in bone mineral density of the appendicular and axial skeleton with aging: relationship to spinal osteoporosis. J Clin Invest 1981;67:328–335.
157. Ettinger B, Genant HK, Cann CE. Postmenopausal bone loss is prevented by treatment with low-dosage estrogen with calcium. Ann Intern Med 1987;106:40–45.
158. Quigley TME, Martin BL, Burnier AM, et al. Estrogen therapy arrests bone loss in elderly women. Am J Obstet Gynecol 1987;156:1516–1523.
159. Savvas M, Studd JWW, Fogelman I, et al. Skeletal effects oral oestrogen compared with subcutaneous oestrogen and testosterone in postmenopausal women. Br Med J 1988; 297:331–333.
160. Lindsay R, Hart DM, MacLean A, Garwood J, Clark AC, Braszweski A. Bone loss during oestriol therapy in postmenopausal women. Maturitas 1979;1:279–285.
161. Nordin BEC, Horsman A, Aaron J, Gallagher JC. Postmenopausal bone loss. Curr Med Res Opin 1975;3:28.

162. Deleted in proof.
163. Deleted in proof.
164. Riis BJ, Thomsen K, Strom V, Christiansen C. The effect of percutaneous estradiol and natural progesterone on bone loss. Am J Obstet Gynecol 1987;156:61–65.
165. Stevenson JC, Cust MP, Genger FF, Hillard TC, Lees B, Whitehead MI. Effects of transdermal versus oral hormone replacement therapy on bone-density in spine and proximal femur in postmenopausal women. Lancet 1990;336:265–269.
166. Al-Azzawi F, Hart DM, Lindsay R. Long-term effect of oestrogen replacement therapy on bone mass as measured by dual photon absorptiometry. Br Med J 1987;294:1261–1262.
167. Lindsay R, Cosman F, Herrington BS. Total bone mass in healthy women. J Bone Min Res 1989;4(suppl):1005.
168. Lindsay R, Hart DM, MacLean A, Clark AC, Kraszewski A, Garwood J. Bone response to termination of oestrogen treatment. Lancet 1978;1:1325–1327.
169. Christiansen C, Christiansen MS, Transbol I. Bone mass in postmenopausal women after withdrawal of estrogen/gestagen replacement therapy. Lancet 1981;1:459–461.
170. Horsman A, Nordin BE, Crilly RG. Effect on bone of withdrawal of oestrogen therapy. Lancet 1979;2:33.
171. Lindsay R, Sweeney A. Urinary cyclic-AMP in osteoporosis. Scott Med J 1976;21:231.
172. Heaney RP. A unified concept of osteoporosis. Am J Med 1965;39:377–380.
173. Cosman F, Shen V, Herrington B, Seibel M, Ratcliffe A, Lindsay R. Estrogen protects against bone resorbing effects of (1-34)hPTH infusion as assessed by biochemical markers. J Bone Min Res 1975;5(suppl 2):A410.
174. Burch JC, Byrd BF, Vaughn WK. Effects of long-term estrogen administration to women following hysterectomy. Front Horm Res 1975;3:208–214.
175. Hutchinson TA, Polansky JM, Feinstein AR. Postmenopausal oestrogens protect against fracture of hip and distal radius. Lancet 1979;2:705–709.
176. Kreiger N, Kelsey JL, Holford TR. An epidemiological study of hip fracture in postmenopausal women. Am J Epidemiol 1982;116:141–148.
177. Weiss NS, Ure CL, Ballard JH. Decreased risk of fractures of the hip and lower forearm with postmenopausal use of estrogen. N Engl J Med 1980;303:1195–1198.
178. Kiel DP, Fallon DT, Anderson JJ. Hip fracture and the use of estrogens in postmenopausal women. N Engl J Med 1987;317:1169–1774.
179. Melton LJ III. Postmenopausal bone loss and osteoporosis. In: Zichella L, Whitehead M, VanKeep PA, eds. The climacteric and beyond. Carnsforth, U.K.: Parthenon, 1987;125–135.
180. Notelovitz M, Martin D, Tesar R, et al. Estrogen therapy and variable-resistance weight training increase bone mineral in surgically menopausal women. J Bone Miner Res 1991;6:583–590.
181. Abdalla H, Hart DM, Lindsay R, Leggate I, Hooke A. Prevention of bone loss in postmenopausal women by norethisterone. Obstet Gynecol 1985;6:789–792.
182. Lindsay R. Skeletal effects of progestogens: clinical studies. Intern Proc J 1989;1:199–204.
183. Prior JC. Progestogen therapy increases trabecular bone in women with endocrine diseases which prevent estrogen treatment. Inter Proc J 1989;1:204–208.
184. Silfverstolpe G, Gustafson A, Samsoe G, et al. Lipid metabolic studies in oophorectomized women. Effects of three different progestogens. Acta Obstet Gynecol Scand 1979;88:89–95.
185. Farish E, Fletcher CD, Hart DM, et al. Lipoprotein and apoprotein levels in postmenopausal women during treatment with norethisterone. Clin Chem Acta 1986;159:147–151.
186. Hammond CB, Jelovser R, Lee KL. Effects of long-term estrogen replacement therapy. II. Neoplasia. Am J Obstet Gynecol 1979;133:537–547.
187. Persson I, Adami HO, Bergkvist L, et al. Risk of endometrial cancer after treatment with

oestogens alone or in conjunction with progestogens: results of a prospective study. Br Med J 1989;298:147–151.
188. Christiansen C, Riis BT, Nilas L, Rodbro P, Deftos L. Uncoupling of bone formation and resorption by combined oestrogen and progestagen therapy in postmenopausal osteoporosis. Lancet 1985;2:800–801.
189. Chesnut CH III, Ivey JL, Gruger HE, Mathews M, Nelp WB, Sisom K, Baylink DJ. Stanozolol in postmenopausal osteoporosis: therapeutic efficacy and possible mechanisms of action. Metabolism 1983;32:577–580.
190. Need AG, Horowitz M, Bridges A, et al. Effect of nandrolone decanoate and antiresorptive therapy on vertebral density in osteoporotic postmenopausal women. Arch Intern Med 1989;149:57–60.
191. Vaishnav R, Gallagher JA, Beresford JM, Poster J, Russell RGG. Direct effects of stanozolol and estrogens on human bone cell in culture. In: Christiansen C, et al. Osteoporosis. Glostrup, Denmark: Aalborg Stiftsbogtrykkeri, 1984;485–488.
192. Steiniche T, Hasling C, Charles P, et al. A randomized study of the effects of estrogen/gestagen or high dose oral calcium on trabecular bone remodeling in postmenopausal osteoporosis. Bone 1989;10:313–320.
193. Munk-Jensen N, Nealsen SP, Obel EB, Eriksen PB. Reversal of postmenopausal vertebral bone loss by oestrogen and progestogen: a double blind placebo controlled study. Br Med J 1988;296:1150–1152.
194. Pacifici R, McMurtry C, Vered I, et al. Coherence therapy does not prevent axial bone loss in osteoporotic women. A preliminary comparative study. J Clin Endocrinol Metab 1988;66:747–753.
194a. Lufkin E, Wahner HW, O'Fallon WM, Hodgson SF, Kotowicz MA, Lane AW, Judd HL, Caplan RH, Riggs BL. Treatment of postmenopausal osteoporosis with transdermal estrogen. Ann Intern Med 1992 (in press).
195. Maresca V. Human calcitonin in the management of osteoporosis: a multicentre study. J Int Med Res 1985;13:311–316.
196. Gennari C, Chierichetti SM, Bigazzi S, et al. Comparative effects on bone mineral content of calcium and calcium plus salmon calcitonin given in two different regimens in postmenopausal osteoporosis. Curr Ther Res 1985;455–464.
197. Gruber HE, Ivey JL, Baylink DJ, et al. Long-term calcitonin therapy in postmenopausal osteoporosis. Metabolism 1984;33:295–303.
198. Mazzuoli GF, Passeri M, Gennari C, et al. Effects of salmon calcitonin in postmenopausal osteoporosis: a controlled double-blind clinical study. Calcif Tissue Int 1986;38:3–8.
199. Wallach S, Cohn SH, Ellish KJ, et al. Effect of salmon calcitonin on skeletal mass in osteoporosis. Curr Ther Res Clin Exp 1977;22:556–572.
200. Polatti F, Montrasio MG, Caprotti M, et al. Bone mineral content after oophorectomy: effects of salmon calcitonin and oral calcium. Min Metab Res 1984;5:159–163.
201. Reginster JY, Albert A, Lecart MP, et al. 1-year controlled randomized trial of prevention of early postmenopausal bone loss by intranasal calcitonin. Lancet 1987;2:1481–1483.
202. Christiansen C. Intranasal calcitonin for prevention and treatment of osteoporosis. Ann Chir Gynaecol 1988;77:229–234.
203. MacIntyre I, Whitehead MI, Banks LM, et al. Calcitonin for prevention of postmenopausal bone loss. Lancet 1988;1:900–901.
204. Franceschini R, Bottaro P, Panapoulos C, et al. Long-term treatment with salmon calcitonin in postmenopausal osteoporosis. Curr Ther Res 1983;34:795–800.
205. Azria M. The calcitonins. Basel: Karger, 1989.
206. Watts NB, Harris ST, Genant HK, et al. Intermittent cyclical etidronate treatment of postmenopausal osteoporosis. N Engl J Med 1990;323:73–79.
207. Smith ML, Fogelman I, Hart DM, et al. Calcif Tissue Int 1989;44:74–79.

208. Storm T, Thamsborg G, Sorensen OH, Lund B. The effects of etidronate therapy in postmenopausal osteoporotic women: preliminary results. In: Christiansen C, Johansen JS, Riis BJ, eds. Osteoporosis. Copenhagen: Osteopres, 1987:1172–1176.
209. Frost HM. The pathomechanics of osteoporosis. Clin Orthop Rel Res 1985;200:198–225.
210. Chan SDH, Chiu DKH, Atkins D. Oophorectomy leads to a selective decrease in 1,25-dihydroxycholecalciferol receptors in rat jejunal villous cells. Clin Sci 1984;66:745–748.
211. Frances RM, Peacock M, Taylor GA, et al. Calcium malabsorption in elderly women with vertebral fractures: evidence for resistance to the action of vitamin D metabolites on the bowel. Clin Sci 1984;66:103–107.
212. Deftos LJ, Weisman MH, Williams GW. Influence of age and sex on plasma calcitonin in human beings. N Engl J Med 1981;302:1251–1353.
213. Greenberg C, Kirkreja SC, Bowser EN, Hargis GK, Henderson WT, Williams GA. Effects of estradiol and progesterone on calcitonin secretion. Endocrinology 1990;118:2594–2598.
214. Stevenson JC, Hillyard CJ, MacIntyre I, Cooper H, Whitehead MI. A physiological role for calcitonin in protection of the maternal skeleton. Lancet 1979;2:767–770.
215. Civitelli R, Agnusdei D, Nardi P, et al. Effects of one-year treatment with estrogens on bone mass, intestinal calcium absorption and 25-hydroxyvitamin D 1-α-hydroxylase reserve in postmenopausal osteoporosis. Calcif Tissue Int 1988;42:77–86.
216. Stevenson JC, White MC, Joplin GF, MacIntyre I. Osteoporosis and calcitonin deficiency. Br Med J 1982;285:1010–1011.
217. Body JJ, Heath H III. Effects of age, sex, calcium and total thyroidectomy on circulating monomeric calcitonin concentrations. Calcif Tissue Res 1983;35:A45.
218. Heath HH III, Sizemore GW. Radioimmunoassay for calcitonin. Clin Chem 1982; 28:1219–1226.
219. Morimoto S, Tsuj M, Okada Y. The effects of oestrogen on human calcitonin secretion after calcium infusion in elderly subjects. Clin Endocrinol 1980;13:135–143.
220. Stevenson JC, Meyers CH, Adjukiewicz AB. Racial differences in calcitonin and kalacalcin. Calcif Tissue Int 1984;36:725–728.
221. Deftos LJ, Weisman MH, Williams GW. Influence of age and sex on plasma calcitonin in human beings. N Engl J Med 1981;302:1351–1353.
222. Hillyard CJ, Stevenson JC, MacIntyre I. Relative deficiency of plasma-calcitonin in women. Lancet 1978;1:961–962.
223. Mulder H, Hackeng WHL, Silberbusch J. Racial difference in serum calcitonin. Lancet 1979;2:154.
224. Stock JL, Coiderre JA, Mallette LE. Effects of a short course of estrogen on mineral metabolism in postmenopausal women. J Clin Endocrinol Metab 1985;61:595–600.
225. Dawson Hughes B, Stern D, Goldman J, Reichlin S. Regulation of growth hormone and somatomedin-C secretion in postmenopausal women: effect of physiological estrogen replacement. J Clin Endocrinol Metab 1986;63:424–432.
226. Wiedemann E, Schwartz E, Frantz AG. Acute and chronic estrogen effects upon serum somatomedin activity, growth, hormone and pralactin in man. J Clin Endocrinol Metab 1976;42;942.
227. Chen TL, Feldman D. Distinction between α-fetoprotein and intracellular estrogen receptors: evidence against presence of estradiol receptors in rat bone. Endocrinology 1978;102:236–240.
228. Ernst M, Schmid C, Froesch ER. Enhanced osteoblast proliferation and collagen gene expression by estradiol. Proc Natl Acad Sci USA 1988;85:2037.
229. Fukayama T, Tashjian FH. Direct modulation by estrodiol of the response of human bone

cells (SaOS-2) to human parathyroid hormone (PTH) and PTH-related protein. Endocrinology 1989;124:397.
230. Rodan GA, Martin TJ. Role of osteoblasts in hormonal control of bone resorption: a hypothesis. Calcif Tissue Int 1981;33:349.
231. Pacifici R, Rifas L, Teitelbaum S, et al. Spontaneous release of interleukin 1 from human blood monocytes reflects bone formation in idiopathic osteoporosis. Proc Natl Acad Sci USA 1987;84:4616–4620.
232. Pacifici R, Rifas L, Vered I, et al. Interleukin-1 secretion from human blood monocytes in normal and osteoporotic women: effect of menopause and estrogen/progesterone treatment. J Bone Min Res 1988;3(suppl):A204.
233. Stock JL, Coderne JA, MacDonald B, Rosenwasser LJ. Effects of estrogen in vivo and in vitro on spontaneous interleukin-1 release by monocytes from postmenopausal women. J Clin Endocrinol Metab 1989;68:364–368.
234. Dewhurst FE, Ago JM, Peros WJ, Stashenko P. Synergism between parathyroid hormone and interleukin-1 in stimulating bone resorption in organ culture. J Bone Min Res 1987;2:127.
235. Feyen JHM, Raisz LG. Prostaglandin production by calvariae from sham operated and oophorectomized rats: effect of 17β estradiol in vivo. Endocrinology 1987;121:819–821.
236. Chen TL, Mallory JB, Chang SL. Effects of transforming growth factor and its interaction with bFGF and EGF in rat osteoblast-like cells. J Bone Min Res 1987;2:256.
237. Ray WA, Downey W, Griffin MR, et al. Long-term use of thiazide diuretics and risk of hip fracture. Lancet 1989;1:687–689.
238. Riggs BL, Hodgson SF, O'Fallon WM, et al. Effect of fluoride treatment on the fracture rate in postmenopausal women with osteoporosis. N Engl J Med 1990;322:802–809.
239. Kleerekoper M, Peterson EL, Nelson DA, et al. A randomized trial of sodium fluoride as a treatment for postmenopausal osteoporosis. Osteoporosis International 1991;1:155–161.
240. Turken S, Siris E, Seldin D, Lindsay R. Effects of tamoxifen on spinal bone density. J Natl Cancer Inst 1989;81:1086–1088.

4

Methods and Role of Bone Densitometry in the Estrogen-Deficient Woman

Charles H. Chesnut III

Estrogen deficiency in women may be caused by a number of factors, most frequently the menopause (natural or artificial, premature or postclimacteric). Menstrual irregularity (amenorrhea due to multiple causes, including excessive exercise; oligomenorrhea), Turner syndrome, anorexia/bulimia, and use of gonadotropin-releasing hormone agonists/antagonists for treating endometriosis or leiomyomata are other possible etiologies of estrogen deficiency. All these estrogen-depleted states are associated with a loss of bone mass (osteopenia), particularly at trabecular (cancellous) bone sites (such as spine, hip, and wrist). This loss of bone mass presumably results in an increased fracture risk (osteoporosis) at these sites. Such fractures, related to estrogen deficiency, are a significant part of the health problem that is osteoporosis: 20 million affected individuals in the United States alone, and an annual cost exceeding $8 billion (U.S. dollars) per year.

To diagnose and treat this most common and expensive disorder of women, it is imperative that techniques be available (*a*) to identify bone loss and predict the risk of fracture; (*b*) to quantitate the severity of such bone loss; and (*c*) to assess the response of bone to various therapeutic programs. In 1992, a number of techniques are available to noninvasively measure bone mass (quantitatively and qualitatively) at multiple skeletal sites composed of both cortical and trabecular bone. This chapter discusses each technique's assets, liabilities, and indications for usage in the estrogen-deficient female.

BASIC PRINCIPLES OF BONE MASS MEASUREMENT

Bone mass is the principal, although not the only, determinant of fracture. Theoretically, therefore, measurements of bone mass would be of value in bone-wasting conditions (such as osteopenia and osteoporosis) to identify and assess fracture risk and to monitor therapy. The spinal x-ray is a relatively insensitive technique for quantitating bone mass: 30 to 35% of bone mass must be lost before demineralization is detected radiographically. Over the past 25 years, a number of considerably more sensitive techniques have been developed to quantitate bone mass at spine, hip, wrist, and virtually any skeletal site. These techniques include single-photon and dual-photon absorptiometry (SPA and DPA), dual-energy x-ray absorptiometry (DEXA), and computed tomography (CT). In addition, the recently developed technique of the measurement of ultrasound velocity at the patella or os calcis may add a new dimension to bone mass assessment, as ultrasound can theoretically both quantitate bone mass *and* assess its quality.

The basic operating principle for the majority of the noninvasive bone mass measurement techniques (SPA at wrist, DPA at spine and hip, DEXA at spine, hip, and total body, and CT at the spine) is the attenuation or absorption of ionizing radiation by bone. Because an exponential relationship exists between bone mass and radiation attenuation, the greater the amount of bone present, the greater the attenuation or absorption of ionizing radiation and the less radiation measured by a detector (Fig. 4.1). For SPA and DPA, radionuclides (iodine-125 and gadolinium-153) are the source of this radiation; for DEXA and CT, x-rays are the source. Ultrasound, on the other hand, utilizes no ionizing radiation, but is based on the theory that the speed at which ultrasound propagates in bone is determined by the mass density and the "elastic modulus" (inherent material quality) of bone. The higher the mass density and the elastic modulus, the higher the speed of ultrasound. Presumably, bone demonstrating high ultrasound velocity is high in strength and will resist fracture, whereas bone with low ultrasound velocity will deform more with force, and consequently will be less able to resist fracture.

THE IDEAL NONINVASIVE TECHNIQUE FOR ASSESSING BONE MASS IN THE ESTROGEN-DEPLETED WOMAN

A number of criteria should be satisfied in assessing bone mass: the ideal noninvasive technique would of course be one capable of predicting an individual woman's risk for osteoporosis, and would be readily applicable to assessing the therapeutic response. The technique should be reasonably precise and accurate, logistically acceptable (i.e., not require excessive patient time nor cause discomfort), relatively inexpensive, and safe (i.e., involve low radiation exposure). It should quantitate primarily trabecular bone, as this is metabolically more active than cortical bone and may be preferentially altered in osteoporosis. Trabecular, or cancellous, bone is also the bone type most

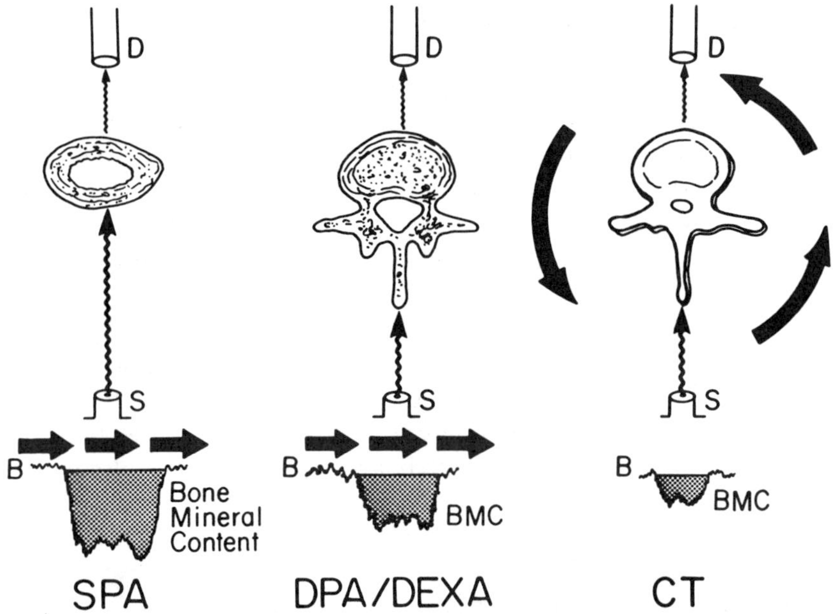

Figure 4.1. Principles of single-photon absorptiometry (SPA), dual-photon absorptiometry (DPA), dual-energy x-ray (DEXA), and computerized tomography (CT). *D,* detection; *S,* source of ionizing radiation (see text); *arrows,* direction of scan (CT, rotary); *B,* baseline count rate; *BMC,* bone mineral content. A scan across the radius (SPA) or vertebra (DPA/DEXA, CT) results in the absorption profile noted, utilizing an exponential relationship between bone mass and radiation attenuation. Computer integration of the area below the baseline is performed with the results compared with calibration standards, providing units of bone mass and/or linear, areal, or formatted volumetric density (grams, g/cm, g/cm^2, mg/cm^3 [CT]). (Chesnut CH. Noninvasive methods for bone mass measurement. In: Avioli LV, ed. The osteoporotic syndrome, 3rd ed. Orlando, FL: Grune & Stratton, in press, 1991.)

affected by medications currently utilized in osteoporosis therapy, including calcitonin, sodium fluoride, bisphosphonates, and estrogen. As seen in Table 4.1, the available noninvasive techniques for assessing bone mass do not uniformly satisfy these ideal criteria.

SPECIFIC TECHNIQUES

Single-Photon Absorptiometry

SPA measurements are most frequently obtained at the wrist, but measurements with a dedicated SPA machine may also be performed at the os calcis. At the wrist, ultradistal, distal, and proximal measurements are available. SPA measurements are obtained in units of grams per centimeter (linear density) and grams per square centimeter (areal density), and are usually compared to laboratory center referent populations. SPA measures primarily cortical bone mass at the wrist (the distal and proximal sites); the ultradistal and os calcis sites are used to measure trabecular bone. Cortical bone of the wrist is neither the type nor the site of bone most frequently involved in osteoporosis (predominantly trabecular bone at spine and hip), nor is it the type of bone most severely affected in such estrogen-depleted states as the menopause, athletic amenorrhea, and so forth. While studies have shown that SPA can generally predict fracture risk, not only at the wrist but also at other skeletal sites, there is no definitive evidence indicating that a measurement of bone mass at the wrist will predict bone mass, or bone mass change, at the spine or hip with clinically acceptable accuracy. Consequently, cortical SPA is of limited value as a primary screening technique for osteoporosis, although the technique may be of value in diseases affecting both cortical and trabecular bone such as hyperthyroidism, hyperparathyroidism, renal osteodystrophy, and certain pediatric clinical situations. SPA may also be of value in following response to therapies affecting cortical and trabecular bone, such as cortisone. Estrogen replacement therapy maintains cortical bone mass, but monitoring response to estrogen therapy is more efficaciously accomplished by measuring trabecular bone at spine or hip.

The SPA ultradistal site and the os calcis sites do assess primarily trabecular bone, but at sites (extreme distal radius and ulna, and calcaneus) subject to mechanical stresses, loading forces, and local hormone interactions quite different from those occurring at spine and hip sites. Although measuring trabecular bone at the os calcis has value in predicting future fracture risk, trabecular bone (as measured at the spine with DPA, DEXA, or CT) may be a more meaningful and specific predictor.

As shown in Table 4.1, SPA does exhibit a reasonable cost, precision, logistic simplicity, and low radiation exposure.

Dual-Photon Absorptiometry and Dual-Energy X-ray Absorptiometry

Both DPA and DEXA measure primarily trabecular bone at hip and spine. Total skeleton evaluations may also be obtained (currently, usually with DEXA). Measurements with both machines are obtained as bone mineral content in grams and bone mineral density (areal density) in grams per square centimeter at the spine, hip, and total skeleton (grams only). These values are automatically compared to age- and sex-matched normal referent populations

Table 4.1.
Noninvasive Techniques for Measuring Bone Mass[a]

Technique	Site Measured	Cortical/Trabecular Bone	Precision/Accuracy	Risk Prediction	Response to Therapy	Radiation Dose	Duration of Procedure	Cost in $US
		%	%			*mrem*	*min*	
SPA	Radius/ulna:							
	Distal	80–95/20–5	±2–4%/±3–4%	+	±[b]	10	10–15	75–125
	Ultradistal	25/75	±2–4%/?	?	?	10	10–15	75–125
	os calcis	20/80	±2–4%/?	+	?	10	10–15	75–125
DPA	Spine: L1–4[c]	35/65	±3–5%/±2–4%	+	+	10	20–30	150–200
	Femur:							
	Neck	75/25	±3–5%/?	?	+[b]	10	20–30	75
	Trochanter	50/50	±3–5%/?	?	?	10	20–30	—
DEXA	Spine: L1–4[c]	35/65	±1%–1.5%/?	+[d]	+[d]	<10	10	150
	Femur:							
	Neck	75/25	±1.5%/?	?	+[d]	<10	10	75
	Trochanter	50/50	±1.5%/?	?	?	<10	10	—
	Total skeleton	80/20	±1%/?	?	?	<5	5–10	?
	Radius-ulna[e]	80–95/20–5	±1.2%/?	+[d]	±[b]	<10	6	?
	Lat spine[e,f]	35/65	±4%/?	?	?	<10	20	?
CT	Single-energy:							
	Spine T12–L3[g]	5/95	±3.5%/6–8%	+	+	300–750	30	150
	Dual-energy							
	Spine T12–L3[g]	5/95	±5–8%/5%	+[d]	+[d]	750	30	150
US	Patella[e]	?5/95	2–3%/?	+	?	—	5	35–50[h]
	Os calcis[e]	20/80	2–3%/?	?	?	—	5	35–50[h]

[a]From Chesnut CH. Non-invasive methods for bone mass measurement. In: Avioli LV, ed. The osteoporotic syndrome. 3rd ed. Orlando, FL: Grune & Stratton, in press, 1991.
[b]? Estrogens.
[c]*Total* vertebral body, including spinous processes, aortic calcification.
[d]Unproven, but probable.
[e]Experimental.
[f]Lateral decubitus (excludes posterior spinous processes, aortic calcification, etc.).
[g]Centrum—area of interest *within* the vertebral body.
[h]Projected.

and to young normal populations, and the resultant bone mass deficit or surplus is quantitated as percentages or standard deviations (Z scores) above or below age-matched or young normal mean values.

At its inception DPA represented a major breakthrough in the evaluation of the osteoporotic patient: for the first time, a measurement of bone mass at spine and hip were available. As seen in Table 4.1, DPA demonstrated a precision and accuracy that was acceptable at the time the technique was introduced, and it could be used to predict the risk of future fracture as well as to follow the response to treatment. However, for reasons discussed below, DPA has largely been replaced by the DEXA technique both for research and clinical purposes. Nevertheless, it should be noted that while DEXA offers many advantages over DPA, the bone mass information obtained by both machines is quite similar, and data obtained by DPA remain quite useful in the clinical management of individuals at risk for or with osteoporosis.

As noted in Table 4.1, DEXA offers a number of advances vis-a-vis DPA. With DEXA, x-rays have replaced the radionuclide gadolinium-153 as a source of ionizing radiation. The greater photon flux available with an x-ray source, combined with DEXA's improved detector configuration and data analysis, results in an improved precision (1 to 1.5% at spine and hip), resolution, and scan time (about 10 minutes) compared to DPA. The radiation exposure (about 5 to 10 mrem) is acceptable, and it is possible that the cost of the study to the patient may be reduced, due to a shorter scan time and a lower maintenance cost (replacing an x-ray tube every 5 to 10 years for perhaps $5,000.00 versus a yearly radionuclide replacement at the same cost). Also, as shown in Table 4.1, multiple skeletal sites and total skeletal bone mass may be easily evaluated with DEXA. Although to date there are little data available, DEXA will undoubtedly prove acceptable for assessing the risk of future fracture, as well as for monitoring the response to treatment (Table 4.1). The improved precision of DEXA, which allows identification of significant changes in bone mass over time with comparatively small bone mass change, will allow a more definitive assessment of treatment over time than has been possible with DPA (DPA precision is 3 to 5%).

The lateral DEXA spine scan has been developed over the past 2 years and is theoretically more accurate than the AP DEXA scan, as it deletes from the measurement the posterior spinous processes, aortic calcification, and severe osteophytes (which the traditional AP projection assesses as bone). In addition, with the lateral scan a measurement of primarily trabecular bone (similar to that obtained with CT; see below) may be provided by an area-of-interest measurement within the vertebral body. However, imprecision due to patient positioning problems and surrounding soft tissue variations have to date been a source of concern, and the lateral scan currently remains a research technique.

As previously discussed, measurement at other sites, including the total skeleton, are also available with DEXA. The measurement of forearm (wrist) bone mass at distal, ultradistal, and midshaft radius and ulna sites is currently under study; the shortened scan time (5 to 6 minutes) and improved precision (1.2%, compared to SPA's 2 to 4%) will undoubtedly result in DEXA x-ray scans at the wrist replacing SPA-radionuclide scans at some time in the near future. Total skeleton bone mass measurements provide an overall assessment of bone mass throughout the skeleton and of various skeletal components. Repetitive measurements differentiate changes throughout the skeletal areas and might be used to identify a differential skeletal response to therapy (i.e., a gain in bone mass at one site at the expense of another site). However, at present the total skeleton measurement remains primarily a research tool. Analyses of body composition (lean body mass, fat composition, etc.), is also available with a number of DEXA machines but is currently for investigational use only. Such measurements could theoretically be of value in assessing body composition in cases of anorexia nervosa, athletic amenorrhea, etc.

There are currently three major DEXA vendors in the United States (Hologic in Waltham, MA; Lunar in Madison, WI; and Norland in Ft. Atkinson, WI). The machines cost, on average, about $75,000 to $95,000.

Computed Tomography

CT measurements are computer-formatted three-dimensional volumetric slices of vertebral bone mass quantitated in milligrams per cubic centimeter. Measurements of primarily trabecular bone within the vertebral body (the "centrum" measurement) or of a mixture of trabecular and cortical bone throughout the entire vertebral body (the "integral" measurement), including transverse processes and posterior elements, are available. The centrum measurement may *hypothetically* provide a more accurate assessment of fracture risk than measurements of the entire vertebral body (as measured with integral CT, DPA, and AP DEXA); it is measuring almost exclusively trabecular bone within the vertebral body, presumably with the preferential loss of such trabecular bone resulting in sacrifice of the structural integrity of the vertebral body and its subsequent fracture. Such a measurement *may* provide a more accurate assessment of fracture risk. Balanced against this presumed asset, however, are a number of logistic liabilities, including problems with accuracy, quality assurance, and radiation dosage (as noted in Table 4.1).

Accuracy with single-energy CT is particularly vulnerable to errors occasioned by marrow fat. The use of dual-energy CT obviates some of this difficulty, but with the liability of reduced precision and increased radiation exposure. As with DPA and DEXA, the accuracy of CT may be adversely affected by pre-existing vertebral compression fractures, vertebral sclerosis, and by scoliosis and kyphosis. Also, significant radiation exposure occurs with CT measurements, particularly compared to DPA and DEXA. The last, and perhaps major, liability of CT is quality assurance. Unless the hospital, office, or laboratory is involved on a day-to-day basis with the utilization of the CT technique to quantitate bone mass, quality assurance may be suspect. Errors in patient positioning, phantom calibration, determination of the location of the CT "slice" through the vertebra, etc., may result in spurious CT bone mass values. While quality assurance in research laboratories with dedicated CT scanners is most acceptable, the clinical radiologist rarely using CT for bone mass assessment may encounter difficulties in achieving an acceptable CT precision and accuracy.

CT has been available for quantitating bone mass, primarily at the spine, for perhaps 10 years. During this period, it has been a most useful technique. At the present time, as with DPA, CT seems much less valuable (in comparison to DEXA) in terms of precision, accuracy, radiation exposure, quality assurance, and day-to-day logistical ease of operation, particularly in a clinical practice setting. The significant radiation exposure may be of particular concern in many women with estrogen deficiency associated with eating disorders, athletic amenorrhea, and exposure to GnRH agonists/antagonists, which may occur at comparatively young ages. A significant radiation exposure associated with repeated CT bone mass measurements may not be indicated in such comparatively young women. Whether the asset of providing a unique trabecular measurement outweighs the above potential liabilities of CT is unclear, but seems doubtful.

Ultrasound

Bone quantity and, presumably, bone quality can be assessed at the patella and os calcis with ultrasound. As shown in Table 4.1, at each of these sites the bone is primarily trabecular, precision is acceptable, and there is no radiation exposure. Recently completed clinical trials utilizing ultrasound at the patella and os calcis have found that discrimination between normal and osteoporotic women is equivalent to that of SPA, DPA, and CT. Ultrasound measurements at the patella also seem to have some utility in predicting fracture risk. Whether ultrasound techniques can be used to follow response to treatment has not been assessed.

Ultrasound has a number of theoretical but potentially great advantages. It putatively measures not only bone quantity but also bone quality. Such an assessment of bone quality (bone microarchitecture, microfractures, etc.) should result in an improved fracture risk assessment for the individual patient. Also, since ultrasound measurement requires only 3 to 5 minutes of patient time, and could be much less expensive than other techniques (perhaps $25 to $50 for examination of the patella or os calcis), ultrasound would be an acceptable screening parameter even if its discriminatory and risk-predicting abilities are no better than those of other techniques that only quantitate bone mass. For the young estrogen-deficient woman, a lack of any radiation exposure would be an asset as a screening technique. However, in 1992 ultrasound remains an experimental technique; more work on this interesting procedure is indicated.

BONE MASS QUANTITATION AND FRACTURE

The techniques described above, with the possible exception of ultrasound, only *quantitate* bone mass. Can a measurement of bone quantity alone accurately predict future fracture risk? This is a most important question, as bone mass quantity is not the only determinant of fracture risk. Propensity for falling, lack of neuromuscular coordination, and bone quality and microarchitecture also contribute to fracture occurrence. However, in 1992, extensive data are available to indicate that bone mass quantitation can indeed predict the risk of fracture. Such data indicate a significant relationship between bone mineral density (BMD) and bone strength, with perhaps 75% of the variance in bone strength provided by BMD. In addition, a significant correlation exists between BMD and fracture risk: a lower bone mass is associated with an increase in fracture risk. Fracture risk can be stratified according to bone mass levels, and fracture risk of hip, spine, or wrist can be predicted by bone mass measurements at these sites. It seems reasonable to assume that measurements of bone quantity alone can predict fracture risk, or lack thereof, in estrogen-deficient women.

It should also be noted that the noninvasive techniques for bone mass quantitation are the only currently available means of assessing fracture risk. The use of risk factors, such as body habitus, calcium intake, activity levels, alcohol and smoking history, etc., to determine fracture risk is not supported by available data. Studies have shown that osteoporosis risk factors derived from history and physical examination can predict neither bone mass nor subsequent fracture risk, at least in individual patients. However, the use of risk factors in combination with bone mass measurements may more fully define an individual's risk for osteoporosis.

Lastly, it should be noted that, while bone mass quantitation may predict fracture risk, the assessment of bone mass quantity may not discriminate between osteoporotic and normal subjects of the same age and sex; there is significant overlapping in bone mass values (as measured by any of the above techniques) between normal and osteoporotic groups. The reason for this finding may lie, again, in the fact that bone mass is not the only determinant of fracture risk (bone quality is another important factor). However, such a lack of discrimination should not be seen as a liability for these techniques; discriminatory ability assesses the value of a technique in diagnosing the presence of osteoporotic fractures. Since spinal x-rays can sensitively diagnose the presence of fracture (though not the degree of demineralization, as previously discussed), there is no need for bone mass measurement techniques to be utilized in fracture diagnosis. Rather, they are utilized in predicting fracture risk, providing considerably more important clinical information than discrimination between normal and diseased individuals.

CLINICAL CONSIDERATIONS IN THE USE OF BONE MASS MEASUREMENT IN THE ESTROGEN-DEFICIENT WOMAN

In which clinical situations would the techniques described above be utilized? Recently, a National Osteoporosis Foundation task force listed a number of clinical indications for bone mass measurements; the following represents an adaptation of this information, as applied specifically to the estrogen-deficient woman:

1. *In estrogen-deficient women, to diagnose significantly low bone mass to make decisions about hormone replacement therapy or about alternatives to hormone replacement therapy (calcitonin, bisphosphonates, etc.).* Women with premature or natural menopause should be evaluated, most efficaciously at the spine, with a technique that for this purpose should be safe, relatively inexpensive, and logistically simple for both the operator and the patient. Also, the measurements obtained should relate to the risk for future fracture. The newer techniques, particularly DEXA, fulfill most of these criteria. The measurements obtained could be utilized clinically as follows:

the presence of positive risk factors associated with normal bone mass after the menopause would indicate a conservative therapeutic program primarily based on an adequate calcium intake plus exercise with bone mass follow-up within 1 to 2 years. On the other hand, positive risk factors associated with low bone mass after the menopause indicate a need for estrogen or its alternatives (potentially nasal-spray calcitonin or the bisphosphonates).

Within the context of this indication for bone mass measurement, women with estrogen deficiency secondary to other causes should also undergo bone mass evaluation. Young women with endometriosis or leiomyomata have been known to experience significant bone loss while being treated with GnRH agonists or antagonists, primarily at the spine and (to a lesser extent) at the hip, although with apparently no loss at primarily cortical sites (such as the wrist). While it has not yet been determined whether bone mass measurement is indicated for all individuals on GnRH therapy or agonists/antagonists, certainly such individuals with multiple risk factors for osteoporosis are well advised to undergo bone mass evaluation, particularly if they are to receive repeated therapy with these agents. Cumulative deficits in bone mass, particularly at the spine, could occur with repeated exposure to GnRH agonists/antagonists.

Women whose estrogen deficiency is a consequence of disorders such as anorexia nervosa and bulimia may experience significant, severe bone loss, not only at trabecular sites (the axial skeleton), but also at cortical sites (the appendicular skeleton). Bone mass measurements at spine and hip, and also at the wrist and, indeed, the entire skeleton, would be particularly valuable in evaluating these individuals. Also, although at present body composition measurement remains an experimental modality, such measurements (including lean body mass) would be of value in individuals with these eating disorders. Treating these conditions is, of course, quite difficult; demonstration of a skeletal disorder, however, could have the positive effect of ensuring compliance with primary therapy (such as increased caloric intake).

Lastly, bone mass measurements, primarily at the trabecular spinal sites, are indicated in young individuals with early or prolonged athletic amenorrhea. Significant spinal bone mass loss has been known to occur in these estrogen-depleted women, and identifying significant bone loss could lead to changes (decreases) in exercise schedules and possibly to the use of such experimental medications as estrogen replacement therapy and nasal spray calcitonin.

2. *In estrogen-deficient women known to have vertebral abnormalities or radiographically detected osteopenia, to diagnose the presence (or absence) of osteoporosis, to make clinical decisions regarding other diagnostic and/or therapeutic evaluations.* It should be remembered that the x-ray is an insensitive demineralization evaluator. Findings obtained with x-ray should be confirmed with bone mass measurements.
3. *In estrogen-depleted women receiving therapy to prevent or treat significant bone loss, or to monitor the response to such therapy.* In postmenopausal women, bone mass assessment is indicated to monitor the response to calcium/exercise programs and the response to such medications as estrogen, calcitonin, and/or the bisphosphonates. Bone mass measurements should be performed at intervals of 1 to 2 years after the onset of therapy, and then, if bone mass is stable, every 3 or 4 years. For premenopausal women treated with gonadotropin-releasing agonist/antagonists, measurements are indicated at perhaps 3-month intervals during the usual 6 months of therapy, to monitor any possibly developing bone mass deficit. Equally spaced measurements are of value in assessing the response to experimental therapies, such as low-dose estrogen, calcitonin, or bisphosphonates, which might combat the deleterious effect of the GnRH agonist on bone mass. In anorexic/bulimic patients, bone mass measurements at yearly intervals can assess the response to such therapies as increased caloric intake. For women with athletic amenorrhea, measurements at 3- to 6-month intervals can be utilized in following any developing bone mass deficit, or in following the response to therapies such as estrogen, nasal spray calcitonin, or bisphosphonates.

The use of these techniques for screening *all* estrogen-deficient women after the menopause is probably not indicated. If a postmenopausal woman has agreed to estrogen replacement therapy, bone mass measurement is probably not necessary.

The practitioner in the osteoporosis field specializing in estrogen depletion is also faced with a number of other clinical questions regarding the noninvasive bone mass measuring techniques. For instance, which site (spine, wrist, hip, os calcis, patella, etc.) and which bone type (cortical, trabecular) should be measured; also, which bone mass measuring technique should be used?

First, each of the above sites seems to provide some information defining risk for future fracture in individual patients; however, an accurate assessment of risk is relatively site-specific. The spine overall seems to be the most reasonable site for measurement, at least in young women and in women up to age 65 or 70. After that age, bone mass measurements at the spine *and* hip may be of value; in young estrogen-depleted women with athletic amenorrhea (age 20 to 40) hip measurements may also be of clinical utility.

Second, for following the response to therapy, the spine again appears to be the preferred site, but certain medications (such as sodium fluoride, estrogen, and cortisone) may affect cortical as well as trabecular bone, and a measurement of cortical bone (usually performed at the wrist) may also be indicated as well.

Last, assuming the spinal site is currently the most important, DEXA seems to be the technique of choice in 1992. Its ease of measurement, greater precision, lower radiation exposure, and excellent quality control reinforces such a choice.

A financial problem in 1992 is that the third-party health care carriers (Medicare/Medicaid, private insurers, etc.) do not uniformly reimburse the costs for these procedures. Given the clinical value of these techniques, such a position seems inappropriate. It is hoped that reimbursement will be available in the future.

CONCLUSIONS

Substantial data support the observation that the risk of bone fracture increases as bone mass decreases. Techniques quantitating bone mass can therefore be used to predict fracture risk. These techniques can and should be used in evaluating estrogen-depleted women at risk for osteoporosis and those with osteoporosis.

Key Points

- Bone mass is the principal determinant of fracture; therefore, a measurement of bone mass would be of value to identify and assess fracture risk and to monitor therapy.
- Dual-energy x-ray absorptiometry (DEXA) is the preferred technique for quantitating bone mass at hip, spine, wrist, and total skeleton.
- DEXA provides a precise(1% precision), logistically simple (10-minute scan time), safe (approximately 10 mrem of radiation exposure, or 1/6 that of a chest x-ray), and efficaceous assessment of bone mass.
- Bone mass may be used to assess risk for subsequent fracture, as an exponential relationship exists between bone mass and fracture risk.

- Women with estrogen depletion from any cause (premature menopause, the postmenopausal state, Turner syndrome, athletic amenorrhea, and anorexia nervosa) should be considered for bone mass measurements to define a lowbone mass state and a subsequent need for estrogen replacement therapy.

Suggested Readings

Consensus Development Conference. Prophylaxis and treatment of osteoporosis. Am J Med 1991; 90:107–110.

Johnston CC Jr, Melton LJ III, Lindsay R, Eddy D. Clinical indication for bone mass measurement. J Bone Min Res 1989; 4 (suppl 2).

Johnston CC, Melton LJ. Bone density measurement in the management of osteoporosis. In: Favus MJ, ed. Primer on metabolic bone diseases and disorders of mineral metabolism. Kelseyville, California, American Society of Bone & Mineral Research, 1990: 93–100.

Physician's resource manual. National Osteoporosis Foundation, 1991, 2nd edition, Washington, D.C.

Chesnut CH. Non-invasive methods for bone mass measurement. In: Avioli LV, ed. The osteoporotic syndrome. 3rd ed. Orlando, FL: Grune & Stratton, in press, 1991.

Genant HK, Foulkner KG, Glüer C-C. Measurement of bone mineral density: current status. Am J Med 1991; 91 (suppl 5B):5B-49S–5B-53S.

Wasnich RD. Bone mass measurements in diagnosis and assessment of therapy. Am J Med 1991; 91 (suppl 5B):5B-54S–58S.

5

Calcium and Exercise: Alternatives or Adjuncts to Estrogen in Preventing Osteoporosis

Bruce Ettinger and Barbara L. Drinkwater

Despite agreement that ovarian hormone replacement is the logical and effective therapy for ovarian deficiency, most women refuse to take it. Concerns over long-term safety, troublesome side effects, cost, and other factors that affect compliance result in about 80% of ovarian-deficient women avoiding long-term replacement therapy. Many women would welcome other ways to prevent bone loss and the ravages of osteoporosis. They seek the counsel of physicians regarding the effect of diet and lifestyle on skeletal health. This chapter examines the roles of enhanced calcium intake and physical exercise as alternatives or adjuncts to hormone replacement therapy (HRT).

CALCIUM AND SKELETAL HEALTH

The Adolescent

Adolescence is a critical time for development of a woman's skeleton. Skeletal mass doubles between the ages of 7 and 14 years (1, 2), increasing about 10% each year between the ages of 9 and 14 years. Longitudinal growth peaks around age 12 years, so skeletal mass can increase 20% per year (2). Adequate ovarian function is necessary for these skeletal changes. In cases of female hypogonadism, peak skeletal mass may reach only one-half to two-thirds of normal, and even subtle reduction in ovarian function, such as a few years' delay in menarche, is associated with reduced peak bone mass (3).

The average daily skeletal calcium accretion for growing girls is about 130 mg. About half this amount is sufficient for periods of slow growth, but two to three times as much may be needed during the peak growth spurt (Fig. 5.1) (1, 2, 4). Given the obligatory losses of calcium from skin and urine (150 to

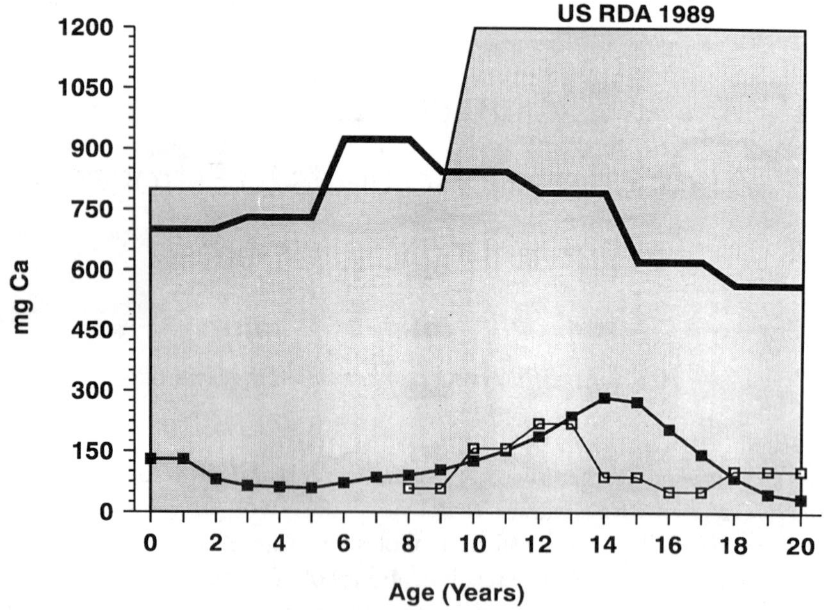

Figure 5.1. Dietary calcium intake and skeletal calcium needs for growing girls. *Shaded background,* U.S. recommended dietary calcium allowances (RDA). *Solid line,* median calcium intake (7) and calculated daily skeletal calcium accretion, for women, by age. *Solid boxes,* daily skeletal calcium accretion, calculated using the method of Leitch and Aitken (4) from annual increments in body weight; assumes skeletal calcium is 30 g at birth and increases to 950 g at age 20 years, in proportion to increments in body weight. *Open boxes,* projected daily skeletal calcium accretion from radial bone mineral content (2); assumes total body calcium at age 20 years is 700 g.

250 mg/day), a net absorption of 400 to 600 mg/day is required to provide for the skeleton's growth. Absorption efficiency in mature women is 25 to 35%; fortunately, young children and adolescents have demonstrated a greatly enhanced capacity to absorb calcium, as much as 40 to 50% of intake (5). Thus, adequate amounts of calcium can be ensured if the dietary calcium is 800 to 1200 mg/day, explaining the longstanding recommendation that adolescents consume 1200 mg of calcium daily (the recommended daily allowance [RDA] is set high enough to provide for the needs of nearly all healthy people). A greater intake of calcium is superfluous, although some have argued that more is better (6). It is undisputed, however, that the diets of many adolescent girls in the United States contain less than the recommended levels of calcium. A national dietary survey of young girls showed shocking

evidence of dietary calcium inadequacy; more than 25% of girls aged 9 to 11 years consumed less than 600 mg/day, and more than 25% of girls aged 12 to 14 years consumed less than 500 mg/day (7).

Adolescent girls ingesting less than 800 mg/day might be expected to suffer poor skeletal development and decreased skeletal mass. Clinical and epidemiologic studies suggest, at most, a modest relationship between calcium intake and skeletal mass at maturity. Women raised on habitually low calcium intakes (typically, no milk or less than 600 to 800 mg/day) appear to have 3 to 5% less skeletal mass than those whose diets are replete with calcium (8–11). This effect could possibly be due to other confounding variables such as total caloric intake, protein intake, body size, or activity level. One frequently quoted epidemiologic study examined the bone mass of persons in two regions of Yugoslavia, an area where dairy products formed an important part of the diet and another area where consumption was lower (8). The average daily calcium intakes of these two regions, 1100 mg and 600 mg, appeared to correlate with the finding of higher bone mass in the young people residing in the high-calcium district. Others have found similar differences in bone mass between adult women who had grown up on lower calcium intakes and those with habitually higher intakes. Kanders et al. (9) examined 24- to 35-year-old women and stratified them by calcium intake above or below 800 mg. The higher-intake group showed 5% more spinal mineral, but there were no discernible differences in cortical bone measured at the distal radius. Sowers et al. (10), applying the same criteria to a group of 20- to 35-year-old women, found 3% greater radial bone mass in the higher-calcium group. Sandler et al. (11) asked 229 recently menopausal women (average age 58 years) if they had regularly consumed milk as a child; those with a history of youthful milk drinking were found to have a 3% greater bone mass in the radius. Not all investigations have concluded that high calcium intake is beneficial to bone health. In a group of 20- to 35-year old Canadian women, similar to the study population of Kanders et al., Brown and coworkers (12) were unable to show any greater bone mass in those who had regular higher calcium consumption compared with those who had lower intakes. Other cross-sectional studies of mature women have also failed to find a statistically significant relationship between bone mass and calcium intake, even when comparing extremes of intake (13–15).

The concept of a threshold for calcium intake makes intuitive sense. We have evolved as efficient scavengers of calcium. When the needs of growth are greatest and availability is reduced, we compensate by enhancing absorption. When calcium is present in excess, we can reduce the efficiency of absorption to protect ourselves from overload. At calcium intakes below a critical level, the needs of growth cannot be satisfied, and a reduced skeletal mass must result. Growing rabbits subjected to calcium intakes one-third of normal and three times normal were compared with those with normal intakes; the spinal density was 8% lower in the group with one-third of normal intake but no greater in the group with a threefold increase in intake (16).

It is not known whether skeletal size and skeletal calcium content must always increase proportionally. For example, under conditions of inadequate calcium supply, can the skeleton increase normally in volume at the expense of reduced density? If so, can density be later restored to normal once calcium is in adequate supply? Rats raised on a calcium-deficient diet grow to normal size but have severely reduced skeletal calcium content; even at sexual maturity, providing a normal calcium intake allows complete restoration of the deficit (17). Until such compensatory mechanisms are demonstrated in humans, public health measures must be taken to guard against low calcium intake, especially during the years of peak growth.

Ultimately, controlled experiments will be required to show the possible benefits of higher calcium intakes in youth. An ongoing clinical trial was designed to test the effect of added calcium, in the form of milk or calcium carbonate, in 14-year-old girls (18). The untreated group had an average daily calcium intake of 700 mg, compared with 1600 and 1700 mg for the milk and calcium carbonate–supplemented groups. After 2 years, the incremental bone mass tended to be greater in the high-calcium groups, but differences did not reach statistical significance. Further studies are needed to test the effect of dietary intake in girls between the ages of 9 and 13 years.

The Mature Woman

Peak density is reached in trabecular bone by the time longitudinal growth ends, but cortical bone density continues to increase through the third decade. During the skeletal consolidation phase, ages 18 to 30 years, cortical bone density increases about 10%. This phase requires a small daily calcium accretion of about 20 to 30 mg. Based on extensive balance studies in mature women, Heaney et al. (19) have calculated that for every 100-mg increase in dietary calcium, there is a 10-mg net absorption and a 6-mg increase in urinary excretion; this yields about 4 mg for the skeleton. A woman consuming 800 mg of calcium can easily achieve the needed amount, even if her fractional gastrointestinal absorption is 15 to 20%. Despite these findings, in 1989, the U.S. National Research Council extended the 1200-mg RDA from ages 11 to 18 years to ages 11 to 24 years. Higher intakes could optimize skeletal consolidation, possibly allowing some women to "catch up" in bone density if their previous calcium intakes had been inadequate for proper skeletal mineralization.

In mature women, once the minimum intake of calcium is achieved, further increases do not offer any advantage. Epidemiologic studies fail to show a relationship between bone density and calcium intake within the range of 260 to 2000 mg/day (20). Skeletal demands for calcium are relatively low during adult life, and homeostatic mechanisms compensate during periods of low intake by increasing fractional gastrointestinal absorption and reducing urinary excretion.

Whereas bone mass is maintained or slightly increases in young women who are estrogen replete, estrogen-deficient women will suffer bone loss. Numerous clinical examples provide convincing evidence; ovariectomy, premature ovarian failure, and secondary hypogonadism all cause aggressive bone loss. Recently, GnRH agonists, used to treat endometriosis or uterine myomas, have provided an experimental tool to study the induction and resolution of bone loss caused by secondary hypogonadism. It was hoped that enhanced calcium intake would reduce the magnitude of skeletal losses in estrogen-deficient young women. Based on short-term experiments in women given GnRH, calcium supplementation did not prevent and may even have increased skeletal losses (21). Athletes (22) and other young women with amenorrhea (23) suffer skeletal losses despite their high calcium intakes. When ovarian function is regained, bone mass improves; stopping GnRH permits full restoration (21). Reducing the level of exercise allows partial restoration of bone mass (24).

There is evidence that endogenous estrogen production begins to fall a few years before menopause. This process is marked by an increase in serum FSH level and a reduction in serum estradiol level. Bone loss, particularly trabecular, begins during this period (25). Analysis of vertebral trabecular bone indicates that 10% may be lost during the transition to menopause (26). Based on findings of a synergistic effect of high-calcium diet with suboptimal doses of estrogen replacement (see below), it might be predicted that raising calcium intake to a level of 1500 mg/day would enhance the osteotrophic effects of low endogenous estrogen levels, thereby reducing bone loss occurring during the few years before menopause.

The Menopausal Woman

The possible bone-sparing effects of calcium in early menopausal women were first suggested by the experiments of Recker (27). Women who were, on the average, 9 years postmenopausal were randomly assigned to take 1000 mg of calcium or placebo. After 2 years, the calcium-treated women had lost 0.2% of initial metacarpal thickness, while those not taking calcium had lost 1.2%. It is rarely mentioned that, in this same study, bone mineral content measured at the radius decreased 2.9% in the calcium-treated women, compared with losses of 2.0% in the control subjects. Nilas et al. (28) compared bone loss rates in women who were 6 to 36 months beyond menopause. When stratified by habitual calcium intakes (less than 550, 550 to 1150, and more than 1150 mg/day), all groups were shown to lose bone at the same rate. In another study of women just beyond menopause, during 3 years of follow-up, there was no relationship between bone loss and level of calcium intake, even over the broad range of 300 to 3000 mg/day (29) (Fig. 5.2). Cumulative losses of skeletal mineral were 15% in the spine and 3% in the peripheral skeleton. Based on a prospective, randomized 2-year study, Riis et al. (30) showed that giving 2000 mg of supplemental calcium to estrogen-deficient women had no effect on bone loss in the spine or distal radius, but this treatment slowed bone loss in the midradius and in the total skeleton. These beneficial effects were minor compared with the complete protection afforded by estrogen in the same study. In another randomized placebo study, Stevenson et al. (15) showed that high calcium intake was ineffective in stopping bone loss in women within 5 years of menopause. Those consuming an average of 1621 mg/day lost as much or more than those consuming an average of 504 mg/day. Measurements in the spine and radius failed to show that any site was protected. A recently completed double-blind, randomized study of early menopausal women showed that bone loss was not prevented by the administration of calcium supplements of 1000 mg/day (31). In this same study, the estrogen users were protected.

It appears that high calcium intake is of little or no use in the immediate postmenopausal years but may become more effective as bone turnover spontaneously slows, 5 to 10 years after menopause. This may be particularly true if the habitual calcium intake is low. Examining the effects of 500 mg of added calcium, given to women whose usual calcium intakes were less than 650 mg/day, Dawson-Hughes and coworkers (32) found no effects in women within 5 years of menopause, but found a 60 to 80% reduction in the rate of bone loss in women who were more than 5 years postmenopausal. The synergism between estrogen and calcium was also suggested by another study of women who were, on the average, 9 years postmenopausal (33). Endogenous estrogen levels and dietary calcium intakes each had statistically significant relationships to bone density. However, the greatest effects on

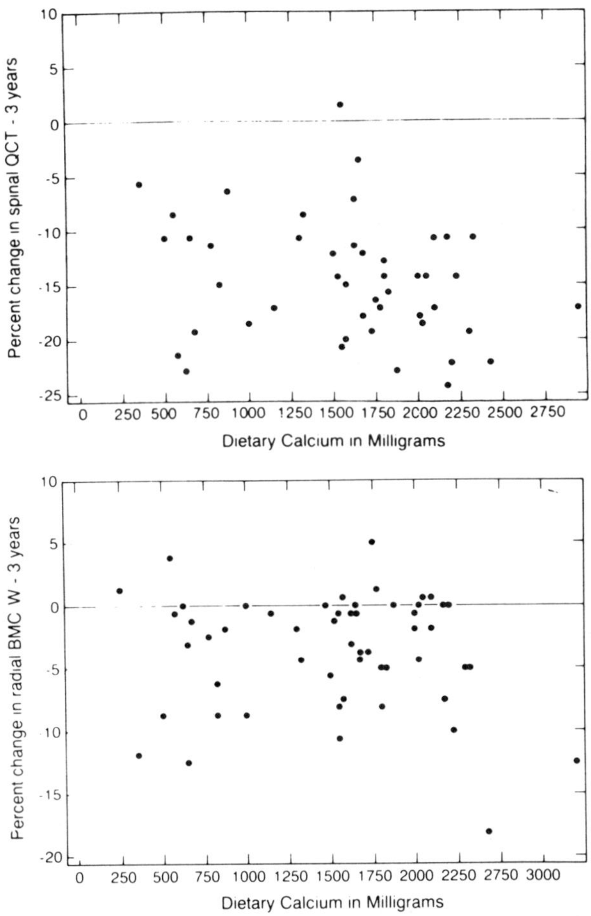

Figure 5.2. Cumulative percent change in mineral content after 3 years compared with daily calcium intake. *Top,* Spinal trabecular mineral content as measured by quantitative computed tomography QCT). *Bottom,* Proximal radius mineral content per width (BMC/W) as measured by single-photon absorptiometry (29). (From Ettinger B, Genant HK, Cann CE. Low-dosage estrogen combined with calcium prevents postmenopausal bone loss: results of a 3-year study. In: Cohn DV, Martin TJ, Meunier PJ, eds. Calcium regulation and bone metabolism: basic and clinical aspects. New York: Elsevier, 1987;9:918–922.)

bone density were observed in those women with both high endogenous estrogen levels and high calcium intakes.

The side effects of estrogen, particularly the resumption of monthly menses, have caused many women to refuse or discontinue hormonal replacement. The prevalence and magnitude of side effects are related to the daily dosage. In the hope of enhancing the bone protection afforded by extremely low doses of estrogen, half the customary dose, 0.3 mg conjugated estrogens, was combined with a calcium intake of at least 1500 mg/day. To reach this intake level, all subjects consumed calcium carbonate supplements; most used 750 to 1000 mg/day. The average daily calcium intake, from all sources, was 1773 mg. The combination proved as effective as 0.6 mg of conjugated estrogen given without calcium supplements (34) (Fig. 5.3). This study was criticized on several counts. It was neither randomized nor double-blinded, three-quarters of subjects used a progestogen for 10 to 12 days per month, and none had been previously ovariectomized. To answer these concerns, a double-blind, randomized study was mounted comparing graded doses of micronized 17β-estradiol to placebo, in women who were also given calcium supplements. All were within 5 years of menopause, 24% were surgically menopausal, and none received concurrent progestogen during the 18 months of the trial (endometrial biopsies were performed to monitor untoward effects of estrogen on the endometrium). Once again, the combination of calcium and low-dose estrogen proved effective in preventing bone loss (31) (Fig. 5.4). Whereas in previous studies, 1.0 to 2.0 mg of micronized estradiol was required in nonsupplemented women (35), as little as 0.5 mg prevented bone loss in these subjects with high calcium intakes. This synergistic effect has now been confirmed for 0.3 mg of conjugated estrogens (36) and has been expanded to piperazine estrone sulfate (37).

Does a woman who uses standard doses of estrogen need to maintain a high-calcium diet? Until recently, trials of the osteotrophic effects of estrogen were performed in women who were not given calcium supplements. In all such trials, estrogen protected 90 to 100% of subjects. When investigators evaluate the occasional "estrogen failure," they do not find a deficiency of dietary calcium. But in a recent report, we observed that during 18 months of treatment with 1.0 mg micronized 17β-estradiol which resulted in an annual change in spinal trabecular bone density of +2.0%, there was a statistically significant positive correlation between total calcium intake and spinal trabecular bone density ($r = 0.37, p = .02$) (37a). It is highly unlikely, given the present climate of osteoporosis research, that anyone will be able to randomly allocate research subjects to calcium deprivation to test the

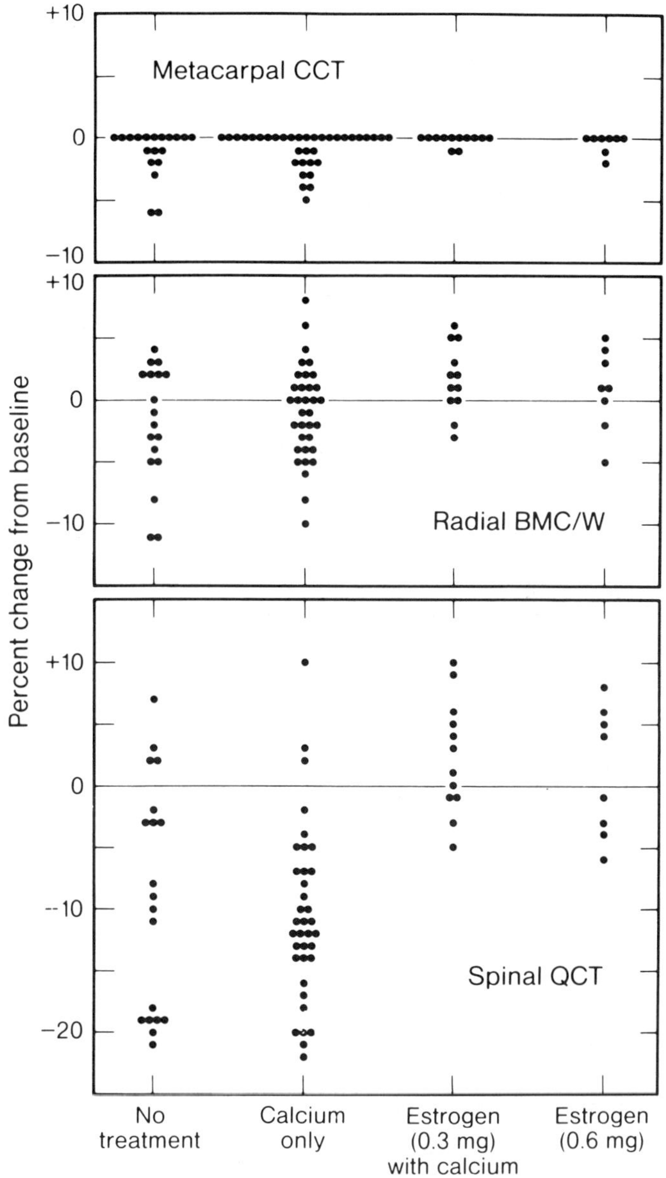

Figure 5.3. Skeletal changes after 2 years, expressed as a percentage of baseline values; metacarpal combined cortical thickness (CCT), radial bone mineral content per width (BMC/W), and spinal trabecular mineral content measured by quantitative computed tomography (QCT) (34). (Reproduced, with permission, from Ettinger B, Genant HK, Cann CE. Postmenopausal bone loss is prevented by treatment with low-dosage estrogen with calcium. Ann Intern Med 1987;106:40–45.)

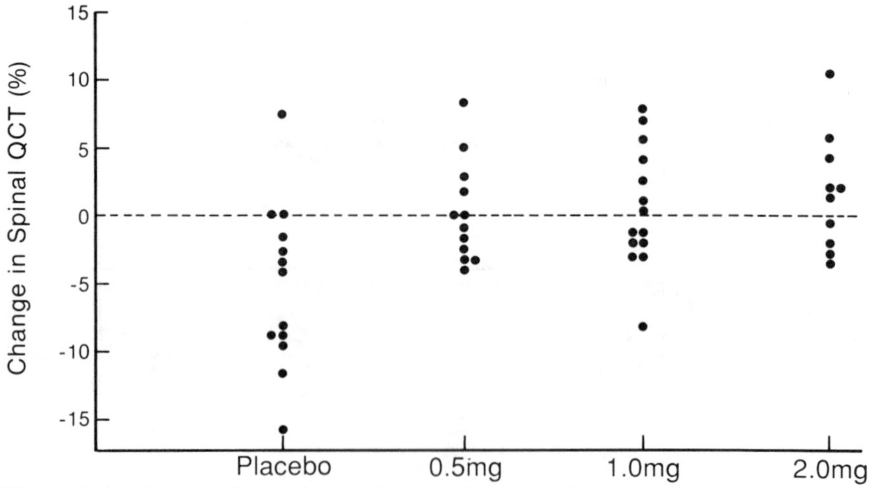

Figure 5.4. Percent change in spinal mineral content after 18 months, measured by QCT (annual rate, expressed as percent of baseline). Treatment was with placebo, 0.5, 1.0, or 2.0 mg micronized 17β-estradiol. All subjects received calcium supplements (31). (Reprinted with permission from the American College of Obstetricians and Gynecologists. Ettinger B. Prevention of osteoporosis: treatment of estradiol deficiency. Obstet Gynecol 1988;72 [suppl]:12S–17S.)

effectiveness of estrogen in calcium-deprived women. Animal experiments in ovariectomized dogs show that estrogen protects equally well against bone loss in calcium-deprived and calcium-replete animals (38).

The Older Woman

With increasing age, especially beyond age 65 years, enhancing calcium intake may again have an important role in bone health. Several mechanisms account for this: (*a*) with reduced bone resorption, there is a lessening of the flux of calcium from bone to blood and a reduced tendency to elevate the serum calcium level and suppress parathyroid hormone; (*b*) intestinal calcium absorption becomes less efficient with age; (*c*) dietary calcium intake may decrease with age, as income and total caloric expenditure decrease; and (*d*) vitamin D activity may diminish with age, in part because of reduced renal mass. The mechanism accounting for bone loss shifts from bone resorption, calcium excess, and low parathyroid hormone level to low bone turnover, calcium deprivation, and a rise in parathyroid hormone level.

What evidence exists that a high calcium intake will prevent bone loss and fractures in the elderly? Matković et al. (8) reexamined their study of

Yugoslavian women mentioned earlier, focusing now on the changes in the two districts with aging; there was no bone loss seen until after menopause, but then bone loss was greater among women living in the high-calcium district (39). There were fewer hip fractures in this district, probably because of the salutary effects of a high bone mass developed in childhood and carried over into old age. Riggs et al. (20) found that habitually higher calcium intake did not affect the rate of bone loss in older people, but in short-term clinical trials, Jensen et al. (40) and Orwoll et al. (41) found high calcium intakes reduced the rates of loss. In a unique 3-year study of nursing home residents with an average age of 81 years, Smith et al. (42) reported that giving women 750 mg/day of calcium increased their radial bone mineral 1.6%, compared with 3.3% loss in those untreated. Men and women living in a retirement community in southern California were evaluated for habitual calcium intake, and subsequent hip fracture incidence was observed (43). Those consuming more than 765 mg/day of calcium had 60% fewer hip fractures than those consuming less than 460 mg/day. Was the apparent salutory effect due to the calcium intake or confounding factors associated with the intake? People consuming more calcium in old age might have also had a higher intake when young, which could be associated with achieving a greater peak bone mass. These and other potentially serious design problems plague this study. In a nonrandomized, nonblinded trial of osteoporotic women, Riggs et al. (44) found new vertebral deformities were half as frequent in those receiving calcium compared to those left untreated. Using a more rigorous experimental design, others have failed to show reductions in the rate of new vertebral deformities when calcium was compared to placebo (45).

Calcium—What Kind and How Much?

Recognizing that high calcium intake cannot prevent bone loss due to estrogen deficiency, it is still prudent to avoid adding the additional insult of calcium deprivation. In counseling patients, we find it useful to make a simplified estimate of dietary calcium intake: to the 300 to 400 mg obtained from a dairy-free diet add 300 mg for each portion of dairy product consumed. If intake is not up to par, the choices are to increase dairy intake, increase calcium-fortified foods, or take calcium supplements.

An increasing number of food products are fortified with calcium. We have recently seen the introduction of fortified juice, punch, soda pop, cereal, and even milk. Calcium supplements are aggressively advertised but should be used only if dietary sources are inadequate. The cost of these supplements varies from 5 to 10 cents to more than 30 cents per day for 1000 mg. Most generic oyster-shell calcium preparations are adequate, although a few have been shown to be poorly absorbed because of an insoluble coating and limited dispersability (46, 47). Absorption of calcium supplements is greatly enhanced by consuming them with food, even a small snack. Achlorhydric patients can adequately absorb calcium from calcium carbonate, provided the supplements are taken with food (48). A simple test for tablet dissolution has been recommended: observe the tablet in household vinegar after intermittently agitating it for 30 minutes.

It is important to know the number of milligrams of elemental calcium contained in a supplement. Calcium carbonate has the highest percentage of elemental calcium, but it is only 40% calcium by weight. Calcium lactate contains 12% and calcium gluconate has 9% elemental calcium; neither of these preparations warrants the expense and the large number of tablets required. Enhanced intake of calcium is safe, thanks to the homeostatic mechanisms that protect most of us against oversupply.

Avoiding calcium undersupply is especially important in late childhood and adolescence, when 1200 mg/day should be consumed. During a woman's mature years, 800 mg is sufficient. In the elderly, 1500 mg is a reasonable prescription. Women who are unwilling or unable to take full doses of hormone replacement and who want protection against bone loss should consider the combination of 1500 mg of calcium with half-strength estrogen. Finally, estrogen-deficient women should be warned that calcium alone is not an alternative to estrogen for preventing osteoporosis.

PHYSICAL EXERCISE AND SKELETAL HEALTH

Weightbearing physical activity is essential for bone health. When mechanical stress or gravitational force on the skeleton is removed as in bed rest (49), space flight (50, 51), immobilized limbs (52), or paralysis (53), bone loss is rapid and extensive. In contrast, athletes, who exercise much more intensely and consistently than the average person, usually have above-average bone mass (54–56). The question that remains unanswered is how these two facts can be applied to the prevention and treatment of osteoporosis. Can women reduce their risk of osteoporotic fractures by increasing their physical activity?

Exercise could have a direct role in preventing osteoporosis by maximizing peak bone mass in young women, maintaining that peak mass throughout the mature adult years, and attenuating the loss of bone in the postmenopausal years. This theoretical benefit would accrue only if osteoporotic fractures are directly related to low bone mass. Although some investigators (57) have questioned the predictive value of bone density in assessing fracture risk, several recent studies (58–60) have reported that fracture risk does increase with a decrease in bone density. Indirectly, exercise may decrease fracture risk in an older population by reducing the risk of falling. Active older people do have better coordination, balance, and muscular strength than their sedentary peers (61, 62). Regardless of age, women can improve these essential aspects of physical fitness by participating in carefully planned exercise programs. A recommendation for an exercise program should include identification of the most effective type of exercise as well as the frequency, duration, and intensity of the exercise sessions. While there is a broad experimental database underlying exercise programs designed to develop cardiovascular fitness or increase muscular strength, there is no such basis for an "exercise prescription" for bone health. Until these definitive studies have been done, women and their physicians must rely on the data at hand. The following sections examine the evidence that exercise can increase bone mass, how exercise interacts with estrogen and calcium, and the potential benefits of exercise at different stages of the life cycle.

Maximizing Bone Mass in the Young Adult

There is a certain logic to the concept that one might decrease the likelihood of osteoporosis in the postmenopausal years by using the consolidation phase of skeletal development to maximize bone mass. If one looks at the fracture risk for various populations relative to their peak bone mass, it is evident that the groups that have the highest bone mass also have the lowest risk of osteoporotic fractures (63). For example, both African-American women and white men have a higher peak bone density and a lower incidence of fractures than white women (64–66). These observations have led to the theory that failure to accumulate adequate bone mass in the early adult years increases the risk of osteoporosis in the postmenopausal years (67). Among the limited options available to young women for increasing bone mass during this period is exercise. Whether the positive effect of physical activity on bone can be compared to the genetic advantage of racial heritage or gender in achieving a high peak bone mass is by no means certain. Unlike the biological advantage, the beneficial effect of exercise is transient unless the physical activity is continued throughout life.

TRAINING PRINCIPLES

General principles of training may also apply to bone. For example, a training program should be designed to attain a specific goal. Aerobic activities such as running, swimming, or cycling are selected if the goal is to improve cardiovascular fitness. The same activities may have little or no effect on bone mass. The effect of exercise on bone appears to be a localized effect, and the specificity principle suggests that the exercise program should involve activities that add mechanical stress to the areas where osteoporotic fractures occur most frequently, such as the spine, femoral neck, distal radius, and humerus.

Another training principle emphasizes the importance of progressive overload. To effect change, the training stimulus must slowly but consistently increase. For example, to increase the strength of a muscle, the weight the muscle is required to lift must be increased. If the same principle applies to bone, the training stimulus cannot remain static. Once the skeleton has become adapted to a specific activity, such as walking, further increases in bone mineral density (BMD) would not be expected unless the exercise stimulus is increased. Whether that progressive overload is best achieved by increasing the intensity, the frequency, or the duration of activities designed to increase bone mass is not known at this time.

Perhaps the most important principle of training is the recognition of individual differences. The effectiveness of any exercise program varies from person to person. Women who have been sedentary most of their lives usually show the greatest improvement, while those who are already active may have a minimal response. Training studies that select only sedentary women as subjects have a built-in bias because they are optimizing their chances for a positive result.

There is a limit to the training effect, and as one approaches this ceiling it requires more time and effort to achieve ever smaller gains. This ceiling is determined for each woman by her own biological endowment. Like other physiological systems, the skeleton "detrains" when the training stimulus is removed. Dalsky et al. (68) showed clearly that when women stop exercising, their BMD reverts to the pretraining level.

COST AND BENEFIT OF EXERCISE

Cost refers to the duration, frequency, and intensity of exercise required to elicit a specific benefit, which in this case is the difference in BMD between active women and their sedentary peers. Data are available from seven cross-sectional studies (69–75) that measured vertebral BMD in active women and a group of sedentary controls (Fig. 5.5). Many of these women were varsity athletes in team or individual sports and practiced an average of 2.5 hours/day at least 5 days/week. Others ran 6 days/week, averaged 1.6

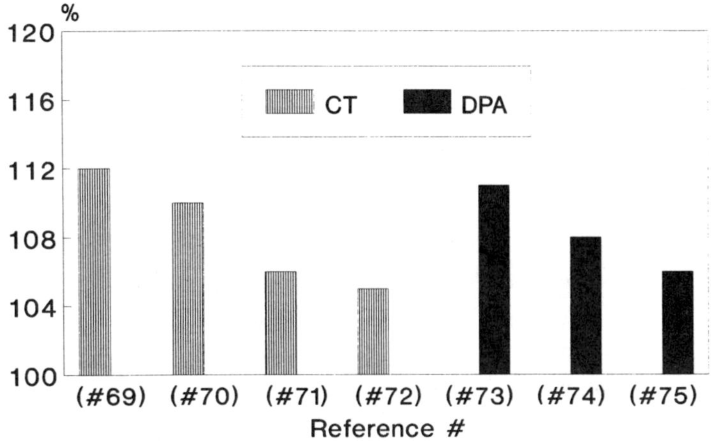

Figure 5.5. The bone mineral density (BMD) of the lumbar spine (L1-L4) of active young women as a percentage of the lumbar density of sedentary women of the same age. Data included those from computed tomography (CT) and dual-photon absorptiometry (DPA).

hours/day, and covered 40 to 60 miles/week. In each case, the BMDs of the active women were higher than those of the inactive group. However, considering the training regimen of these young athletes, the difference between the two groups is relatively small (range, 5 to 12%; mean, 8.3%).

If the average lumbar BMD of 165.8 mg/cm^3 reported by Cann et al. (76) for premenopausal women (n = 50) is used to calculate the potential benefit of an exercise program for a woman who is two standard deviations below the mean, 107 mg/cm^3, a 12% increase in BMD would still leave her spinal density (119.8 mg/cm^3) well below average. Even a woman only one standard deviation below the mean, 136.4 mg/cm^3 would need a 21.5% improvement to reach the average BMD.

EXERCISE AND ESTROGEN

The positive effect of exercise on the skeletons of young women is dependent on the presence of normal levels of endogenous estrogen. Several studies (22, 70, 71, 76–78) have reported statistically significant lower lumbar BMDs in amenorrheic athletes (Fig. 5.6). Unlike their eumenorrheic teammates, these women have a lower vertebral BMD than sedentary women of the same age. Interestingly, the spine is the only skeletal site where this difference is apparent.

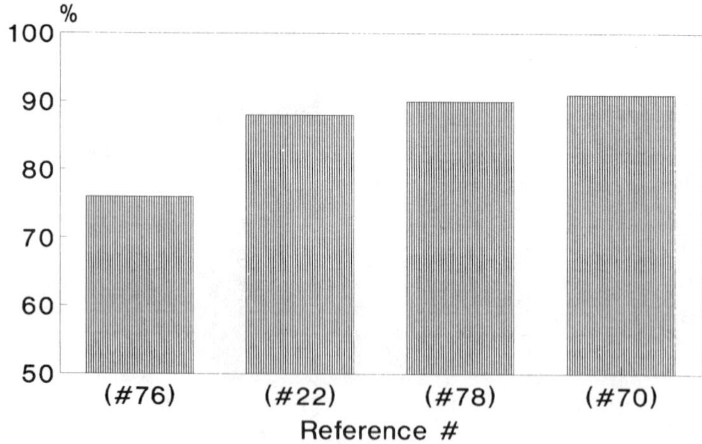

Figure 5.6. The bone mineral density of the lumbar spine (L1-L4) of amenorrheic athletes as a percentage of the lumbar density of sedentary women of the same age.

Although women who resume normal menses do regain some bone (24, 74), there appears to be a residual loss from periods of menstrual irregularities (79, 80). Women with a history of amenorrhea or oligomenorrhea have a lower vertebral density than women who have always had regular periods. This suggests a need for the physician to consider some form of intervention when a woman presents with hypoestrogenic amenorrhea associated with strenuous physical activity. Exercise alone will not protect her from bone loss. Some preliminary results suggest that young women respond to HRT as postmenopausal women do. There is no further decrease in bone density, but neither is there a significant gain (Fig. 5.7). If these observations are confirmed, they suggest that treatment should be initiated as soon as the diagnosis of anovulatory hypothalamic amenorrhea is confirmed (81).

Preventing Bone Loss in the Mature Woman

Cross-sectional studies may give an erroneous estimate of age-related bone loss (82). Not only is the date of birth related to skeletal size, but the lifestyle of women has changed dramatically since today's postmenopausal women were young. Women are more physically active both in leisure activities and in the workplace. Whether the epidemiological estimates of bone loss in the premenopausal years are truly an aging effect or the cumulative result of lifestyle choices such as smoking, excessive consumption of alcohol, inadequate calcium intake, and inactivity has not been determined. Although

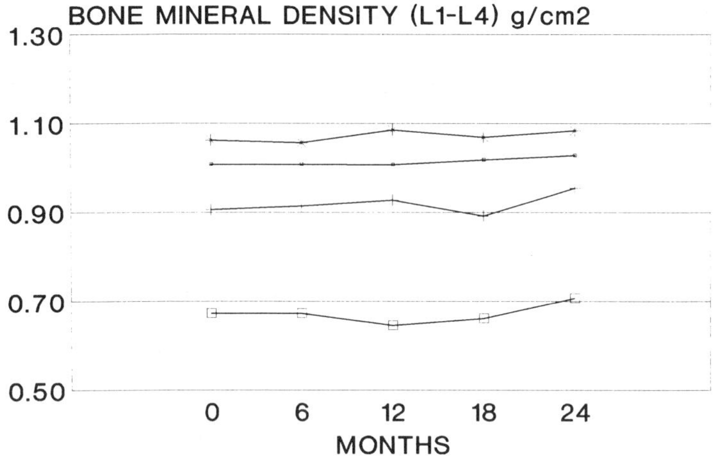

Figure 5.7. The changes in bone mineral density of the lumbar spine in four amenorrheic athletes treated with conjugated estrogens (Premarin, 0.625 mg. Ayerst Laboratories, New York, NY) and a progestin (Provera, 10 mg, Upjohn, Kalamazoo, MI) for 24 months.

women in this age group (35 to 50 years) are past the age when bone mass apparently reaches its peak, data from the few studies (83–85) that have examined the effect of physical activity in this age range suggest that active women have a higher BMD than sedentary women and that an exercise training program does increase bone mass.

None of the studies can be considered truly definitive. The two cross-sectional studies (83, 84) have the usual problem of selection bias. Brewer et al. (83) compared sedentary women to a group of runners who were training for a marathon. Although the runners had been running an average of 5 years and averaged 40 miles/week, their average os calcis density was 6.8% less than those of the inactive women. The greater body weight (+7.5 kg) of the sedentary group was apparently more effective than running in determining the density of this weight-bearing bone. The runners did have higher values for the midshaft of the radius (+4.7%) and the middle phalanx of the fifth finger (+12.3%). The meaning of these observations is a bit obscure, since neither site receives the benefit of mechanical loading during running. Quite likely women who run marathons are active in other ways as well.

In the second study, Aloia et al. (84) correlated total body calcium (TBCa) and vertebral density with activity as measured by a motion sensor. A statistically significant relationship was found between these measures of bone mass and estimates of physical activity in a group of 24 sedentary women; the authors concluded that exercise might be a major determinant of bone mass. Unfortunately, they did not report regression equations so the advantage of increasing activity could be quantified. A correlation coefficient of .41 between spinal BMD and activity would account for only about 16% of the variability in BMD among the women, leaving 83% of the variability unaccounted for. Smoking was negatively associated with vertebral density and also accounted for 16% of the variability in BMD. It would be interesting to determine if eliminating cigarettes and adding exercise would have an additive effect on bone mass.

The only longitudinal study to measure spinal BMD did not include a control group, making the report of a 6.5% increase in density in a group of 16 regular runners suspect (85). The pervasive problem of calibration drift in dual-photon absorptiometry (DPA) machines makes a control group a necessity.

Other studies of this age group also include younger and older women as well and are discussed under Fitness and Bone Loss Throughout Life.

Until data from well-designed prospective studies are available that clearly define the role of exercise in maintaining or increasing bone mass in the mature adult female, the conservative approach is to recommend that all women incorporate some form of moderate activity into their lives. The well-established benefits of regular exercise on cardiovascular fitness, muscular strength and endurance, flexibility, and body composition can be enjoyed while we await the final word on the effect of exercise on the skeletal system.

THE POSTMENOPAUSAL WOMAN

By far, the greatest number of studies examining the effect of exercise on bone have involved postmenopausal women. It should be stated at the outset that there is no evidence that exercise can offset the deleterious effect the decrease in endogenous estrogen production has on bone mass. To the contrary, the experience of young amenorrheic athletes suggests that prolonged intensive training programs cannot protect the skeleton from the hypoestrogenic state. However, there are women for whom HRT is contraindicated, and some decide against HRT for other reasons. For these women, any protection against bone loss, no matter how small, is an advantage.

It is also possible that estrogen and exercise may act synergistically in older women, as in young women. Active young women with normal estrogen levels, for example, have statistically significantly greater vertebral BMD than sedentary women with normal menses (69–75). Once past the early postmenopausal years and into the eighth and ninth decades, even small gains in bone mass may be protective for older women. If an osteoporotic fracture can be delayed by even a few years, the result may be a shorter period of dependency.

CROSS-SECTIONAL STUDIES

Taken in their entirety, these studies raise more questions than they answer. Differences in subject selection, definitions of activity, measurement sites and techniques, use or nonuse of estrogen, and activity history make it difficult to isolate the effect of exercise per se on bone mass. In general, women defined as active had higher bone mass than those described as sedentary, although the differences between active and inactive groups varied widely. In one case, the more active group was reported to be losing bone at a faster rate than inactive women (86). The active women were younger (51 to 65 years), however, and likely to be in the stage of rapid bone loss associated with onset of menopause, whereas the inactive women were older (70 to 91 years) and in a more stable phase.

Two other studies (55, 87) drew from the same subject pool, a 50-Plus Runners Association, but reported quite different results. Lane et al. (55) reported a lumbar vertebral density of 139 mg/cm^3 for six runners and 103.2 mg/cm^3 for their matched controls, a 35% advantage for the active women. Michel et al. (87) found an average lumbar density of 112.5 mg/cm^3 for 28 women from the same association and only a 9.2% difference between runners and the controls. In each case, the values are well below those of young women measured by the same computed tomography technique (165.8 mg/cm^3) (76), suggesting that running had not completely prevented bone loss.

Chow et al. (88) and Oyster et al. (89) divided women into two groups on the basis of estimated aerobic power ($\dot{V}O_2$max) and a physical activity profile, respectively. The more fit or active women were about 18% higher in the cortical width of the second metacarpal (89) or in calcium bone index measured at the trunk and proximal femur by neutron activation (88). This effect is much larger than is usually seen in a longitudinal study of training and suggests either selection bias or the cumulative effect of years of activity compared with the relatively short period of a training study. When Åström et al. (90) examined the level of physical activity in groups of older women with and without a femoral neck fracture, they found women without fracture had been more active between the ages of 15 and 45 years than the fracture group.

No bone density measurements were presented for this relatively small sample of 49 matched pairs.

A number of studies have suggested a close relationship between strength or muscle mass and bone mass (91–95). Young men who had been weight training an average of 3.6 days/week for 6.1 years had higher densities in the lumbar vertebrae (+10.6%), trochanter (+15.1%), and femoral neck (+15.7%) than a matched control group but had no difference at the midradius (91). A positive benefit in femoral neck (+9%) and vertebral integral density (+18%) between young male weightlifters and a control group was also reported by Block et al. (92). As in other studies (93, 96), a statistically significant relationship was found between muscle size or strength and bone density in men.

It is uncertain whether a similar relationship exists for older women. While some investigators (94, 95) have reported statistically significant correlations between strength measures and bone density for women, others (88) have failed to find that strength training increases BMD, and still others (96) have reported mixed results. In one study, a relationship that was statistically significant for premenopausal women was not significant for postmenopausal women (95). A fact often overlooked in evaluating the interaction of strength with bone mass is that strength is directly related to muscle mass, which in turn is related positively to body weight and negatively to age. Caution is warranted in considering the results of any study that does not take these factors into consideration in the experimental design or statistical analysis.

Strength training satisfies many of the training principles discussed above. Mechanical loading can be directed to specific skeletal sites, and the workload can be slowly but consistently increased. The program can be individualized for each woman, who can progress at her own pace. Theoretically, this type of activity has the potential to have a positive effect on bone mass. Whether it will be effective in the absence of HRT is not known at this time.

LONGITUDINAL STUDIES

Three separate studies (97–99) have reported that a walking program of 6 months to 3 years does not prevent bone loss in women with an average age in the mid to late 50s. The decrease in bone mass in the two studies that selected the radius as the measurement site may represent an application of the specificity principle (97, 98). Walking is expected to place more mechanical and gravitational force on the legs than on the arms. However, Cavanaugh et al. (99) reported a loss of even greater magnitude (−5.6%) in the trabecular area of the lumbar vertebrae. None of the investigators measured bone mass changes in the femur, tibia, or fibula. Because walking is a popular choice of exercise for many older women and a relatively safe exercise prescription with its low risk for musculoskeletal injuries, the value of this weightbearing activity for preserving bone mass needs to be investigated in more detail.

Studies that have used a more varied exercise program that included aerobics (100), calisthenics (42, 100–102), stair climbing (68), or activities designed to load specific bones (100, 103, 104) have reported a more positive result. The average increase in lumbar density has been 6.0% (68, 102, 104); in the radius, 1.4% (42, 101, 103, 104). Notelovitz et al. (104) were the only group to look at the additive effect of exercise plus estrogen, and they reported the largest increases in spinal density (+8.4%). They were also the only group to use a resistance-circuit weight-training program. Both of these variables, the effect of estrogen plus exercise and the value of resistance training, need to be examined further.

Any increase in bone mass during these postmenopausal years has to be considered a benefit. Although the relative increase is modest, the gain must be weighed against the continued loss of bone mass (−1.8%/year) in the respective control groups. The overall benefit for the active women is the sum of the increase in bone mass plus the estimated loss of bone if they had remained inactive. This estimated total benefit is in the range of 4 to 8%, depending on the skeletal site and the exercise program. The effect of this attenuation in bone loss on the probability of an osteoporotic fracture in this age group is not known.

Fitness and Bone Loss Throughout Life

A number of cross-sectional studies have examined the relationship between bone mass and exercise across a wide age range. Some have used an activity questionnaire to divide their subjects into active and sedentary groups; others have related BMD to some measure of physical fitness such as aerobic power ($\dot{V}O_2max$). There are problems with both techniques. For example, $\dot{V}O_2max$ is a measure of cardiorespiratory fitness and may not represent participation in activities that augment bone mass. It also has a significant genetic component and when expressed as liters/minute is directly related to body size, which in turn is related to bone mass. When submaximal tests are used to predict $\dot{V}O_2max$, the validity of the results is open to question. According to McArdle et al. (105) the error in prediction is 10 to 20%. They state unequivocally that this amount of error is not acceptable for research purposes.

Activity levels measured by questionnaire are generally used to categorize women into activity groups, but they are seldom validated and are subject to selective recall. There has been no attempt to discriminate between activities that do or do not place mechanical stress on the specific skeletal sites being measured. As in all cross-sectional studies, the data are subject to selection bias. Differences in bone density between these self-selected groups cannot be attributed solely to differences in activity levels.

The results of studies in this category are inconclusive. Pocock et al. (106) reported a statistically significant relationship between predicted $\dot{V}O_2max$ in liters/minute and both femoral neck (r = .60) and lumbar spine (r = .54) BMD in women aged 20 to 75 years. It would be interesting to know how the relationship would be affected if the women were divided by menopausal status, because two other groups of investigators (69, 96) found no statistically significant relationship between spinal density and $\dot{V}O_2max$ (measured directly and expressed relative to body weight [$ml \cdot kg^{-1} \cdot min^{-1}$]) in postmenopausal women. In fact, Kirk et al. (69) reported no difference in lumbar density between older women who ran 37 miles/week and sedentary women of the same age, whereas the difference between younger runners and their control group was significant.

Two other studies (107, 108) also suggest that the beneficial effect of exercise on bone may be somewhat attenuated in older women. Stillman et al. (107) measured radial BMD in women aged 30 to 85 years and made two important observations: the positive effect of physical activity on bone was observed only in the premenopausal women and only in the high-activity group, after the means were adjusted for age and menstrual status. In the only longitudinal study involving a wide range of ages, 35 to 65 years, Smith et al. (108) found that women who exercised 45 minutes, 3 days a week, for 4 years continued to lose bone at the radius, ulna, and humerus. However, the rate of loss was significantly less than in the sedentary group. Premenopausal women who exercised averaged a −0.32 rate of loss per year in density at the three sites; postmenopausal women (not on hormone replacement therapy) had an average annual rate of −1.24%. Apparently, the exercise routines were unable to prevent an increased rate of bone loss following menopause.

When BMD measurements are taken for large numbers of women of a wide age range and correlated with some measure of physical activity or fitness, the results may be statistically significant but physiologically meaningless. For example, a correlation of .23 between lumbar BMD and hours spent walking each day was significant in a large group of women (109). However, R^2, the amount of variation in BMD that could be predicted from walk time, was only

5%. In other words, 95% of the variability in lumbar density in this group of 123 women could not be explained by the number of hours they spent walking. As noted earlier, other investigators (97–99) have been unable to document a positive effect on bone from walking programs in early postmenopausal women.

Exercise Prescription for Bone Health

TYPES OF ACTIVITIES

No randomized, prospective study has systematically examined the effect of various activities or sports on bone mass. Tentative recommendations can be made based on the cross-sectional and longitudinal studies that have shown that certain types of activities are associated with a higher than average BMD. However, the effectiveness of each activity in increasing bone mass or decreasing the rate of loss in the general population requires further investigation.

Recommended activities: Running, jogging; weight training; aerobics; stair climbing; field sports (soccer, lacrosse, field hockey); racquet sports (tennis, squash, racquetball); court sports (basketball, volleyball); dancing (folk, square, modern, ballet).

Questionable activities (both positive and negative results have been reported): Swimming, walking.

No data available: Cycling, skiing, skating.

It should be kept in mind that any increase in physical activity may have a positive effect on bone mass for women who have been sedentary. Theoretically, a plateau will eventually be reached and no further benefit will occur unless the physical demands on the skeletal system are increased.

DURATION, FREQUENCY, AND INTENSITY OF ACTIVITY

No study has examined how the length of the training session affects the magnitude of the response. Studies that have reported a positive effect of exercise on bone have used periods that varied in length from 30 to 60 minutes. The body responds as an integrated whole to the training stimulus, and it seems reasonable to suggest that aerobic activities be continued for at least 30 minutes to achieve cardiovascular as well as skeletal benefits. Workouts with weights or resistance equipment are structured by repetitive lifts using various muscle groups, and the duration of a session depends in part on the ability of the individual. The usual protocol for developing muscular strength and endurance should be followed because departures from the accepted protocol could result in injury.

Once again, recommendations must be based on what has been shown to be successful instead of on results of experimental studies. At present, it appears that exercising 3 to 4 days per week results in an increase in BMD; the effect of increasing frequency to 5 to 7 days is unknown. Some active women find that a combination of 3 days of aerobic exercise interspersed with 3 days of weight training provides the benefits of both yet allows each "system" a rest period between training sessions.

No one has quantified the intensity of exercise required to elicit a training effect on the human skeleton. The principle of progressive overload suggests that the intensity must be greater than that normally placed on the bone and that it must be gradually increased to maintain a training effect. This is relatively easy to do in weight training; it is more difficult to accomplish in other activities. Running, jogging, and stair climbing all place more stress on the skeleton than walking, but the bones will eventually become habituated to the demands of those activities. It is not known if increasing the frequency or duration of the exercise sessions can substitute for an increase in intensity.

The increase in bone mass reported for formerly sedentary women who have participated in the exercise studies reviewed in this chapter is encouraging but should not be taken as an indication that physical activity is an alternative to HRT for postmenopausal women. Exercise is an adjunct therapy. The beneficial effects on the skeletal system will last only as long as the women continue their exercise program. Because moderate physical activity has so many positive effects on physiological function, all women should be encouraged to include exercise as a vital part of their daily routine.

Key Points

- During adolescence skeletal mass will double—girls ingesting less than 800 mg of calcium a day could suffer poor skeletal development.
- In the mature, estrogen-replete woman, high calcium intake does not offer any advantage.
- Estrogen deficiency, regardless of etiology, causes aggressive bone loss. High calcium intake is of little or no use in the woman who has recently become estrogen deficient.
- High calcium intake potentiates the bone protection of low-dosage estrogens.

- The woman who uses standard doses of estrogen does not need to maintain a high-calcium diet.
- With increasing age, especially beyond age 65, enhancing calcium intake may help to prevent bone loss.
- To make a simplified estimate of dietary calcium intake: to the 300–400 mg obtained from a dairy-free diet, add 300 mg for each portion of dairy product consumed.
- Calcium intake during late childhood and adolescence should be 1200 mg/day. During a woman's mature years, 800 mg is sufficient. In the elderly, 1500 mg is reasonable.
- Estrogen-deficient young women should be warned that calcium alone is not an alternative to estrogen for prevention of osteoporosis.
- Physical activity is an important factor in maximizing bone mass in young women and attenuating bone loss later in life.
- Exercise should be considered an adjunct therapy for the preservation of skeletal integrity. There is no evidence that exercise alone can prevent bone loss in hypoestrogenic women.
- The positive effect of exercise on bone is most evident at the specific skeletal site where mechanical stress is applied.
- There must be a progressive increase in the amount of stress applied to the bone for further increments in bone mass.
- The positive effect of exercise on bone will be lost if the exercise program is discontinued.
- Increases in bone density reported in prospective training studies average about 6%; control groups continue to lose bone.
- The benefits of exercise may also be indirect; improved coordination, balance, and muscular strength may decrease the likelihood of falls.
- The overall benefits of regular physical activity are so pervasive that all women should be encouraged to remain physically active throughout life.

References

1. Mazess RB, Cameron JR. Growth of bone in school children: comparison of radiographic morphometry and photon absorptiometry. Growth 1972;36:77–92.
2. Christiansen C, Rödbro P, Thöger Nielsen C. Bone mineral content and estimated total

body calcium in normal children and adolescents. Scand J Clin Lab Invest 1975;35:507–510.

3. Rosenthal DI, Mayo-Smith W, Hayes CW, et al. Age and bone mass in premenopausal women. J Bone Min Res 1989;4:533–538.
4. Leitch I, Aitken FC. The estimation of calcium requirement: a re-examination. Nutr Abstr Rev 1959;29:393–411.
5. Matkovic V, Heaney RP, Chesnut C. Absorption of calcium in adolescent females [Abstract]. J Bone Min Res 1989;4(suppl 1):S381.
6. Heaney RP. High calcium intake is important in preventing osteoporosis in women. Affirmative. Hegsted DM. Negative. In: Gitnick G, ed. Debates in medicine. Chicago: Year Book, 1988;1:166–191.
7. National Center for Health Statistics, Carroll MD, Abraham S, Dresser CM. Dietary intake source data: United States, 1976–80. Vital Health Stat[11]:231. DHHS Pub. No. (PHS) 83-1681. Washington, DC: U.S. Government Printing Office, 1983.
8. Matković V, Kostial K, Šimonović I, Buzina R, Brodarec A, Nordin BEC. Bone status and fracture rates in two regions of Yugoslavia. Am J Clin Nutr 1979;32:540–549.
9. Kanders B, Dempster DW, Lindsay R. Interaction of calcium nutrition and physical activity on bone mass in young women. J Bone Min Res 1988;3:145–149.
10. Sowers MF, Wallace RB, Lemke JH. Correlates of forearm bone mass among women during maximal bone mineralization. Prev Med 1985;14:585–596.
11. Sandler RB, Slemenda CW, LaPorte RE, et al. Postmenopausal bone density and milk consumption in childhood and adolescence. Am J Clin Nutr 1985;42:270–274.
12. Brown JP, Chevalier M, Friede J, Breton M, Blanchet MF. Beneficial effects of a lifelong dietary calcium intake on premenopausal bone mass [Abstract]. J Bone Min Res 1989;4(suppl 1):S229.
13. Johnell O, Nilsson BE. Life-style and bone mineral mass in perimenopausal women. Calcif Tissue Int 1984;36:354–356.
14. Dawson-Hughes B, Jacques P, Shipp C. Dietary calcium intake and bone loss from the spine in healthy postmenopausal women. Am J Clin Nutr 1987;46:685–687.
15. Stevenson JC, Whitehead MI, Padwick M, et al. Dietary intake of calcium and postmenopausal bone loss. Br Med J 1988;297:15–17.
16. Gilsanz V, Roe T, Antunes J, Carlson M. Effect of calcium intake on peak bone density of growing rabbits [Abstract]. J Bone Min Res 1989;4(suppl 1):S384.
17. Thomas ML, Ibarra MJ, Simmons DJ. Dietary calcium intake and bone mineralization during sexual maturation in the female rat [Abstract]. J Bone Min Res 1988;3(suppl 1):S190.
18. Matkovic V, Tominac C, Fontana D, Chestnut C. Influence of calcium on peak bone mass: a 24-month follow-up [Abstract]. J Bone Min Res 1988;3(suppl 1):S85.
19. Heaney RP, Recker RR, Stegman MR, Moy AJ. Calcium absorption in women: relationships to calcium intake, estrogen status, and age. J Bone Min Res 1989;4:469–475.
20. Riggs BL, Wahner HW, Melton LJ III, Richelson LS, Judd HL, O'Fallon WM. Dietary calcium intake and rates of bone loss in women. J Clin Invest 1987;80:979–982.
21. Cann CE, Henzl M, Heinrichs I, Burry K. Calcium aggravates GnRH agonist-induced bone loss [Abstract]. J Bone Min Res 1987;2(suppl 1):no 333.
22. Drinkwater BL, Nilson K, Chestnut CH III, Bremner WJ, Shainholtz S, Southworth MB. Bone mineral content of amenorrheic and eumenorrheic athletes. N Engl J Med 1984;311:277–281.
23. Klibanski A, Biller BMK, Rosenthal DI, Schoenfeld DA, Saxe V. Effects of prolactin and estrogen deficiency in amenorrheic bone loss. J Clin Endocrinol Metab 1988;67:124–130.
24. Lindberg JS, Powell MR, Hunt MM, Ducey DE, Wade CE. Increased vertebral bone mineral in response to reduced exercise in amenorrheic runners. West J Med 1987;146:39–42.

25. Falch JA, Oftebro H, Haug E. Early postmenopausal bone loss is not associated with a decrease in circulating levels of 25-hydroxyvitamin D, 1, 25-dihydroxyvitamin D, or vitamin D-binding protein. J Clin Endocrinol Metab 1987;64:836–841.
26. Block JE, Smith R, Glueer C-C, Steiger P, Ettinger B, Genant HK. Models of spinal trabecular bone loss as determined by quantitative computed tomography. J Bone Min Res 1989;4:249–257.
27. Recker RR, Saville PD, Heaney RP. Effect of estrogens and calcium carbonate on bone loss in postmenopausal women. Ann Intern Med 1977;87:649–655.
28. Nilas L, Christiansen C, Rødbro P. Calcium supplementation and postmenopausal bone loss. Br Med J 1984;289:1103–1106.
29. Ettinger B, Genant HK, Cann CE. Low-dosage estrogen combined with calcium prevents postmenopausal bone loss: results of a 3-year study. In: Cohn DV, Martin TJ, Meunier PJ, eds. Calcium regulation and bone metabolism: basic and clinical aspects. Amsterdam: Elsevier, 1987;9:918–922.
30. Riis B, Thomsen K, Christiansen C. Dose calcium supplementation prevent postmenopausal bone loss?: a double-blind, controlled clinical study. N Engl J Med 1987;316:173–177.
31. Ettinger B. Prevention of osteoporosis: treatment of estradiol deficiency. Obstet Gynecol 1988;72(suppl):12S–17S.
32. Dawson-Hughes B, Dallal G, Tannenbaum S, Sahyoun N, Krall E. Effect of two calcium supplements on postmenopausal bone loss from the spine [Abstract]. J Bone Min Res 1989;4(suppl 1):S390.
33. Cauley JA, Gutai JP, Kuller LH, et al. Endogenous estrogen levels and calcium intakes in postmenopausal women: relationships with cortical bone measures. JAMA 1988;260:3150–3155.
34. Ettinger B, Genant HK, Cann CE. Postmenopausal bone loss is prevented by treatment with low-dosage estrogen with calcium. Ann Intern Med 1987;106:40–45.
35. Christensen MS, Hagen C, Christiansen C, Transbøl I. Dose-response evaluation of cyclic estrogen/gestagen in postmenopausal women: placebo-controlled trial of its gynecologic and metabolic actions. Am J Obstet Gynecol 1982;144:873–879.
36. Gallagher JC, Goldgar D, Kable WT. Comparison of estrogen and progestin therapy on cortical and trabecular bone using SPA, DPA and QCT [Abstract]. Calcif Tissue Int 1989;44:153.
37. Genant HK, Harris ST, Steiger P, Melnikoff S, Kurkjian B, Block JE. The efficacy of estrone sulfate (Ogen) in preserving spinal and peripheral bone density in early post-menopausal women: preliminary results [Abstract]. J Bone Min Res 1989;4(suppl 1):S376.
37a. Ettinger B, Genant HK, Steiger P, Madvig P. Low-dosage micronized 17B-estradiol prevents bone loss in postmenopausal women. Am J Obstet Gynecol 1992;166:479–488.
38. Schot LPC, Geusens P, Nijs J, Dequeker J, Schuurs AHWM. Effect of 17β-oestradiol on bone metabolism of ovariectomised dogs fed with a calcium deficient diet [Abstract]. J Bone Min Res 1988;3(suppl 1):S189.
39. Matkovic V, Dekanic D, Kostial K. The rate of cortical bone loss according to age, sex and calcium intake [Abstract]. J Bone Min Res 1988;3(suppl 1):S88.
40. Jensen GF, Transbøl I. Calcium therapy for bone preservation in elderly females. In: Cohen DV, Martin TJ, Meunier PJ, eds. Calcium regulation and bone matabolism, basic and clinical aspects. Amsterdam: Excerpta Medica, 1987;9:965.
41. Orwoll ES, McClung MR, Oviatt SK, Recker RR, Weigel RM. Histomorphometric effects of calcium or calcium plus 25-hydroxyvitamin D3 therapy in senile osteoporosis. J Bone Min Res 1989;4:81–88.
42. Smith EL Jr, Reddan W, Smith PE. Physical activity and calcium modalities for bone mineral increase in aged women. Med Sci Sports Exerc 1981;13:60–64.

43. Holbrook TL, Barret-Connor E, Wingard DL. Dietary calcium and risk of hip fracture: 14-year prospective population study. Lancet 1988;2:1046–1049.
44. Riggs BL, Seeman E, Hodgson SF, Taves DR, O'Fallon WM. Effect of the fluoride/calcium regimen on vertebral fracture occurrence in postmenopausal osteoporosis. N Engl J Med 1982;306:446–450.
45. Boyle IT, Davis BS, Boyce BF, et al. The effect of oral calcium supplements on bone turnover and skeletal integrity in postmenopausal osteoporosis [Abstract]. J Bone Min Res 1989;4(suppl 1):S371.
46. Burros M. Calcium supplements are not all equal. New York Times 1988;January 27:C1,C8.
47. Brennan MJ, Duncan WE, Wartofsky L, Butler VM, Wray HL. In vitro dissolution of calcium carbonate preparations. J Bone Min Res 1988;3(suppl 1):S160.
48. Recker RR. Calcium absorption and achlorhydria. N Engl J Med 1985;313:70–73.
49. Krølner B, Toft B. Vertebral bone loss. Clin Sci 1983;64:537–540.
50. Vogel JM. Bone mineral measurement: Skylab experiment N-078. Acta Astronautica 1975;2:129–139.
51. Vogel JM, Whittle MW. Bone mineral changes: the second manned Skylab mission. Aviat Space Environ Med 1976;47:396–400.
52. Andersson SM, Nilsson BE. Changes in bone mineral content following ligamentous knee injuries. Med Sci Sports 1979;11:351–353.
53. Whedon GD. Disuse osteoporosis: physiological aspects. Calcif Tissue Int 1984;36(suppl):S146–S150.
54. Dalén N, Olsson KE. Bone mineral content and physical activity. Acta Orthop Scand 1974;45:170–174.
55. Lane NE, Bloch DA, Jones HH, Marshall WH Jr, Wood PD, Fries JF. Long-distance running, bone density, and osteoarthritis. JAMA 1986;255:1147–1151.
56. Nilsson BE, Westlin NE. Bone density in athletes. Clin Orthop 1971;77:179–182.
57. Ott SM, Kilcoyne RF, Chesnut CH III. Ability of four different techniques of measuring bone mass to diagnose vertebral fractures in postmenopausal women. J Bone Min Res 1987;2:201–210.
58. Brienza RS, Kleerekoper M, Schultz LR, Johnson CC. History of fracture associated with low bone density irrespective of site of measurement [Abstract]. J Bone Min Res 1989;4(suppl 1):S328.
59. Cummings SR, Black D, Arnaud C, et al. Appendicular densitometry predicts hip fractures: a prospective study [Abstract]. J Bone Min Res 1989;4(suppl 1):S327.
60. Hui SL, Siemenda CW, Johnston CC Jr. Baseline measurement of bone mass predicts fracture in white women. Ann Intern Med 1989;111:355–361.
61. Rikli R, Busch S. Motor performance of women as a function of age and physical activity level. J Gerontol 1986;41:645–649.
62. Hettinger T. Physiology of strength. Springfield, Ill: C C Thomas, 1961.
63. Cummings SR. Epidemiology of hip fractures. In: Christiansen C, Johansen JS, Riis BJ, eds. Osteoporosis 1987. Copenhagen: Osteopress, 1987.
64. Smith RW Jr, Rizek J. Epidemiologic studies of osteoporosis in women of Puerto Rico and southeastern Michigan with special reference to age, race, national origin and to other related or associated findings. Clin Orthop 1966;45:31–48.
65. Riggs BL, Melton LJ. Evidence for two distinct syndromes of involutional osteoporosis. Am J Med 1983;75:899–901.
66. Bell NH, Spicer KM, Shary J, Liel Y. Effects of body habitus and race on bone mineral density of the hip and spine in women [Abstract]. J Bone Min Res 1987;2(suppl 1):No 383.
67. Riggs BL, Melton LJ III: Involutional osteoporosis. N Engl J Med 1986;314:1676–1686.
68. Dalsky GP, Stocke KS, Ehsani AA, Slatopolsky E, Lee WC, Birge SJ Jr. Weight-bearing

exercise training and lumbar bone mineral content in postmenopausal women. Ann Intern Med 1988;108:824–828.

69. Kirk S, Sharp CF, Elbaum N, et al. Effect of long-distance running on bone mass in women. J Bone Min Res 1989;4:515–522.
70. Marcus R, Cann C, Madvig P, et al. Menstrual function and bone mass in elite women distance runners: endocrine and metabolic features. Ann Intern Med 1985;102:158–163.
71. Baker E, Demers L. Menstrual status in female athletes: correlation with reproductive hormones and bone density. Obstet Gynecol 1988;72:683–687.
72. Buchanan JR, Myers C, Lloyd T, Leuenberger P, Demers LM. Determinants of peak trabecular bone density in women: the role of androgens, estrogen, and exercise. J Bone Min Res 1988;3:673–680.
73. Jacobson PC, Beaver W, Grubb SA, Taft TN, Talmage RV. Bone density in women: college athletes and older athletic women. J Orthop Res 1984;2:328–332.
74. Drinkwater BL, Nilson K, Ott S, Chestnut CH III. Bone mineral density after resumption of menses in amenorrheic women. JAMA 1986;256:380–382.
75. Westfall C, Going S, Parmenter R, Perry C, Boyden T, Lohman T. Femur and spine bone mineral of eumenorrheic female body builders, swimmers, runners, and controls [Abstract]. Med Sci Sports Exerc 1988;20(suppl):S60.
76. Cann CE, Martin MC, Genant HK, Jaffe RB. Decreased spinal mineral content in amenorrheic women. JAMA 1984;251:626–629.
77. Lindberg JS, Fears WB, Hunt MM, Powell MR, Boll D, Wade CE. Exercise-induced amenorrhea and bone density. Ann Intern Med 1984;101:647–648.
78. Nelson ME, Fisher EC, Catsos PD, Meredith CN, Turksoy RN, Evans WJ. Diet and bone status in amenorrheic runners. Am J Clin Nutr 1986;43:910–916.
79. Cann CE, Cavanaugh DJ, Schnurpfiel K, Martin MC. Menstrual history is the primary determinant of trabecular bone density in women runners [Abstract]. Med Sci Sports Exerc 1988;20(suppl 2):S59.
80. Drinkwater BL, Bruemner B, Chesnut CH III. Menstrual history as a determinant of current bone density in young athletes. JAMA 1990;263:545–548.
81. Drinkwater BL, Davajan V. The amenorrheic athlete and conception. In: Artal R, Wiswell RA, Drinkwater BL, eds. Exercise in pregnancy. Baltimore: Williams & Wilkins, 1990.
82. Recker RR, Davies KM, Kimmel DB, Heaney RP. Cross-sectional studies overestimate age-related bone loss [Abstract]. J Bone Min Res 1989;4(suppl 1):S327.
83. Brewer V, Meyer BM, Keele MS, Upton SJ, Hagan RD. Role of exercise in prevention of involutional bone loss. Med Sci Sports Exerc 1983;15:445–449.
84. Aloia JF, Vaswani AN, Yeh JK, Cohn SH. Premenopausal bone mass is related to physical activity. Arch Intern Med 1988;148:121–123.
85. King CR, Lukert B, Robinson RG. Increased bone mineral content (BMC) in adult female recreational runners [Abstract]. Med Sci Sports Exerc 1987;19(suppl):S13.
86. Smith DM, Khairi MRA, Norton J, Johnston CC Jr. Age and activity effects on rate of bone mineral loss. J Clin Invest 1976;58:716–721.
87. Michel BA, Bloch DA, Fries JF. Weight-bearing exercise, overexercise, and lumbar bone density over age 50 years. Arch Intern Med 1989;149:2325–2329.
88. Chow RK, Harrison JE, Brown CF, Hajek V. Physical fitness effect on bone mass in postmenopausal women. Arch Phys Med Rehabil 1986;67:231–234.
89. Oyster N, Morton M, Linnell S. Physical activity and osteoporosis in post-menopausal women. Med Sci Sports Exerc 1984;16:44–50.
90. Åström J, Ahnqvist S, Beertema J, Jónsson B. Physical activity in women sustaining fracture of the neck of the femur. J Bone Joint Surg 1987;69-B:381–383.
91. Colletti LA, Edwards J, Gordon L, Shary J, Bell NH. The effects of muscle-building exercise

on bone mineral density of the radius, spine, and hip in young men. Calcif Tissue Int 1989;45:12–14.
92. Block JE, Friedlander AL, Brooks GA, Steiger P, Stubbs HA, Genant HK. Determinants of bone density among athletes engaged in weight-bearing and non-weight-bearing activity. J Appl Physiol 1989;67:1100–1105.
93. Doyle F, Brown J, Lachance C. Relation between bone mass and muscle weight. Lancet 1970;1:391–393.
94. Sinaki M, Offord KP. Physical activity in postmenopausal women: effect on back muscle strength and bone mineral density of the spine. Arch Phys Med Rehabil 1988;69:277–280.
95. Pocock N, Eisman J, Gwinn T, et al. Muscle strength, physical fitness, and weight but not age predict femoral neck bone mass. J Bone Min Res 1989;4:441–448.
96. Bevier WC, Wiswell RA, Pyka G, Kozak KC, Newhall KM, Marcus R. Relationship of body composition, muscle strength, and aerobic capacity to bone mineral density in older men and women. J Bone Min Res 1989;4:421–432.
97. Cauley JA, Sandler R, LaPorte RE, Kriska A, Hom D, Sashin D. Physical activity and postmenopausal bone loss: results of a three-year randomized clinical trial [Abstract]. Am J Epidemiol 1986;124:525.
98. White MK, Martin RB, Yeater RA, Butcher RL, Radin EL. The effects of exercise on the bones of postmenopausal women. Int Orthop 1984;7:209–214.
99. Cavanaugh DJ, Cann CE. Brisk walking does not stop bone loss in postmenopausal women. Bone 1988;9:201–204.
100. Chow R, Harrison JE, Notarius C. Effect of two randomised exercise programmes on bone mass of healthy postmenopausal women. Br Med J 1987;295:1441–1444.
101. Aloia JF, Cohn SH, Ostuni JA, Cane R, Ellis K. Prevention of involutional bone loss by exercise. Ann Intern Med 1978;89:356–358.
102. Krølner B, Toft B, Nielsen SP, Tøndevold E. Physical exercise as prophylaxis against involutional vertebral bone loss: a controlled trial. Clin Sci 1983;64:541–546.
103. Ayalon J, Simkin A, Leichter I, Raifmann S. Dynamic bone loading exercises for postmenopausal women: effect on the density of the distal radius. Arch Phys Med Rehabil 1987;68:280–283.
104. Notelovitz M, Martin D, Tesar R, Khan AK, Probart C, Fields C, McKenzie L. Estrogen therapy and variable resistance weight training increase bone mineral in surgically menopausal women. J Bone Min Res 1991;6:583–591.
105. McArdle WD, Katch FI, Katch VL. Exercise physiology: energy, nutrition, and human performance. Philadelphia: Lea & Febiger, 1981.
106. Pocock NA, Eisman JA, Yeates MG, Sambrook PN, Eberl S. Physical fitness is a major determinant of femoral neck and lumbar spine bone mineral density. J Clin Invest 1986;78:618–621.
107. Stillman RJ, Lohman TG, Slaughter MH, Massey BH. Physical activity and bone mineral content in women aged 30 to 85 years. Med Sci Sports Exerc 1986;18:576–580.
108. Smith EL, Gilligan C, McAdam M, Ensign CP, Smith PE. Deterring bone loss by exercise intervention in premenopausal and postmenopausal women. Calcif Tissue Int 1989;44:312–321.
109. Zylstra S, Hopkins A, Erk M, Hreshchyshyn MM, Anbar M. Effect of physical activity on lumbar spine and femoral neck bone densities. Int J Sports Med 1989;10:181–186.

6

Cardiovascular Effects of Menopause and Estrogen Replacement: The Epidemiological Evidence[a]

Graham A. Colditz and Meir J. Stampfer

Despite a steady decline over the past 2 decades, coronary heart disease (CHD) remains the leading cause of death in women in the United States, as it is among men. The mortality is low in younger women; for example, among women aged 30 to 34 years, the rate was 2.0 per 100,000 in 1986, only about 28% the rate among men of the same age. In contrast, among middle-aged women aged 55 to 59 years, the rate was 105.7 per 100,000 (1). The marked degree of protection from coronary disease enjoyed by younger women and the sharp rise in rates among older women led many to speculate that the hormonal milieu of premenopausal women was beneficial and that the occurrence of menopause led to an increase in coronary risk. In this chapter we review the evidence for an association between menopause, both natural and surgical, and risk of heart disease. We then review the epidemiological evidence regarding the association between postmenopausal estrogen replacement and atherosclerosis and CHD.

MENOPAUSE AND HEART DISEASE

Rates of Heart Disease in Women at Different Ages

As shown in Figure 6.1, it is obvious that coronary mortality rises very sharply with age among both men and women. The biggest apparent increase in women occurs around age 50, approximately the time of menopause. Moreover, although at every age men have a higher rate than women, the

[a]Supported by Public Health Service grants CA40935 and CA40356 from the National Cancer Institute, National Institutes of Health, Department of Health and Human Services. This chapter is adapted from material presented in a review in the *Annals of the New York Academy of Sciences* and from material presented at a workshop on tamoxifen and prevention of breast cancer, Wisconsin, October 1989.

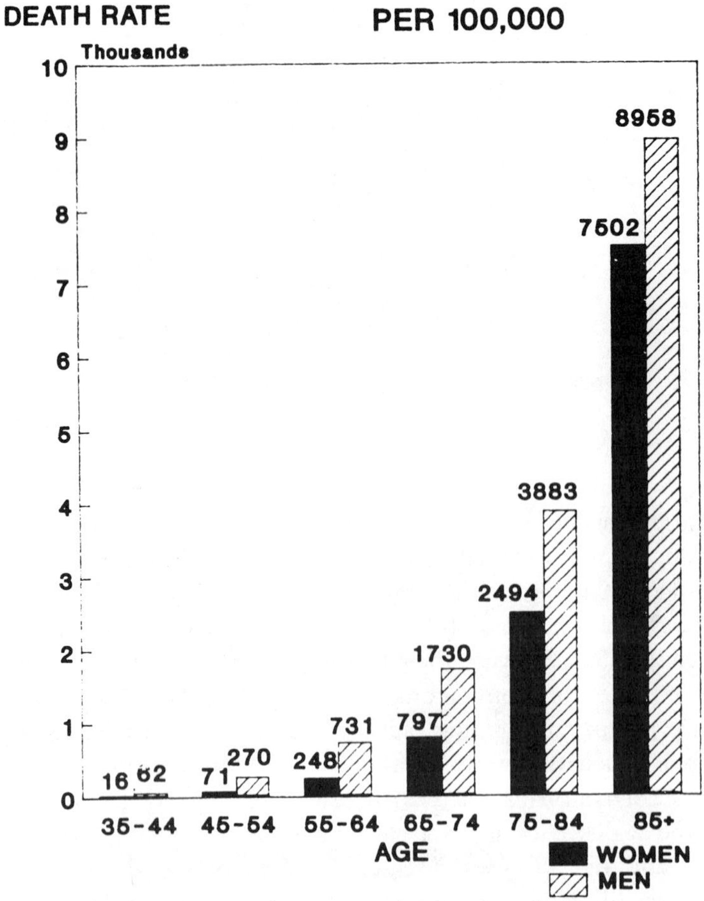

Figure 6.1. Mortality from CHD in white men and women in the United States. (From U.S. vital statistics, 1986. Washington, DC: U.S. Department of Health and Human Services, 1987.)

disparity is greatest at younger ages, when most of the women are premenopausal. However, a closer look at these statistics is instructive. By plotting on a log scale, one can evaluate the rate of increase in coronary mortality with increasing age. Tracy (2) demonstrated that there is no shift in the rate of increase at the time of menopause as there is for breast cancer (2). Virtually identical results were observed by Winkelstein and Rekate (3) using data from New York State and by Heller and Jacobs in an analysis of data from England and Wales (4). The decreasing disparity in the rates between men and women at older ages is not due to a shift in women's rates at menopause, but rather to a slowing of the rate of increase in men. Hence, the rates of heart disease in the general population do not offer strong support for the hypothesis that menopause is accompanied by a sharp rise in the risk of coronary disease.

These findings are supported by Ackerman et al. (5), who assessed the degree of coronary atherosclerosis in 100 consecutive autopsies in women at each of six decades of age, 600 autopsies in all. They found that the degree of atherosclerosis rose steadily from about 5% with severe stenosis in the 30- to 40-year age group, to about 60% among those 70 to 80 years of age. There was no suggestion of a sharp increase to coincide with the age of menopause, but these investigators did not specifically assess menopause. Because age at natural menopause varies over about 1 decade, a moderate effect of menopause could easily be blurred in these data and in population statistics. Studies of individuals of known menopause status provide much more persuasive evidence.

Coronary Risk Factors That Influence Occurrence of Menopause

In evaluating the effect of natural menopause on the risk of heart disease, one must consider potential confounding factors that are associated both with the occurrence of menopause and with heart disease. There are three important coronary risk factors that affect the occurrence of menopause; age, cigarette smoking, and obesity. Age is obvious but not trivial. Natural menopause occurs over a rather limited age range, with about two-thirds of women passing through menopause between ages 48 and 53 years (6). Thus, even in a narrow age group, say 5 years, the postmenopausal women will tend to be older than the premenopausal women. As shown in Figure 6.1, the risk of heart disease rises sharply with age; a difference of 5 years, between 47 and 52, corresponds to an increase of 103% in coronary mortality (1). Hence, close control for age is essential to avoid mixing the potential effects of menopause with the effects of age alone. Inadequate control for age would tend to artificially increase the risk of heart disease associated with menopause.

Obesity and cigarette smoking are two other coronary risk factors that influence menopause; overweight women tend to have menopause at a later age (7–9) and smokers tend to have earlier menopause (7, 10, 11). These factors must be considered together because smokers tend to be leaner than nonsmokers, and although both are independent coronary risk factors, it is difficult to distinguish their effect on menopause. Willett et al. (7) examined these interrelationships by prospectively evaluating the experience of 66,663 Nurses' Health Study participants who were premenopausal in 1976. The Nurses' Health Study is a prospective cohort of 121,700 U.S. women 30 to 55 years of age in 1976 who are observed to study relations between lifestyle and health. Over the following 2 years, 5,004 became naturally postmenopausal. The effect of smoking was quite pronounced, with a strong dose-response effect: the relative risk for occurrence of natural menopause rose from about 1.3 for smokers of 1 to 14 cigarettes per day to 2.0 for smokers of 35 + per day, compared with "never-smokers" (women who indicated on the 1976 questionnaire that they had never smoked cigarettes) (Figure 6.2). Overall, the relative risks (comparing current smokers with never-smokers) for menopause ranged from 2.16 (95% confidence interval, 1.73 to 2.69) for

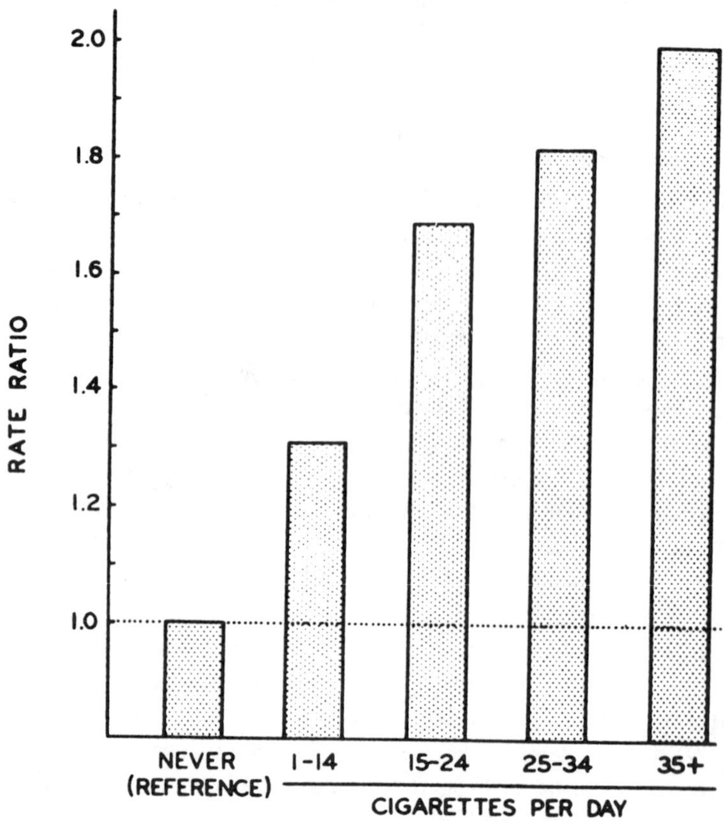

Figure 6.2. Rate ratios for menopause by number of cigarettes smoked per day among a sample of female U.S. nurses who were aged 40 to 49 years in 1976. Test for trend, $P<.001$. (Reproduced, with permission, from Willett WC, Stampfer MJ, Bain C, et al. Cigarette smoking, relative weight, and menopause. Am J Epidemiol 1983;117:651–658.)

women 40 to 44 years, to 1.20 (95% confidence interval, 1.12 to 1.28) for women 50 to 55 years. These relative risks were only very slightly attenuated after adjustment for body mass index. For example, in the 40- to 44-year group, the relative risk changed from 2.16 to 2.13, and for the 50- to 55-year group, from 1.20 to 1.19. These changes indicate that differences in body mass index can explain almost none of the effect of smoking on the occurrence of menopause. The median age at natural menopause for never-smokers (derived from life table analyses) was 52.4 for never-smokers, 51.0 for smokers of 15 to 24 cigarettes per day, and 50.4 for smokers of 35 and more per day.

In contrast, the effect of obesity was weaker. In a comparison of women in the leanest quintile of the distribution of relative weight (mean weight, 116 pounds) with those in the heaviest quintile (mean weight, 181 pounds), the relative risks of menopause ranged from 1.43 (95% confidence interval, 0.74 to 2.78) among women 30 to 39 years to 1.09 (95% confidence interval, 0.99 to 1.19) among women 50 to 55 years of age. The effect of obesity was apparent only among smokers. When nonsmokers were examined separately, there was no significant trend of increased delay of menopause with increased body mass index. These findings suggest that of the two factors, cigarette smoking is far likelier to be an important confounder than obesity. This is particularly so because cigarette smoking is a stronger risk factor for heart disease than is obesity. Among middle-aged women in the United States, fully half of the heart disease is attributable to smoking, and the relative risk for smoking 15 to 24 cigarettes per day is 4.2 (12). Thus, whereas failure to control for obesity will have little impact on assessing the effect of menopause on the risk of heart disease, failure to adjust for smoking will tend to artificially increase the apparent risk associated with menopause. The degree of distortion could be substantial if the population includes a large proportion of smokers.

Natural Menopause and Risk of Heart Disease

Because of the sharp increase in coronary disease with age and the fact that, on average, postmenopausal women are older than premenopausal women, rates of heart disease are higher in postmenopausal women. Studies that do not adjust for difference in age are uninformative and are not discussed. Also not considered in this chapter are reports of case series that compare age at infarction within various categories of menopausal status. Without reference to an appropriate control population, such studies are difficult to interpret.

Several studies provide data on menopause and heart disease but do not distinguish between natural and artificial menopause. This distinction is important, because women with surgical menopause are clearly at higher risk for coronary disease than premenopausal women, as discussed in detail below.

In a recent study, Witteman et al. (13) reported on the prevalence of calcification of the abdominal aorta observed in a cross-sectional survey of 676 women 45 to 55 years of age. After adjustment for age and other risk factors, the relative risk of such calcifications in naturally postmenopausal women was 3.4 (95% confidence interval, 1.2 to 9.7). The estimates are unstable because only 8 of 294 premenopausal women in the reference group had calcifications.

The case-control study of oral contraceptives and myocardial infarction in women under age 45 reported by Mann et al. (14) also includes some data on natural menopause. Six patients (10.2% of cases) were postmenopausal, compared with 8.8% of controls, giving a relative risk of 1.2 (95% confidence interval, 0.4 to 3.2). The data were not age adjusted, though overall cases and controls had a similar age distribution, and there was no control for cigarette use.

In a hospital-based case-control study, Abramov (15) found that among 96 myocardial infarction (MI) patients aged 40 to 60 years without hysterectomy, 79 were naturally postmenopausal, as compared with 57 of 84 controls, giving a relative risk of 2.4 (95% confidence interval, 1.2 to 4.7). Unfortunately, age was not adequately controlled for in this analysis, and smoking was not considered. Also, it is always difficult to choose appropriate diagnoses for selection of controls in a hospital-based study. Diagnoses must not be related to the exposure of interest, a particular problem when considering menopause or replacement estrogen therapy.

A case-control study of menopause and nonfatal MI was conducted by Rosenberg at al. (16) among women under age 56. Cases and controls were identified from the Nurses' Health Study cohort baseline questionnaire, sent in 1976. Cases with MI were matched on exact year of birth with controls without such a history, with a 20:1 matching ratio. There were 156 infarctions among premenopausal women and 25 among women with natural menopause. The relative risk for women with natural menopause (compared with premenopausal women) was 0.9 (95% confidence interval, 0.6 to 1.3). After multivariate analysis to adjust for cigarette smoking and a variety of other coronary risk factors, the relative risk was even lower. There was a suggestion of a higher risk for women with natural menopause under age 35, with a multivariate relative risk of 2.8, but this finding was not statistically significant and was based on only a single case and seven controls. At other ages, the multivariate relative risks ranged from 1.1 to 0.5.

The Mayo Clinic case-control study of incidence of coronary disease among women under age 60 yielded analogous findings (17). For women with natural menopause, there was no significant increase in risk for women reporting that menopause occurred before age 50 compared with those reporting menopause after age 50 (the median age for menopause). The observed relative risk, 1.3 (95% confidence interval, 0.7 to 2.1), was not adjusted for smoking; such adjustment almost certainly would have further attenuated the relative risk. Prospective cohort studies have two major advantages over the case-control approach: elimination of possible recall bias and the sometimes knotty problem of appropriate control selection. The population-based cohort study of women in Gothenburg provided an opportunity to examine this issue. Lapidus et al. (18) observed a cohort of 1,462 women for 12 years. The relative risks were somewhat elevated for women with early natural menopause, but they did not approach statistical significance for any of a variety of cardiovascular endpoints. Age groupings were within 5-year categories, and no adjustment was made for the effects of cigarette use.

The Framingham Heart Study examined the effects of natural menopause by observing the occurrence of coronary disease among 1,934 women who had a natural menopause during the course of follow-up and comparing these rates with those of premenopausal women of similar age (19). This paper is widely cited as showing an increase in risk of coronary disease after menopause. The women were examined every 2 years for up to 24 years. Those who both became postmenopausal and had their coronary event in the same 2-year interval between examinations were analyzed separately. Despite the long follow-up, only 18 cases of major coronary disease (myocardial infarction, coronary insufficiency, and coronary death) occurred among women with natural menopause, and only five such cases occurred among premenopausal women. Hence, the findings are statistically unstable. The authors quote an age-adjusted (in 5-year age groups) relative risk of 2.7, but this figure was attained only by including angina pectoris as an endpoint. Moreover, the authors assigned this elevated risk a P value of $<.01$, but a reanalysis of the data from their table confirms the relative risk of 2.7 (including angina) but with a P value of borderline significance. $P = .07$ (20). For major coronary disease excluding angina pectoris, the relative risk was 2.0 (95% confidence interval, 0.6 to 6.3; $P = .26$).

Normally in a prospective analysis, one allocates the endpoint according to the most recently ascertained exposure status. Thus, women who had become menopausal and had a coronary event in the same interval would normally be analyzed as premenopausal. This basic principle of prospective analysis avoids the possibility that the diagnosis could affect the exposure status or its reporting. The logic of this procedure becomes clear when one considers that a woman who is premenopausal at the beginning of the interval and had a fatal infarction would be considered premenopausal even if her menses had ceased before the infarct, because there would be no opportunity to report this at the next follow-up. If one follows this principle, the data from the Framingham Heart Study become even less persuasive in supporting an effect of menopause, with a relative risk for major coronary events of 0.8 (95% confidence interval, 0.4 to 1.7; $P = .65$). Although these analyses are age-adjusted by 5-year age groups, within each such group the premenopausal women are younger, and hence at lower risk by virtue of age, than the postmenopausal women within that 5-year age group. Moreover, the results do not take into account the effect of cigarette smoking.

In an update of the Framingham data that includes 26 years of follow-up, natural menopause was associated with a 4.1-fold higher 10-year incidence of CHD compared with rates in premenopausal women aged 50 to 59 years, but no adjustment for age or cigarette use was made (21).

The largest prospective study of natural menopause and heart disease is from the Nurses' Health Study cohort (22). In this study, 116,258 female nurses aged 30 to 55 years who were free from diagnosed coronary disease at baseline in 1976 were observed for 6 years through biennial questionnaires for the occurrence of nonfatal myocardial infarction and fatal CHD. The questionnaire provided information on a wide array of coronary risk factors as well as menopausal status. The accuracy of the self-reported information on coronary risk factors and menopausal status has been well documented (23, 24). Coronary endpoints were documented by medical records, and follow-up was high: for fatal outcomes follow-up was at least 98.3% and for nonfatal, 95.4%. At baseline, there were 14,732 women with a natural menopause, and with each subsequent 2-year period, additional women became postmenopausal. In all, 105 cases of major coronary disease (84 nonfatal MIs and 21 coronary deaths) occurred in 102,114 person-years of follow-up among women with a natural menopause. This experience was compared with that of premenopausal women, in whom there were 88 cases in 436,003 person-years of follow-up (Figure 6.3). After adjustment for age in 5-year categories, the rate of heart disease was significantly elevated in the postmenopausal women,

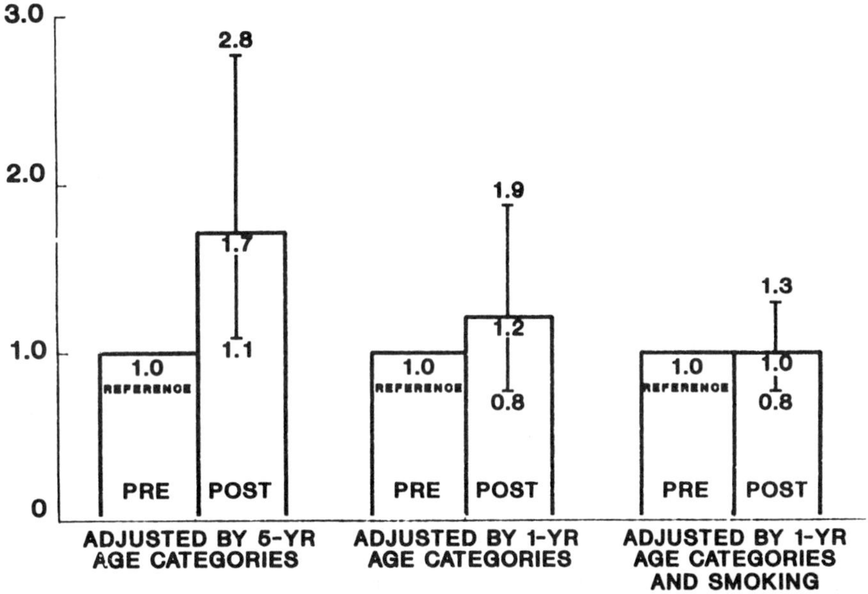

Figure 6.3. Relative risk of nonfatal MI and fatal coronary disease, comparing postmenopausal to premenopausal women in the Nurses' Health Study, after adjustment for age by 5-year groups, by 1-year groups, and by 1 year of age and current cigarette use. (Adapted from data of Colditz GA, Willett WC, Stampfer MJ, et al. Menopause and the risk of coronary heart disease in women. N Engl J Med 1987;316:1105–1110.)

with a relative risk of 1.7 (95% confidence interval, 1.1 to 2.8), results similar to those of the Framingham Study cited above. However, when the analysis was repeated using 1-year age groups, the relative risk was reduced to 1.2 (95% confidence interval, 0.8 to 1.9), thus demonstrating the need for close control of age. After further control for cigarette smoking, which is related to both coronary disease and age at menopause, there was no difference in the rates between premenopausal and naturally postmenopausal women; the relative risk was 1.0 (95% confidence interval, 0.8 to 1.3).

CHD Following Bilateral Oophorectomy

The data on the effects of bilateral oophorectomy stand in sharp contrast to the generally null findings for natural menopause. Evidence for an increase in risk in those women is based on studies using a number of different approaches, including autopsy surveys, case-control studies, and prospective cohort studies. These studies do not share the same methodologic issues as those of natural menopause because surgical menopause is not as closely correlated with age (so that very close control for age is not critical), and there is no known close link between oophorectomy and coronary risk factors as there is for natural menopause.

Several of the studies of natural menopause also examined the risk among women with bilateral oophorectomy, and all observed significantly elevated relative risks compared with premenopausal women. The cross-sectional survey of calcification of the abdominal aorta showed higher prevalence among women with bilateral oophorectomy, with a relative risk of 5.5 (95% confidence interval, 1.9 to 15.8) (13). Rosenberg et al. found a relative risk of 2.9 (95% confidence interval, 2.1 to 4.0) overall, with a pronounced trend toward higher risk among women who had bilateral oophorectomy at younger ages (16). The Mayo Clinic study likewise observed a significantly higher risk in premenopausal-aged women with both ovaries removed (17). In the Framingham study, such women also appeared to have an elevated risk, but the estimates are quite unstable, with just six cases apart from angina, and only one case in the reference group of premenopausal women (19).

Most, but not all other studies have found an excess risk in women with bilateral oophorectomy (25). Ritterband et al. observed the same rate of heart disease in women with bilateral oophorectomy as in those with simple hysterectomy (26). However, both groups had more than twice the rate of a control group without gynecological survey. Another follow-up study of 102 women with bilateral oophorectomy had different results, with a significantly elevated risk of coronary disease compared with controls with a simple hysterectomy (27). A similar study, comparing 36 women with bilateral with 31 women with unilateral oophorectomy also found more coronary disease in those with both ovaries removed, but the number of cases was small, with one infarction and eight of nine anginas in the bilateral oophorectomy group (28). In an autopsy series, Novak and Williams observed no important differences in the extent of atherosclerosis between women with bilateral oophorectomy and those without such surgery (29). Similarly, there was no significant difference in atherosclerosis at angiography between 20 women with bilateral oophorectomy and 65 controls (30). In contrast, two other autopsy series found increased atherosclerosis in women with bilateral oophorectomy (31, 32). In one of those studies, an increasing risk of coronary disease was apparent with increasing time since the ovaries were removed (32).

In the Nurses' Health Study investigation described earlier (22), the effects of bilateral oophorectomy were also assessed. A total of 41 cases of coronary disease arose in 51,929 person-years of follow-up among women with

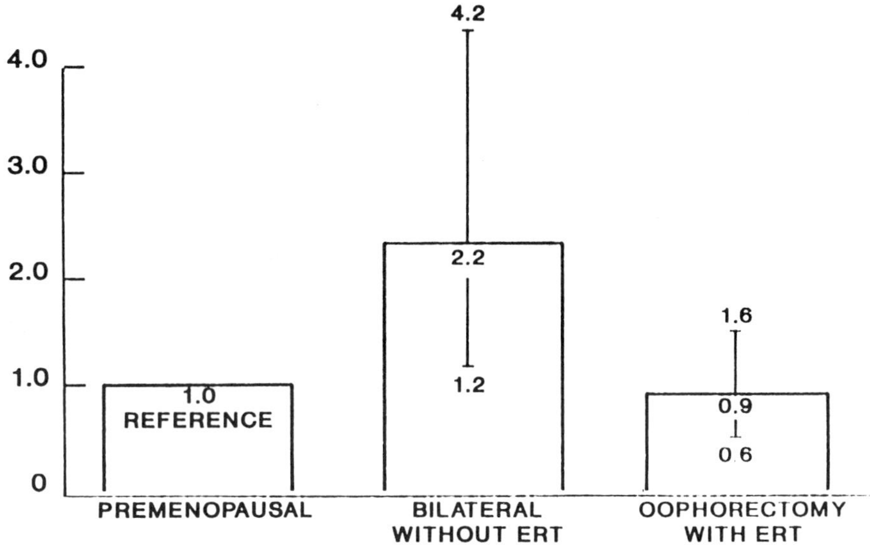

Figure 6.4. Relative risk of nonfatal MI and fatal coronary disease, comparing premenopausal women to women with bilateral oophorectomy either without or with estrogen replacement therapy in the Nurses' Health Study. The data are adjusted for age and cigarette smoking. (Adapted from data of Colditz GA, Willett WC, Stampfer MJ, et al. Menopause and the risk of coronary heart disease in women. N Engl J Med 1987;316:1105–1110.)

bilateral oophorectomy. Most of these women were given postmenopausal estrogens. During 9,630 person-years of follow-up among women with bilateral oophorectomy who never took hormones, 14 cases of coronary disease were confirmed. After adjustments for age and smoking, the relative risk compared with that of premenopausal women was 2.2 (95% confidence interval, 1.2 to 42.). In contrast, the women with bilateral oophorectomy who were given estrogen ("ever-users") had no increase in risk compared with premenopausal women, with a relative risk of 0.9 (95% confidence interval, 0.6 to 1.6) (Figure 6.4).

CHD Following Hysterectomy

The weight of evidence supports the view that bilateral oophorectomy is associated with increased risk of coronary disease, but controversy remains over the effect of other forms of surgical menopause (33). In the Framingham Study, elevated risks were observed for all forms of menopause, even simple hysterectomy. However, as discussed earlier, this study was too small to examine this issue in detail. For example, in the analysis reported by Gordon et al. (19), only four cases of coronary disease other than angina occurred among premenopausal women with a simple hysterectomy. Even with the 26-year analysis, there were only six cases, and no age adjustment within the 10-year age group (21). The case-control study reported by Rosenberg et al. (16), described earlier, also examined the risk of nonfatal MI among women with hysterectomy without bilateral oophorectomy and observed a moderately but significantly elevated relative risk of 1.6 (95% confidence interval, 1.1 to 2.1). In the Mayo Clinic case-control study (17), hysterectomy was associated with a nonsignificantly elevated relative risk of 1.5 (95% confidence interval, 0.9 to 2.3). The effect of hysterectomy without bilateral oophorectomy on the risk of coronary disease was examined prospectively in the Nurses' Health Study (22). Overall, for such women who had never used postmenopausal estrogens, the relative risk (compared with that of premenopausal women) was 1.0, but the 95% confidence interval was broad, 0.3 to 2.6.

In attempting to explain a possible effect of simple hysterectomy on raising CHD risk, Shelton (34) proposed that the uterus may produce prostacyclin, which could reduce the risk of coronary disease. However, the physiologic effect of prostacyclin in reducing the risk of heart disease is unknown, and, in any event, it apparently does not act as a circulating hormone (35). Moreover, the evidence that the uterus does, in fact, produce prostacyclin is quite meager. A more plausible explanation has recently been advanced by Siddle et al. (36), who argue that surgery for hysterectomy promotes earlier ovarian failure. In a careful study of 90 women with hysterectomy but with ovaries left intact, these investigators observed that the mean age at ovarian failure (defined as onset of persistent estrogen-deficiency symptoms) was 4.1 years earlier than that in a nonhysterectomized control group, and there was a high correlation between age at hysterectomy and age at ovarian failure for women with hysterectomy under age 44 (Spearman $r = 0.6, P < .001$). This finding is consistent with the observation that hysterectomy increases the frequency of consultations for symptoms of estrogen deficiency (37).

The previous literature on ovarian function after hysterectomy was summarized by Siddle et al. (36), and it is clear that a subgroup of women (ranging from 17 to 58%) experience earlier ovarian failure. The authors offer two possible explanations for this phenomenon: one is the effect of surgery itself, in possibly compromising the blood supply to the ovaries. Supporting this view are the findings of reduced ovarian blood flow (38) and decreased estradiol production (39) after surgery for hysterectomy. Similarly, Cattanach

(40) found decreased estrogen levels following tubal ligation in four of seven women. The other possibility raised by Siddle et al. (36) is that the uterus may make an important endocrinologic contribution to ovarian function.

ESTROGEN REPLACEMENT THERAPY

The finding of an increased risk of atherosclerosis and CHD among women with bilateral oophorectomy (41) supports the view that estrogen replacement therapy after menopause might decrease the risk of heart disease. A substantial body of evidence has accumulated, including cross-sectional studies, hospital and community-based case-control studies, prospective cohort studies, and a single small clinical trial.

Cross-Sectional Studies

Table 6.1 summarizes the findings from three important cross-sectional studies (42–44). These studies compare the degree of coronary artery occlusion between users and nonusers of postmenopausal estrogens among women having coronary arteriography. In the study reported by Sullivan et al.

Table 6.1.
Results of Cross-Sectional Surveys of Coronary Artery Occlusion in Women with and without Postmenopausal Estrogen Who Had Coronary Angiography

Study	Age of Patients	Number of Patients	Percentage Estrogen Users/ Type of Use	Age and Risk Factor-Adjusted Relative Risks (95% CI)[a]
	yr			
Sullivan et al. (42)	Mean, 62.8	2,188	4.4/current	0.4 (0.3–0.7) for occlusion 70 + % vs no stenosis
Gruchow et al. (43)	Range, 50–75	933	15.5/current	0.6 (0.5–0.7) moderate vs low occlusion score 0.4 (0.3–0.5) severe vs low occlusion score
McFarland et al. (44)	Range, 35–59; Mean, 52.3	283	41/ever	0.5 (0.3–0.8) for occlusion 70 + vs no stenosis

[a]CI, confidence interval.

(42), women with congenital heart defects, valvular disorders, or primary myocardial disease were excluded, as were women with mild or moderate (less than 70%) stenosis. Current estrogen usage was assessed among the 1,444 postmenopausal women with greater than 70% occlusion and the 744 women with no stenosis evident at angiography. Among women with coronary artery disease, 2.7% were estrogen users, compared with 7.7% among women with no stenosis ($P < .01$). After adjustment for age, diabetes, hypertension, cholesterol level, and cigarette smoking, the relative risk for coronary artery disease among estrogen users was 0.58, with a 95% confidence interval of 0.35 to 0.97.

In a smaller study among 283 younger postmenopausal women McFarland et al. (44) used the same design as Sullivan et al. (42). Estrogen use was defined as ever-use of 6 months or more, but it is likely that most usage was current because the women were young (mean age, 52.3; range, 35 to 59). McFarland et al. observed a relative risk of 0.5 (95% confidence interval, 0.3 to 0.8) for severe stenosis compared with no stenosis.

The study reported by Gruchow et al. (43) employed a similar design. They examined the records of 933 postmenopausal women with coronary angiography, including 154 current estrogen users. For each woman, an occlusion score was assessed ranging from 0 (no occlusion) to 300 (complete occlusion of three main coronary arteries). The mean occlusion score among estrogen users was 65.7, compared with 103.5 among the nonusers ($P < .01$). After adjustment for age, current smoking status, exercise, and body mass index, the relative risk for severe coronary occlusion (an occlusion score greater than 150) for current estrogen users was 0.37, with a 95% confidence interval of 0.46 to 0.29. For moderate occlusion (occlusion score 50 to 150), the relative risk for estrogen users was 0.59,with a 95% confidence interval of 0.48 to 0.73. Estrogen use was the single strongest independent predictor of the occlusion score. When total cholesterol and triglyceride levels were included in the regression model, there was no material alteration in the significant inverse association between estrogen use and coronary occlusion.

Inclusion of high-density lipoprotein (HDL) cholesterol in the regression equation substantially reduced the association between estrogen use and the occlusion score and rendered it statistically nonsignificant. This finding is consistent with elevations in HDL (and a decrease in low-density lipoprotein [LDL] cholesterol as the most likely mechanism of action for the apparent benefit of estrogen. Because changes in lipids are apparently part of the causal chain, it is generally not appropriate to adjust for lipid levels in the analysis. To do so is tantamount to assessing the effect of estrogen on the risk of heart disease apart from its effects on lipids.

Case-Control Studies

Table 6.2 summarizes the findings from hospital-based case-control studies (45–48). In this design, estrogen usage is ascertained among patients hospitalized for MI. This usage is compared with that among other patients. Although this design has the advantages of convenience and usually a high participation rate, there are some important disadvantages. One is that it is largely limited to nonfatal disease. Also, there is the possibility of recall bias. Another more difficult problem is proper selection of controls. It is essential to select controls from among women diagnosed with diseases that are unrelated to estrogen use. This can be difficult. For example, in one study (47), a substantial fraction of controls were chosen from among patients who entered the hospital because of fracture. That study was designed before it was widely appreciated that postmenopausal estrogen therapy reduces osteoporosis and fracture. Inclusion of those controls—who would be less likely to be estrogen users—would tend to attenuate the apparent inverse association between estrogens and risk of heart disease; the controls are no longer representative of the pattern of estrogen use in the population from which the cases arose, but rather they would selectively be less likely to be estrogen users.

Even the exclusion of diseases that are biologically related to estrogen use may not be sufficient. In some instances, physicians may be reluctant to prescribe estrogens to women who are undergoing therapy for other illness to avoid possible interactions with other medications or simply to avoid overburdening the patient with many different medications. Thus, even a nonbiological behavioral link between disease status among the controls and the likelihood of estrogen usage could potentially bias the results. In most instances, the bias would be such that estrogen usage in the controls would be reduced. Hence, one would expect that hospital-based case-control studies might underestimate the reduction in the risk of heart disease due to estrogen. The relative risks observed in these case-control studies range from 4.2 to 0.6 (45–48). Two of these studies yielded essentially null results (46, 47), and in a third, an elevated relative risk was observed (46).

Both of the hospital-based case-control studies with null findings were conducted by Rosenberg et al. In the first study (45), the investigators initially observed a relative risk of 0.7 for estrogen use. After adjustment for an array of variables, the relative risk was changed to 1.0. Of the 336 cases in that study,

Table 6.2.
Hospital-Based Case-Control Studies of Estrogen Use among Patients Hospitalized for MI

Study	Age of Patients	Number of Patients	Percentage Estrogen Users	Endpoint	Exposure to Estrogen	Relative Risk (95% CI)	
						Age-Adjusted	Risk Factor-Adjusted
	yr						
Rosenberg et al. (45)	40–75; median age of exposed cases, 54	336	2.4	Nonfatal MI	Current use	0.7 (0.3–1.4)[a]	1.0 (0.5–2.0)
Jick et al. (46)	39–45	14	50	1st nonfatal MI	Current use	4.2 (1.0–18.8)[a]	
Rosenberg et al. (47)	30–49; median, 45	99 postmenopausal	18	1st MI	Current use	1.4 (0.7–2.7)[a]	
Szklo et al. (48)	35–64	39	28	1st MI	Ever-use	0.8	0.6 (0.2–1.9)

[a]These figures were derived from data given in the chapter.

only eight were current users of estrogen. The second study (47) was limited to women under age 50. Hence, the generalizability to other postmenopausal women is uncertain. Moreover, in this study, a substantial proportion of the controls were women who entered the hospital because of fracture.

The only case-control study that reported an increased risk of coronary disease for estrogen users was conducted by Jick et al. (46), who observed a relative risk of 7.5 for estrogen use. When the findings were limited to postmenopausal women under age 46 (14 cases, 21 controls), the relative risk was 4.2 with a 95% confidence interval of 1.0 to 18.8. Of the 14 patients who entered the analysis, at least 13 were current cigarette smokers. The small size of this study and the restriction of cases to women under age 46 render the findings difficult to interpret.

Table 6.3 summarizes the findings from population or community-based case-control studies (49–55). Although this design shares the methodological limitations of retrospective studies, it does have the advantage of avoiding the use of hospital controls. Hence, one would not expect a systematic underestimate of the effect of estrogens. The relative risks from studies using this design range from 0.3 to 0.9. These studies are consistent in observing an apparent protective effect of estrogen, but in only one of the six studies was this inverse association statistically significant. A seventh case-control study (55) of a combined endpoint of MI and stroke yielded essentially null results for past estrogen use.

The largest study, with 171 cases, was conducted by Pfeffer et al. in a California retirement community (50). For current use of estrogens, they observed a relative risk of 0.7 (95% confidence interval, 0.3 to 1.4). For assessment of estrogen use, these investigators relied on pharmacy records that were thought to be nearly complete. However, in a later analysis (51), it was noted that many women had estrogen usage noted on their medical records without any record in the retirement community pharmacy. Such misclassification, if random with respect to case status, would tend to bias the results toward the null.

Ross et al. conducted another case-control study in the same retirement community but used the medical records to ascertain estrogen usage (51). They observed a statistically significant 60% reduction in the risk of fatal MI compared with living controls and a 40% reduction compared with deceased controls.

In the two studies (50, 52) that examined ever and current use of estrogen, a greater apparent benefit was observed for current use.

Table 6.3.
Community/Population-Based Case-Control Studies of the Effects of Estrogen Use on Risk of Heart Disease

Study	Age of Patients	Number of Patients	Endpoint	Exposure to Estrogen	Percentage Estrogen Users	Relative Risk (95% CI) Age-Adjusted	Relative Risk (95% CI) Risk Factor-Adjusted
	yr						
Talbott et al. (49)	25–64	64 (unknown number post-menopausal	Sudden death	Current-use	5	0.3 (0.1–1.3)[a]	
Pfeffer et al. (50)	50–98 mean = 75	171	1st MI	Ever-use	30		0.9 (0.5–1.4) 0.7 (0.3–1.4)
				Current use	8.7		
Ross et al. (51)	under 80	133	Fatal CHD	Ever-use	Not given	Living control	No change
	mean = 73					0.4 (0.2–0.8)	
						Dead controls	No change
						0.6 (0.3–1.0)	
Bain et al. (52)	30–55	120	1st MI	Ever-use	53	0.9 (0.6–1.2)	0.8 (0.6–1.3)
				Current use	27	0.7 (0.5–1.1)	0.7 (0.4–1.1)
Adam et al. (53)	50–59	76	Fatal MI	Ever-use	12	0.6 (0.3–1.4)[a]	
Beard et al. (54)	40–59	108	MI or sudden death	Ever-use	28		0.6 (0.2–1.3)
Thompson et al. (55)	45–69	603	MI and stroke	Ever-use	Estrogen alone	1.1 (0.8–1.6)	1.1 (0.7–1.8)
				94% past use	Estrogen and progesterone	0.9 (0.4–1.7)	1.2 (0.4–3.1)

[a]These figures represent the crude relative risk.

Prospective Studies

The results of 13 prospective studies (56–69) are summarized in Table 6.4. All but one of these are observational studies. Apart from the Framingham Study, all of these have observed a protective effect of estrogens for risk of CHD. The findings from several of these studies, including the Framingham Study, are reviewed in detail below.

In a landmark study, Bush et al. (65) reported on findings from the Lipid Research Clinics follow-up of 2,270 women aged 40 to 69 at the outset, who were observed for an average of 8½ years. Estrogen use in this study was ascertained at baseline and was not further updated. The age-adjusted relative risk of cardiovascular death among current estrogen users compared with that among nonusers was 0.34 (95% confidence interval, 0.12 to 0.81). Further adjustment for other potential confounding factors, including age, blood pressure, smoking, and prior cardiovascular disease, had little impact on the apparent protective effect of estrogen. However, when HDL and LDL cholesterol were included in the model, the coefficient for estrogen use was markedly reduced and was no longer statistically significant. This finding lends support to the view that the effect of estrogen is mediated primarily through alterations in HDL and LDL cholesterol.

Prospective data from the Nurses' Health Study also address the relation between current use of estrogen therapy, past use, and risk of CHD (62). The Nurses' Health Study was established in 1976 when 121,700 married female registered nurses aged 30 to 55 years completed a mailed questionnaire that inquired about health status, medical history, and a variety of lifestyle practices. That same questionnaire elicited information on hormone use and a variety of coronary risk factors. This information was updated by a follow-up questionnaire sent in 1978. A total of 32,317 postmenopausal women without prior CHD were followed for an average of 3½ years for a total follow-up of 105,786 person-years. Nonfatal MI was reported by the participants on the 1978 and 1980 follow-up questionnaire. (Only cases documented by medical records or other confirmatory information are included in the analysis). Follow-up for nonfatal outcomes was approximately 92% complete. Fatal outcomes were reported by relatives or the postal service. The state vital records were searched for all nonrespondents to the questionnaire so that follow-up for fatal outcomes was nearly complete. Deaths from CHD were documented by medical records. The incidence of nonfatal MI and fatal coronary disease was compared among current users, past users, and never-users of postmenopausal estrogens. Current users of estrogens had a

Table 6.4.
Prospective Studies

Study	Age at Baseline (Mean or Range)	Number in Population	Percentage Estrogen Users at Baseline	Follow-up Period (Mean or Range)	Endpoint (Number of Cases)	Exclusion for Prior CHD	Relative Risk (95% CI)	
							Age-Adjusted	Risk Factor-Adjusted
	yr			*yr*				
Potocki (56)		198			All CVD	No	0.33	
Burch et al. (57)		737	100%	13.4	Fatal CHD (9)	No	0.43 (0.2–0.8)	
MacMahon (58)	49	1,891	100%	12	CHD death	No	0.3[a]	
Hammond et al. (59)	46.3	619	49%	1.3	CHD (58)	No	0.3 (0.2–0.6)[b]	
Nachtigall et al. (60)	55	168	50%	10	MI (4)	Yes	0.3 (0.1–2.8)[b]	
Lafferty and Helmuth (61)	45–60 (53.7)	124	49%	3–16	MI (6)	Yes	0.2 (0.03–1.1)[b]	
Stampfer et al. (62)	30–55 (48.8)	32,317	Past 18% Current 35%	8.6	Nonfatal MI & CHD death (90)	Yes	Past 0.7 (0.4–1.2) Current 0.3 (0.2–0.6)	0.6 (0.3–1.1) 0.3 (0.1–0.6)

Framingham Heart Study:								
Wilson et al. (63)	50–84	1,234	Past 14% Current 10%	8	All CVD (194)	?	1.8 ($P<.01$)[c]	
					CVD death (48)		1.9 ($P>.05$)[c]	
					MI (51)		1.9 ($P>.05$)[c]	
Eaker and Castelli (64)	50–59	695	15%	10	CHD excluding angina (35)	Yes	0.3 (0.1–0.8)	0.4 ($P>.05$)[d]
	60–69	602	8%		(51)			2.2 ($P>.05$)[d]
Bush et al. (65)	40–69	2,270	26%	8.5	CVD death (44)	No[e]	0.3 (0.1–0.8)	0.4 (0.2–0.9)
Petitti et al. (66)	18–54	6,093	Ever 44%	10–13	CVD death (40)	No	0.9 (0.2–3.3)	0.6 (0.3–1.1)
Criqui et al. (67)	50–79	1,868	39%	12	CHD death (87)	No	0.8 (0.5–1.2)	1.0 (0.6–1.7)
Henderson et al. (68)	40–101 (median about 73)	8,807	Past 43% Current 14%	4.6	MI deaths (149)	No	Past 0.6 (0.4–0.9)	No change
							Current 0.5 (0.2–1.1)	No change
							Ever 0.6 (0.4–0.8)	No change
					Total MI	No	Ever 0.7 (0.5–1.0)	No change
Croft and Hannaford (69)	20–60[b]	Nested case-control	Ever 6.5%	19	MI (9)	Yes	0.8	0.8 (0.3–1.8)

[a]These data are compared with expected rates in the general population.
[b]The crude odds ratio and confidence intervals are derived from data given in the paper.
[c]These results are taken as the average of findings using examination 11 and examination 12 as baseline.
[d]This includes HDL in the regression analysis.
[e]After exclusion for CHD, the age-adjusted relative risk is 0.4 (0.1–1.1).

relative risk of 0.3 (95% confidence interval, 0.2 to 0.6). Among past users, there was a trend toward protection with a relative risk of 0.7, but this did not attain statistical significance. Adjustment for a variety of coronary risk factors, including hypercholesterolemia, family history of heart disease, hypertension, diabetes, obesity, and smoking, did not alter these relative risk estimates. Extended follow-up of this cohort through 1986 showed that these results persisted (70). Current users had an adjusted relative risk of 0.56 (0.40 to 0.80) for major coronary disease compared to never-users. Results from the Leisure World Study were reported by Henderson et al. (68). In this study 8,841 women aged 40 through 101 years completed a health survey in 1981. After 5½ years of follow-up (40,919 person–years), 1,019 deaths (149 due to MI) had occurred. For all-cause mortality, the relative risk was 0.8 (95% confidence interval, 0.70 to 0.91) for ever-users of estrogen, compared with never-users. Much of this reduction in total mortality was attributable to a decrease in fatal myocardial infarction. For ever-users of estrogens, the relative risk was 0.59 (95% confidence interval, 0.42 to 0.82). Estrogen use was defined as current or past on the baseline questionnaire and was not updated. The relative risk for past users was 0.62 and for current users, 0.47. Adjustment for a number of coronary risk factors, including prior coronary disease, hypertension, smoking, obesity, and exercise did not appreciably change the relative risk for estrogen users. The mean age in the Leisure World Study was over 75 years. The large number of endpoints led to substantial statistical power and precise estimates of effect in this study.

A cohort of 6,093 women aged 18 to 54, members of the Northern California Kaiser Permanente Medical Care Program, were observed for an average of 10 to 13 years (66). The mortality from cardiovascular disease was lower in women who reported noncontraceptive estrogen use, with a relative risk of 0.9 (95% confidence interval, 0.2 to 3.3). After adjustment for a variety of cardiovascular risk factors, including age, hypertension, obesity, and smoking, the apparent protective effect was more marked, with a relative risk of 0.6 (95% confidence interval, 0.3 to 1.1). In this study, estrogen use was defined at the baseline in 1968–1972 and was updated through 1977. After 1977, follow-up of the cohort continued for mortality but without further updating of estrogen use.

In contrast to findings from all other cohort studies, Wilson et al. (63) reported an increase in the risk of cardiovascular disease associated with estrogen use by women in the Framingham Heart Study. A participant was classified as a user of estrogen if estrogen was included on the medication form during an 8-year period. Follow-up began at the end of that 8-year interval for

1,234 women who were postmenopausal and 50 years of age or older. Of these, 302 had used estrogens at some time. They were followed for an additional 8 years. After adjustment for age, hypertension, obesity, total cholesterol, HDL cholesterol, smoking, and alcohol consumption, the relative risk for all cardiovascular disease among ever-users of estrogen was 1.8, compared with that among never-users. The rubric to total cardiovascular disease included CHD, angina pectoris, intermittent claudication, transient ischemic attack, MI, congestive heart failure, and coronary and sudden death. Despite the apparent elevation in risk, there was no effect on total mortality, with a relative risk of 1.0. The apparent elevation in risk was not statistically significant when only MI was considered.

A reanalysis of the Framingham data with more specific endpoints—CHD without angina—observed a nonsignificant protective effect among women aged 50 to 59 with a relative risk of 0.4; in that reanalysis, there was a nonsignificant adverse effect among older women, in whom the relative risk was 2.2 (64). Both Framingham analyses presented findings adjusted for HDL cholesterol, which is probably inappropriate, as that is the most plausible mechanism of action for estrogen.

There has been only one clinical trial of estrogen use and coronary disease (60). Eighty-four pairs of women matched for age and medical condition were randomly assigned to take 2.5 mg of conjugated estrogen daily and 10 mg of medroxyprogesterone for 7 days a month or placebos. The women were all residents of a long-term chronic care hospital. After 10 years of follow-up, the relative risk for estrogen users was 0.33 for fatal and nonfatal MI. The 95% confidence interval was 0.1 to 2.8; there were only four MIs in this small trial, so the results, while intriguing, are difficult to interpret.

Interpretation of These Epidemiologic Data

Although the findings from the epidemiologic studies are not completely consistent, the preponderance of evidence strongly suggests that women receiving postmenopausal estrogen therapy are at decreased risk for CHD. The consistency of the findings is more apparent in the better-designed and better-analyzed studies. In particular, of the 12 prospective studies, only one, the Framingham Study, reported an adverse effect (63). Even in that study, the elevated relative risk did not attain statistical significance, and a reanalysis of the data using more specific endpoints showed a protective effect among younger postmenopausal women (64).

A positive association does not necessarily imply cause and effect. Physicians and their patients decide on estrogen therapy, and in many instances the health status of the patient will have an important influence. The only randomized trial (60) was far too small to come to a firm conclusion. It is possible that estrogen use is merely a marker rather than a cause of good health, though the evidence for this position is weak. In the Nurses' Health Study, the distribution of established coronary risk factors was quite similar among current-users and never-users of estrogens (62). In the report by Bush et al. (65), multivariate control for a wide array of risk factors had little impact on the relative risk, and in the study of Petitti et al. (66), such control revealed an even stronger protective effect, implying that estrogen users had a somewhat higher underlying risk. In the smaller study of Lafferty and Helmuth (61), all the patients were judged eligible for and were offered estrogen therapy; the risk of coronary disease was marginally higher among those who declined.

The most likely biological mechanism for the apparent protective effect of estrogens is the beneficial impact on the lipid profile. Estrogens tend to raise levels of HDL cholesterol and lower the levels of LDL cholesterol (71) (see Chapter 8 for a more detailed discussion). Both of these changes are associated with a reduced risk of heart disease. The impact of estrogens on each of these lipid fractions is substantial. In their review of the experimental work, Bush and Miller found that, on average, a standard dose of 0.625 mg/day of conjugated estrogens led to a 10% increase in HDL cholesterol and a 4% decrease in LDL cholesterol (71). Because a 1-mg/dl increase in HDL cholesterol is associated with approximately a 3 to 5% decrease in risk of coronary disease (71), and a 1-mg/dl decrease in LDL cholesterol is associated with about a 2% decline in risk, the changes induced by estrogen could lead to a relatively large decrease in risk.

The effects of estrogen on the lipid profile are apparent within weeks of initiation of therapy and do not persist after therapy is terminated. This may explain the consistent finding of a stronger protective effect for current use compared with ever-use or past use. Only a few of the prospective studies reclassified the subjects' estrogen use during follow-up. To the extent that subjects ceased their estrogen use, we would expect to find misclassification and an underestimate of the magnitude of protection. This point is discussed clearly by Criqui et al. in the analysis of their findings (67).

In nearly all of the epidemiologic studies, the use of progestins was very uncommon. Progestins are now commonly recommended to reduce or eliminate the excess risk of endometrial cancer due to unopposed estrogen. Unfortunately, progestins tend to have an effect on lipids opposite to that of estrogen: progestins tend to lower HDL cholesterol and raise LDL cholesterol. Although one can devise regimens in which some of the estrogen benefit on lipids remain apparent, that benefit is nonetheless attenuated by the addition of progestin. There are no published data on the effect of added progestins on the risk of coronary disease. One of the important challenges in this area is to develop a progestin regimen or formulation that will maintain the protection for the uterus yet not impair the benefits of estrogen on lipids.

SUMMARY AND CONCLUSIONS

A large number of studies of disparate design are reasonably consistent in demonstrating that women with early bilateral oophorectomy are at increased risk of CHD. The evidence for an increase in risk among women with a surgical menopause but without bilateral oophorectomy is inconclusive, but such an effect, if any, could be plausibly explained by decreased ovarian function in many of these women as a consequence of the surgery. These findings, taken together with the lack of excess risk in women with bilateral oophorectomy who take replacement estrogen, support the view that the increased risk is due to estrogen deficiency. This view is further supported by the improvement in the lipid profile induced by estrogen replacement therapy in postmenopausal women. Because ovarian function begins to decline well before menopause and continues to decline after menopause, it is not surprising that the moment of menopause is not associated with an abrupt increase in the risk of heart disease. Moreover, some time is required for the adverse changes in coronary risk factors that occur during the climacteric (41) to be reflected in increased rates of coronary disease. Although natural menopause does not cause an immediate increase in the risk of heart disease, it does signal a period of increasing risk that is probably related to both age and estrogen deficiency.

Of the 12 prospective studies of estrogen replacement therapy and risk of CHD, only one, the Framingham Heart Study, shows an adverse effect. The bulk of the evidence strongly supports a protective effect of estrogen replacement that is unlikely to be explained by confounding factors. This benefit is consistent with the effect of estrogens to lower LDL and raise HDL cholesterol.

Key Points

- Age at natural menopause is not related to risk of coronary heart disease after controlling for cigarette smoking (which is related to both age at menopause and risk of coronary disease).

- Bilateral oophorectomy is associated with increased risk of coronary heart disease.
- Women who take estrogen replacement after bilateral oophorectomy return to the risk of a premenopausal woman of the same age.
- The preponderance of evidence indicates that women taking estrogen therapy are at decreased risk of coronary heart disease.
- The overall reduction in risk is approximately 50%.
- Possible mechanisms include the protective effect of estrogen therapy on the lipid profile.
- Progestins added to estrogen therapy may reduce the beneficial effect of estrogen therapy; data are limited as to the magnitude of this effect on the risk of coronary heart disease.

Acknowledgment

We thank Stephanie Bechtel and Chris Pappas, who assisted in the preparation of this manuscript.

References

1. U.S. Department of Health and Human Services, Public Health Service, Centers for Disease Control, National Center for Health Statistics. Vital statistics of the United States 1986. Volume II—Mortality, Part A. Hyattsville, MD: U.S. Department of Health and Human Services, 1988.
2. Tracy RE. Sex difference in coronary disease: two opposing views. J Chron Dis 1966; 19:1245–1251.
3. Winkelstein W Jr, Rakate AC. Age trend of mortality from coronary artery disease in women and observations on the reproductive patterns of those affected. Am Heart J 1964;67:481–488.
4. Heller RF, Jacobs HS. Coronary heart disease in relation to age, sex, and the menopause. Br Med J 1978;1:472–474.
5. Ackerman RF, Dry TJ, Edwards JE. Relationship of various factors to the degree of coronary atherosclerosis in women. Circulation 1950;1:1345–1354.
6. Gosden RG. Biology of menopause. The causes and consequences of ovarian aging. London: Academic Press, 1985:8–10.
7. Willett WC, Stampfer MJ, Bain C, Lipnick R, Speizer FE, Rosner B, Cramer D, Hennekens CH. Cigarette smoking, relative weight, and menopause. Am J Epidemiol 1983;117:651–658.
8. Macmahon B, Worcester J. Age at menopause. Washington, DC: National Center for Health Statistics (Vital and Health Statistics, Series II, No. 19) (PHS Publication No. 1000-Series 11-No. 19), 1966.
9. Sherman B, Wallace R, Bean J, et al. Relation of body weight to menarchal and menopausal age: implications for breast cancer risk. J Clin Endocrinol Metab 1981;52:488–493.
10. Lindquist D, Bengtsson C. Menopausal age in relation to smoking. Acta Med Scand 1979;205:73–77.

11. Kaufman DW, Slone D, Rosenberg L, et al. Cigarette smoking and age at natural menopause. Am J Public Health 1980;70:420–422.
12. Willett WC, Green A, Stampfer MJ, Speizer FE, Colditz GA, Rosner B, Monson R, Stason W, Hennekens CH. Relative and absolute excess risks of coronary heart disease among women who smoke cigarettes. N Engl J Med 1987;317:1303–1309.
13. Witteman JCM, Grobbee DE, Kok FJ, Hofman A, Valkenburg HA. Increased risk of atherosclerosis in women after the menopause. Br Med J 1989;298:642–644.
14. Mann JI, Vessey MP, Thorogood M, Doll R. Myocardial infarction in young women with special reference to oral contraceptive practice. Br Med J 1975;2:241–245.
15. Abramov LA. Sexual life and sexual frigidity among women developing acute myocardial infarction. Psychosom Med 1976;38:418–425.
16. Rosenberg L, Hennekens CH, Rosner B, Belanger C, Rothman KJ, Speizer FE. Early menopause and the risk of myocardial infarction. Am J Obstet Gynecol 1981;139:47–51.
17. Beard CM, Fuster V, Annegers FJ. Reproductive history in women with coronary heart disease: a case-control study. Am J Epidemiol 1981;120:108–114.
18. Lapidus L, Bengtsson C, Lindquist O. Menopausal age and risk of cardiovascular disease and death. Acta Obstet Gynecol Scand Suppl 1985;130:37–41.
19. Gordon T, Kannel WB, Hjortland MC, McNamara PM. Menopause and coronary heart disease. The Framingham study. Ann Intern Med 1978;89:157–161.
20. Rothman KJ, Boice JD. Epidemiologic analysis with a programmable calculator. (NIH publication no. 79-1649). Washington DC: Public Health Service, 1979.
21. Lerner DJ, Kannel WB. Patterns of coronary heart disease morbidity and mortality in the sexes: a 26-year follow-up of the Framingham population. Am Heart J 1986;111:383–390.
22. Colditz GA, Willett WC, Stampfer MJ, Rosner B, Speizer FE, Hennekens CH. Menopause and the risk of coronary heart disease in women. N Engl J Med 1987;316:1105–1110.
23. Colditz GA, Martin P, Stampfer MJ, Willett WC, Sampson L, Rosner B, Hennekens CH, Speizer FE. Validation of questionnaire information on risk factors and disease outcomes in a prospective cohort study in women. Am J Epidemiol 1986;123:894–900.
24. Colditz GA, Stampfer MJ, Willett WC, Stason WB, Rosner B, Hennekens CH, Speizer FE. Reproducibility and validity of self-reported menopausal status in a prospective cohort study. Am J Epidemiol 1987;126:319–325.
25. Roberts WC, Giraldo AA. Bilateral oophorectomy in menstruating women and accelerated coronary atherosclerosis: an unproved connection. Am J Med 1979;67:363–365.
26. Ritterband AB, Jaffe IA, Densen PM, Magagna JF, Reed E. Gonadal function and the development of coronary heart disease. Circulation 1963;28:237–251.
27. Robinson RW, Hihano N, Cohen WD. Increased incidence of coronary heart disease in women castrated prior to menopause. Arch Intern Med 1959:104:908–913.
28. Oliver MF, Boyd GS. Effect of bilateral ovariectomy on coronary-artery disease and serum-lipid levels. Lancet 1959;2:690–694.
29. Novak ER, Williams TJ. Autopsy comparison of cardiovascular changes in castrated and normal women. Am J Obstet Gynceol 1960;80:863–872.
30. Manchester JH, Herman MV, Gorlin R. Premenstrual castration and documented coronary atherosclerosis. Am J Cardiol 1971;28:33–37.
31. Wuest JH, Dry TJ, Edwards JE. The degree of coronary atherosclerosis in bilaterally oophorectomized women. J Am Heart Assoc 1953;7:801–809.
32. Parrish HM, Carr CA, Hall DG, King TM. Time interval from castration in premenopausal women to development of excessive coronary atherosclerosis. Am J Obstet Gynecol 1967;99:155–162.
33. Centerwall BS. Premenopausal hysterectomy and cardiovascular disease. Am J Obstet Gynecol 1981;139:58–61.

34. Shelton JD. Prostacyclin from the uterus and woman's cardiovascular advantage. Prostaglandins Leukotrienes Med 1982;8:459–466.
35. Blair IA, Barrow SE, Waddell KA, Lewis PJ, Dollery CT. Prostacyclin is not a circulating hormone in man. Prostaglandins 1982;23:279–289.
36. Siddle N, Sarrel P, Whitehead M. The effect of hysterectomy on the age at ovarian failure: identification of a subgroup of women with premature loss of ovarian function and literature review. Fertil Steril 1987;47:94–100.
37. Roos NP. Hysterectomies in one Canadian province: a new look at risks and benefits. Am J Public Health 1984;74:39–46.
38. Janson PO, Jansson I. The acute effect of hysterectomy on ovarian blood flow. Am J Obstet Gynecol 1977;127:349–352.
39. Stone SC, Dickey RP, Mickal A. The acute effect of hysterectomy on ovarian function. Am J Obstet Gynecol 1975;121:193–197.
40. Cattanach J. Oestrogen deficiency after tubal ligation. Lancet 1985;1:847–849.
41. Stampfer MJ, Colditz GA, Willett WC. Menopause and heart disease: a review. Ann NY Acad Sci 1990;592:193–203.
42. Sullivan JM, Zwagg RV, Lemp GF, Hughes JP, Maddock V, Kroetz FW, Ramanathan KB, Mirvis DM. Postmenopausal estrogen use and coronary atherosclerosis. Ann Intern Med 1988;108:358–363.
43. Gruchow HW, Anderson AJ, Barboria JJ, Sobocinski KA. Postmenopausal use of estrogen and occlusion of coronary arteries. Am Heart J 1988;115:954–963.
44. McFarland KF, Boniface ME, Hornung CA, Earnhardt W, Humphries JO. Risk factors and noncontraceptive estrogen use in women with and without coronary disease. Am Heart J 1989;117:1209–1214.
45. Rosenberg L, Armstrong B, Jick H. Myocardial infarction and estrogen therapy in postmenopausal women. N Engl J Med 1976;294:1256–1259.
46. Jick H, Dinan B, Rothman KJ. Noncontraceptive estrogens and nonfatal myocardial infarction. JAMA 1978;239:1407–1408.
47. Rosenberg L, Stone D, Shapiro S, Kaufman P, Stolley PD, Miettinen OS. Noncontraceptive estrogens and myocardial infarction in young women. JAMA 1980;244:339–342.
48. Szklo M, Tonascia J, Gordis L, Bloom I. Estrogen use and myocardial infarction risk: a case-control study. Prev Med 1984;13:510–516.
49. Talbott E, Kuller LH, Detre K, Perper J. Biologic and psychosocial risk factors of sudden death from coronary disease in white women. Am J Cardiol 1977;39:858–864.
50. Pfeffer RI, Whipple GH, Kurosaki TT, Chapman JM. Coronary risk and estrogen use in postmenopausal women. Am J Epidemiol 1978;107:479–487.
51. Ross RK, Paganini-Hill A, Mack TM, Arthur M, Henderson BE. Menopausal oestrogen therapy and protection from death from ischaemic heart disease. Lancet 1981;1:858–860.
52. Bain C, Willett WC, Hennekens CH, Rosner B, Belanger C, Speizer FE. Use of postmenopausal hormones and risk of myocardial infarction. Circulation 1981;64:42–46.
53. Adam S, Williams V, Vessey MP. Cardiovascular disease and hormone replacement treatment; a pilot case-control study. Br Med J 1981;282:1277–1278.
54. Beard CM, Kottke TE, Annegers JF, Ballard DJ. The Rochester Coronary Heart Disease Project: effect of cigarette smoking, hypertension, diabetes, and steroidal estrogen use on coronary heart disease among 40–59 year old women, 1960–82. Mayo Clin Proc 1989;64:1471–1480.
55. Thompson SG, Meade TW, Greenberg G. The use of hormonal replacement therapy and the risk of stroke and myocardial infarction in women. J Epidemiol Community Health 1989;43:173–178.

56. Potocki J. Wplyw leczenia estrogenami na niewydolnose wiencowa u kobiet po menopauzie. Pol Tyg Lek 1971;26:1812–1815.
57. Burch JC, Byrd BF Jr, Vaughn WK. The effects of long-term estrogen on hysterectomized women. Am J Obstet Gynecol 1974;188:778–782.
58. MacMahon B. Cardiovascular disease and noncontraceptive oestrogen therapy. In: Oliver MF, ed. Coronary heart disease in young women. New York: Churchill Livingstone, 1978:197–207.
59. Hammond CB, Jelovsek FR, Lee KL, Creasman WT, Parker RT. Effects of long-term estrogen replacement therapy. I. Metabolic effects. Am J Obstet Gynecol 1979;133:525–536.
60. Nachtigall LE, Nachtigall RH, Nachtigall RD, Beckman EM. Estrogen replacement therapy II: a prospective study in the relationship to carcinoma and cardiovascular and metabolic problems. Obstet Gynecol 1979;54:74–79.
61. Lafferty FW, Helmuth DO. Postmenopausal estrogen replacement: the prevention of osteroporosis and systemic effects. Maturitas 1985;7:147–159.
62. Stampfer MJ, Willett WC, Colditz GA, Rosner B, Speizer FE, Hennekens CH. A prospective study of postmenopausal estrogen therapy and coronary heart disease. N Engl J Med 1985;313:1044–1049.
63. Wilson PW, Garrison RJ, Castelli WP. Postmenopausal estrogen use, cigarette smoking, and cardiovascular morbidity in women over 50: the Framingham Study. N Engl J Med 1985;313:1038–1043.
64. Eaker ED, Castelli WP. Coronary heart disease and its risk factors among women in the Framingham Study. In: Eaker E, Packard B, Wenger NK, Clarkson TB, Tyroler HA, eds. Coronary Heart Disease in Women. New York: Haymarket Doyma Inc., 1987:122–132.
65. Bush TL, Barrett-Connor E, Cowan LD, Criqui MH, Wallace RB, Suchindran CM, Tyroler HA, Rifking BM. Cardiovascular mortality and noncontraceptive use of estrogen in women: results from the Lipid Research Clinics Program Follow-up Study. Circulation 1987; 75:1102–1109.
66. Petitti DB, Perlman JA, Sidney S. Noncontraceptive estrogens and mortality: long-term follow-up of women in the Walnut Creek Study. Obstet Gynecol 1987;70:289–293.
67. Criqui MH, Suarez L, Barrett-Connor E, McPhillips J, Wingard DL, Garland C. Postmenopausal estrogen use and mortality. Am J Epidemiol 1988;128:606–614.
68. Henderson BE, Paganini-Hill A, Ross RK. Estrogen replacement therapy and protection from acute myocardial infarction. Am J Obstet Gynecol 1988;159:312–317.
69. Croft P, Hannaford PC. Risk factors for acute myocardial infarction in women: evidence from the Royal College of General Practitioners' oral contraceptive study. Br Med J 1989;298:165–168.
70. Stampfer MJ, Colditz GA, Willett WC, Manson JE, Rosner B, Speizer FE, Hennekens CH. Postmenopausal estrogen therapy and cardiovascular disease. Ten year follow-up from the Nurses' Health Study. N Engl J Med 1991;325:756–762.
71. Bush TL, Miller VT. Effects of pharmacologic agents used during menopause. Impact on lipids and lipoproteins. In: Mishell D, ed. Menopause: physiology and pharmacology. Chicago: Year Book Medical Publishers, 1986:187–208.

7

Estrogen Replacement Therapy and Cardiovascular Disease: Effects on Plasma Lipid Risk Markers

David Crook, John C. Stevenson, and Malcolm I. Whitehead

While the protection against osteoporotic fracture conferred by estrogens is rightly considered to be important, it is now clear that the major public health benefit of estrogen replacement therapy (ERT) is a reduction of at least 50% in the incidence of coronary heart disease (CHD) (1–3). The precise mechanisms through which estrogens exert their beneficial actions are not fully understood. Although effects on blood flow and arterial tone may contribute (4, 5), the role of plasma lipoproteins is thought to be of primary importance in mediating the cardioprotective effects of estrogen (1).

Estrogens decrease levels of the potentially atherogenic low-density lipoprotein (LDL) fraction and increase those of the potentially protective high-density lipoproteins (HDLs). These changes in lipoprotein levels would be consistent with a decrease in CHD risk (6, 7), and long-term users of estrogen do indeed have the predicted pattern of low LDL and high HDL levels (1). Although oral estrogens may *increase* risk by raising plasma triglyceride levels, the benefits of raising HDL and lowering LDL would appear to outweigh this potentially unfavorable change.

In non-hysterectomized women, estrogen replacement therapy (ERT) is usually administered as a combination of estrogen with progestin. The addition of a 10 to 14 day cycle of progestin has become widespread due to concern over the long-term effects of unopposed estrogen on the endometrium (8, 9). Progestins induce both symptomatic and metabolic side effects (10). In particular, progestins can oppose many of the effects of estrogens on lipoprotein metabolism, and this has led to concern that such combination therapy will not provide the cardioprotection offered by estrogen alone. While this hypothesis remains to be tested, it would seem prudent to formulate a combined regimen that approximates the lipoprotein profile seen with unopposed estrogen.

The purpose of this chapter is to review the actions of estrogens and progestins on lipoprotein metabolism and to indicate how the potentially adverse impact of progestins on the lipoprotein profile may be minimized.

OVERVIEW OF PLASMA LIPOPROTEIN METABOLISM

An understanding of the basics of lipoprotein metabolism is required to appreciate the role of plasma lipids as risk markers for CHD. Lipids—triglycerides, cholesterol, phospholipids and free fatty acids—are defined as biological substances that are poorly soluble in water. Newspaper stories of the "killer french fries" category obscure the essential metabolic roles of these compounds. Triglycerides and free fatty acids are efficient sources of energy and are the preferred fuel of organs such as the heart. Phospholipids and cholesterol are essential for the structure and function of mammalian cell membranes, and thereby cell function. Lipids also play important roles in the coagulation and immune systems and at interfaces such as gas/liquid transfer in lung alveoli. Cholesterol is essential for the synthesis of steroid hormones. Finally, dietary fat provides essential fatty acids and vitamins.

Lipids per se are poorly soluble in plasma and circulate bound to various proteins. Free fatty acids are bound by albumin, whereas other lipids bind to one or more members of a group of at least 12 specific proteins called *apolipoproteins*. Apolipoproteins not only bind and increase the solubility of lipids but they also modulate the activity of enzymes responsible for lipoprotein metabolism, and provide the signal for receptor-mediated uptake by cells. These complexes of lipids and specific proteins are called *lipoproteins*. Lipids such as triglycerides are more polar (water-soluble) than lipids such as phospholipids. Cholesterol is an alcohol and has limited polar characteristics, but the majority of cholesterol in the body is present in the *esterified* form, i.e., it possesses a fatty acid chain bonded to the steroid ring structure. The presence or absence of this chain affects the solubility of cholesterol, with cholesteryl esters being virtually insoluble in water. The simplest model of plasma lipoprotein structure (Fig. 7.1) shows that nonpolar lipids such as triglycerides and cholesteryl esters form a central hydrophobic ("water-hating") core, whereas hydrophilic ("water-loving") lipids such as phospholipids and free (nonesterified) cholesterol integrate with apolipoproteins to form a surface coat.

Not all apolipoproteins are found on all lipoproteins, but all lipoproteins

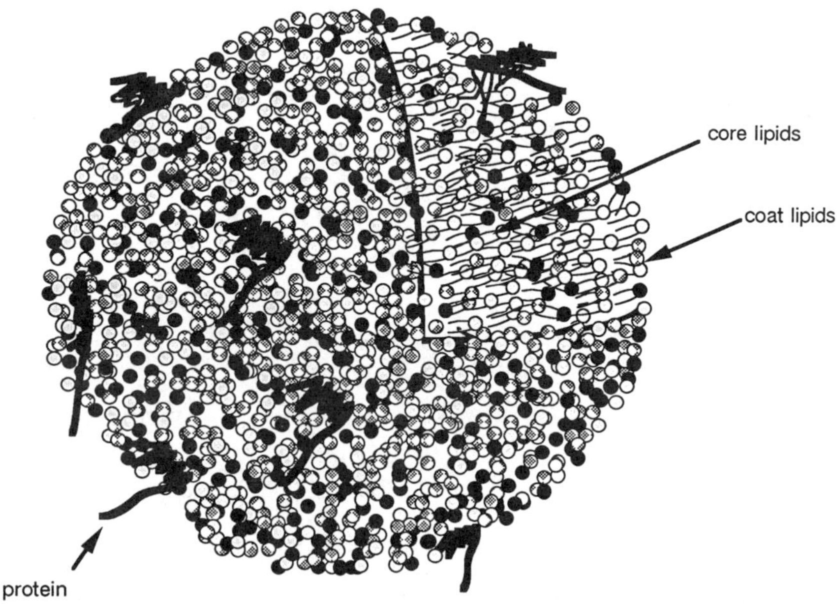

Figure 7.1. Schematic view of lipoprotein structure. Cutaway view of lipoprotein reveals protein and polar lipids (nonesterified cholesterol and phospholipids) forming a surface coat that covers a core of nonpolar lipids such as esterified cholesterol and triglycerides.

contain cholesterol, triglycerides, and phospholipids. The percentage contribution of the lipid and protein components varies widely, causing the density of the particles to vary. These differences have been exploited to produce a classification system for plasma lipoproteins.

The largest lipoprotein particles, responsible for the turbidity of postprandial plasma, are chylomicrons. These are globules of dietary fat (mainly triglyceride), stabilized by a thin film of apolipoproteins and phospholipids. Chylomicrons are synthesized by the small intestine, entering the blood via the lymphatic system. Once in the plasma compartment (Fig. 7.2), they undergo a stepwise delipidation cascade in which the triglyceride content is systematically stripped out of the particle by the action of enzymes called *lipases,* which are bound to the inside surface of the capillary endothelium. The lipases hydrolyze triglycerides, breaking them down into fatty acids and glycerol. This process results in the formation of "remnant" particles. These remnants, containing most of the dietary cholesterol but only 10 to 20% of dietary triglycerides, are then taken up by the liver. Chylomicrons are rapidly

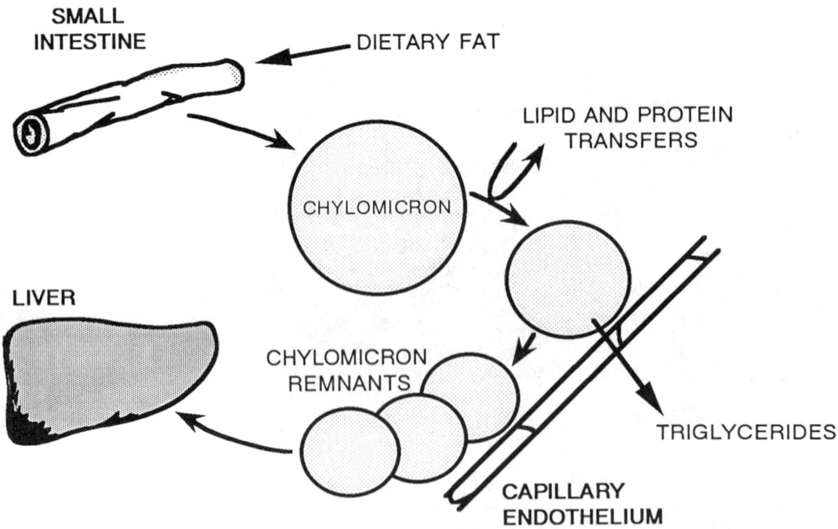

Figure 7.2. Overview of chylomicron metabolism. Dietary fat is secreted from the small intestine in the form of chylomicrons. These large globules accept apolipoproteins from other lipoproteins and then undergo a lipolysis cascade. Triglycerides are sequentially stripped out of the particle core to be taken up by adipose tissue and peripheral cells. The resulting "remnants" are taken up by the liver and catabolized.

catabolized and are not normally present in plasma from fasted subjects. Some of the fatty acids released by the degradation of chylomicrons remain in the plasma compartment and act as fuel for other tissues. The remainder is taken up by adipocytes, re-esterified to form triglycerides, and then stored as fat droplets.

The simplest classification of the plasma lipoproteins typical of fasted subjects (Table 7.1) is based on differences in particle density, due to differing lipid/protein ratios, which can be exploited using ultracentrifugation procedures. In practice, such density-based separations have been superseded by more simple techniques. However, the nomenclature—very low-density lipoproteins (VLDLs), low-density lipoproteins (LDLs), and high-density lipoproteins (HDLs)—has been retained.

The liver synthesizes triglycerides both as a source of energy for peripheral tissues and for storage in adipose tissues. This triglyceride is combined with an apolipoprotein, apoB, and with cholesterol and other lipids to form VLDLs. VLDLs are smaller than chylomicrons and contain the bulk of triglycerides in fasting plasma. Like chylomicrons, they undergo a cascade of degradation in

Table 7.1.
Composition of Human Plasma Lipoproteins[a,b]

Lipoprotein	Density Range	%PROT	%CHOL	%TRIG	%PL	Apolipo-proteins
	g/ml					
Chylomicrons	<1.006	1–2	1–4	**86–94**	3–8	**C, B,** AI
VLDL	<1.006	5–10	16–22	**55–65**	12–18	**B,** C, E
LDL	1.006–1.063	20–24	**40–50**	8–12	20–25	**B**
HDL	1.063–1.21	**45–50**	17–22	3–6	20–30	**AI,** AII, C, E

[a]Adapted from Assmann G. Lipid metabolism and atherosclerosis. New York: Schattauer, 1982.
[b]Major lipids and apoproteins are shown in bold. %PROT, CHOL, TRIG, PL = percentage protein, cholesterol, triglycerides or phospholipid (by weight).

which core triglycerides are hydrolyzed by lipase enzymes on the capillary endothelium (Fig. 7.3). In humans, about one-half of the VLDL remnants are taken up by the liver. The remainder undergo further remodeling to form LDLs.

LDLs are the most cholesterol-rich of all lipoproteins and are the most prominent class of lipoproteins in human plasma. They are taken up predominantly by peripheral cells and hepatocytes through a high-affinity pathway involving the apo_{B100}, E receptor. By this tightly controlled mechanism, cells obtain cholesterol for membrane and steroid hormone synthesis. LDLs may also be catabolized by other cells, such as macrophages. The role of LDL oxidation may be important in these processes (11).

HDLs contain approximately 50% protein and are the most dense class of plasma lipoproteins. They are synthesized and secreted by the liver (and perhaps the small intestine) as protein-rich discoidal bilayers. These "nascent" particles undergo extensive intravascular remodeling (Fig. 7.4), involving exchange of lipids and proteins with other lipoproteins and with the cholesterol-rich membranes of peripheral tissues. Under the influence of the enzyme *lecithin cholesterol acyl transferase* (LCAT), these exchanges result in larger, spherical particles known as HDL subfraction 3 (HDL_3). Further uptake of lipid results in the formation of HDL subfraction 2 (HDL_2); these are catabolized primarily in the liver. As part of this metamorphosis, specific proteins called *transfer proteins* exchange lipids between HDLs and other lipoproteins.

HDL particles have two key functions. They act as a reservoir for key apolipoproteins and structural components required for the hydrolysis of chylomicrons and VLDLs. They also accept "used" cholesterol from periph-

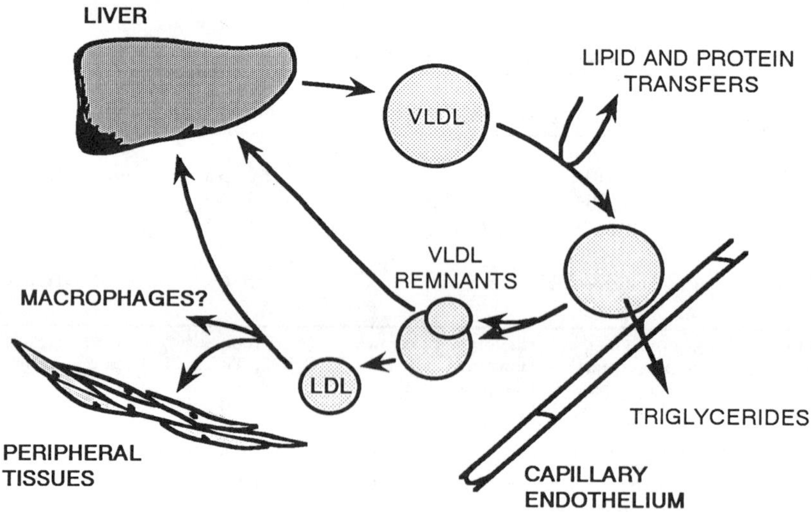

Figure 7.3. Overview of VLDL and LDL metabolism. Endogenous lipids are secreted by the liver in the form of very low-density lipoproteins (VLDLs). VLDLs undergo a lipolysis cascade analagous to chylomicron degradation. Some VLDL remnants are removed by the liver; the remainder discard lipids and apolipoproteins and develop into low-density lipoproteins (LDLs). LDSs interact with high-affinity binding sites on peripheral cells and on hepatocytes, where they are taken up and catabolized. LDLs may be catabolized by other cells such as macrophages.

eral tissues and transfer it (directly or indirectly) to the liver for eventual excretion in bile. This scavenging or "reverse cholesterol transport" is of crucial importance in maintaining cholesterol homeostasis. Although virtually all mammalian tissues can synthesize cholesterol, they are unable to degrade this lipid.

For the reader wishing to understand plasma lipoprotein metabolism in greater detail, excellent reviews of the subject are available (12–14).

Gonadal hormones are powerful modulators of plasma lipoprotein metabolism (15, 16). Gender differences in plasma lipoproteins emerge during puberty, due primarily to changes in testosterone, and continue throughout life. In general, young women have less triglycerides, less LDL cholesterol, and more HDL cholesterol than do men of similar age. The sex difference in HDL levels, due almost exclusively to higher levels of the HDL_2 subfraction (15), continues throughout life. However, LDL levels increase with age in both sexes, and by the sixth decade women have higher LDL levels. Because LDLs are the major class of cholesterol-carrying lipoproteins, older women also have higher plasma total cholesterol levels than men of similar age.

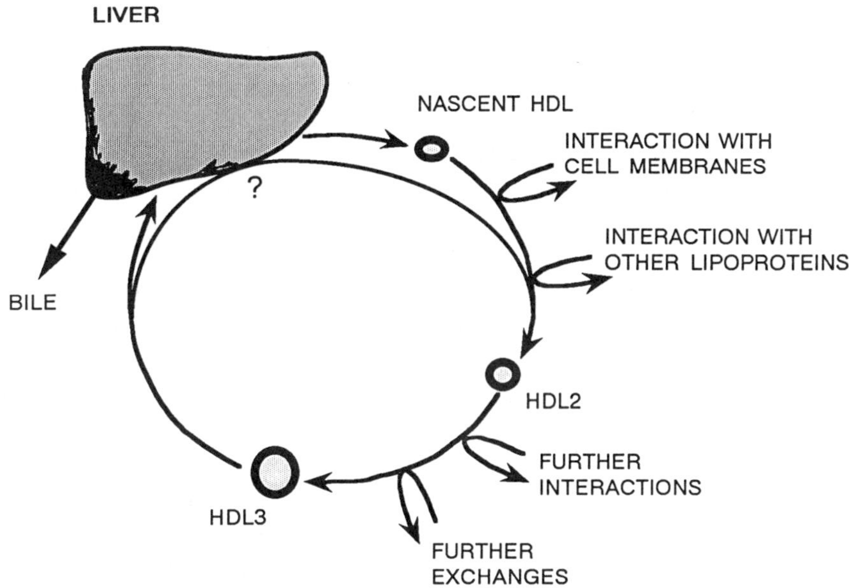

Figure 7.4. Overview of HDL metabolism. High-density lipoproteins (HDLs) are secreted by the liver as nascent discs. These interact with peripheral cells and with other lipoproteins. In this way, excess cholesterol is taken up as the particles increase in size, forming first HDL_3 and subsequently HDL_2. Larger HDL particles such as HDL_2 may be taken up by the liver or may transfer their cholesterol to other lipoproteins.

Oral estrogens increase hepatic secretion of VLDL (and thus plasma triglyceride levels), whereas progestins (especially those with androgenic characteristics) increase VLDL catabolism and have the opposite effect. These effects would seem to conflict with observations that, in untreated subjects, women have lower levels of triglycerides than men. The explanation for this discrepancy lies in the "first-pass" effect of oral estrogens, particularly oral synthetic estrogens. The first-pass effect is the result of the unphysiologic bolus seen with orally administered drugs. The acute impact of this bolus is to increase the hepatic synthesis of various proteins, including apoB, the principal protein of VLDL. This effect is well recognized with the synthetic estrogens used in the combined oral contraceptive pill, but is also seen with the natural estrogens prescribed for ERT.

Estrogens, both exogenous and endogenous, lower plasma LDL levels by increasing the number of $apoB_{100}$, E receptors in tissues, especially the liver. This results in enhanced clearance of LDLs from the plasma. The effects of progestins on LDL metabolism are unclear. Studies in rat liver have shown that progestins will affect the activity of *hydroxy-methyl-glutaryl-transferase coenzyme A (HMGCoA) reductase,* the rate-limiting step in cholesterol synthesis, but only if estrogens are coadministered (17). Increasing the activity of this enzyme would accelerate intracellular synthesis of cholesterol. To prevent an excessive buildup of intracellular cholesterol, the activity of apoB_{100}, E receptors is therefore downregulated so that less LDL is taken up from the plasma, leading to increased plasma levels of LDL cholesterol.

Gonadal hormones may affect HDL metabolism in a number of ways. Hepatic lipase, the enzyme responsible for the catabolism of HDL particles, is exquisitely sensitive to hormonal control, being inhibited by estrogens and activated by progestins, especially those with androgenic properties. The activity of this enzyme will influence the plasma levels of HDL_2 in particular. In addition, estrogens increase the hepatic secretion of apoAI, the major protein of HDL. The precise mechanisms by which pharmacologic administration of estrogens increases plasma HDL levels—increased synthesis, reduced catabolism, or both—are poorly understood. The relative importance of these mechanisms will become apparent when we consider the role of plasma HDL in cardiovascular disease.

PLASMA LIPOPROTEINS AND CARDIOVASCULAR RISK

Numerous epidemiologic, clinical, and experimental studies have shown that plasma total cholesterol levels in both sexes correlate positively with the incidence of CHD and that this relationship is due to the levels of LDL cholesterol, the major carrier of cholesterol in the plasma. Furthermore, levels of HDL have been shown to correlate negatively with the incidence of CHD, consistent with their proposed role in removing cholesterol from peripheral tissues. There is limited evidence that the HDL_2 subfraction is more closely related to cardioprotection than HDL_3. These issues have recently been reviewed (11, 18, 19).

The relative contributions of LDL and HDL to the disease process are poorly understood. In the recent Helsinki Heart Study (20, 21), the authors concluded that the increases in HDL cholesterol levels induced by LDL-lowering therapy accounted for as much of the observed protection from CHD as the fall in LDL cholesterol levels (the primary target of the study).

Other aspects of plasma lipoproteins may have an impact on the development of CHD. There is intriguing evidence that chylomicron remnants may be atherogenic (22), but the role of VLDLs (and thus plasma triglycerides) is less certain (23, 24). Although subjects with CHD frequently have raised triglyceride levels, these may be secondary to reduced levels of HDL cholesterol, and there is disagreement over whether this latter abnormality is the primary source for the increased risk.

In the past, many gynecologists have been concerned that our knowledge of the risk of CHD associated with plasma lipoproteins is based mainly on studies of middle-aged hypercholesterolemic men. However, evidence that plasma lipoproteins are similarly important in women is accumulating (25). Recent epidemiologic studies have shown that plasma lipoproteins, particularly HDLs, are predictors of cardiovascular disease in women (26, 27). Furthermore, analysis of recent data from the Framingham Heart Study (28) indicates that triglycerides are a strong independent predictor of CHD in older women.

The lack of data on risk factors in women is due to many factors, especially the lower incidence of the disease in young women compared to young men. Consequently, epidemiologic studies of cardiovascular disease in women have needed to be much larger to possess sufficient statistical power to allow valid conclusions to be drawn. Because of this restriction, epidemiologists have in the past concentrated on middle-aged men, knowing that a reasonable number of events will be seen within the projected time frame of the study. Thus, studies of lipoproteins and CHD in men are not matched by studies in women.

Despite the restricted nature of the data, we know that women with high LDL and low HDL levels will develop more CHD than their counterparts with normal levels of these lipoproteins. There is no evidence that altering the plasma lipid risk profile in a potentially *adverse* direction, that is increasing LDL and decreasing HDL, will increase the incidence of CHD. Such studies would be unethical, and so the relevance of lipid risk factors in women has to be assessed from studies in which the lipid profile has been altered in a theoretically beneficial manner: by estrogen, which decreases LDL and increases HDL (1) or by phenytoin and other inducers of hepatic enzymes, which increase HDL (29). In both these studies, "improving" the lipoprotein profile decreased the incidence of CHD in women.

EFFECTS OF CHANGES IN OVARIAN FUNCTION

Given the sex differences in plasma lipoproteins, it might be expected that substantial changes in plasma estradiol levels would be associated with marked alterations in plasma lipoprotein concentrations. However, analysis of studies of both natural and artificially induced menopause indicate that estrogen deficiency has surprisingly little effect (15). Postmenopausal women have more LDL and triglycerides than do premenopausal women (30), but such studies may be confounded by the influence of age. When women of similar age have been compared, postmenopausal women have similar levels of HDL cholesterol and higher levels of LDL cholesterol than do their premenopausal counterparts (31). There is some evidence that the LDL particles isolated from postmenopausal women are smaller than those isolated from premenopausal women (32). Such small LDL particles have been implicated in the development of premature CHD (33).

However, such cross-sectional studies are difficult to interpret because they may simply reflect characteristics of women who have undergone an early menopause, rather than the effects of loss of ovarian function. In one of the few prospective studies, Matthews et al. (34) observed a cohort of middle-aged women for 2½ years and compared their changes in plasma lipoprotein profiles with those seen in an age-matched control group of women who remained premenopausal. HDL cholesterol levels fell by 6% in the women who underwent the menopause, but were unchanged in those who remained premenopausal. The fall of HDL levels appeared to be due to reductions in both HDL_2 and HDL_3. LDL cholesterol levels increased in both groups, but more so in those who became postmenopausal. However, measurement of plasma apolipoproteins failed to confirm all of these changes.

There are obvious difficulties in studying such a gradual process as the climacteric, especially when the onset of this process is difficult to define and predict. Women who have experienced premature menopause may help our understanding of estrogen/lipoprotein interactions, because they can be compared to closely age-matched premenopausal controls. In such a study, Sznadjerman and Oliver (35) observed increases in serum cholesterol and triglycerides in women who had undergone a spontaneous premature menopause compared to age-matched controls. Our own studies have shown that this increase in total cholesterol is due to an increase in LDL cholesterol, with no change in HDL cholesterol (Cust, Crook, and Stevenson, unpublished observations). However, this lack of change in HDLs conceals a potentially adverse shift in the HDL subfraction distribution in these women, with lower levels of HDL_2 (a subfraction more closely related to protection from CHD) being matched by higher levels of HDL_3. Thus, while total HDL levels (i.e, the cholesterol content of the entire HDL class) may not be altered as a consequence of loss of ovarian function, important changes may be occurring in HDL subfractions. Because these changes cancel each other out, measurement of the total HDL fraction (and not the subfractions) may, at best, be of little value and, at worst, may fail to detect clinically relevant changes in HDL metabolism.

Studies of plasma lipoproteins in women undergoing bilateral oophorectomy are contradictory and have rarely been of sufficient size to give unequivocal results. The majority fail to demonstrate any effects of acute loss of ovarian function on plasma lipoproteins, although increases in triglycerides have been reported (36, 37). However, it is not known whether these increases reflect the effects of operative procedures themselves, rather than the loss of ovarian function.

An alternative approach to understanding the effects of loss of ovarian function on plasma lipoproteins has been to study women rendered temporarily postmenopausal through treatment for conditions such as endometriosis with luteinizing hormone–releasing hormone (LHRH) supra-agonists. Despite dramatic reductions in plasma estradiol levels, these drugs have virtually no effect on plasma lipoprotein levels (38, 39).

Another phenomenon that conflicts with present concepts is the absence of an effect on plasma lipoproteins during the elevation in plasma estradiol levels associated with female puberty (40). Taken together, these findings indicate that the endocrine control of plasma lipoprotein metabolism requires further study.

EFFECTS OF POSTMENOPAUSAL ESTROGENS AND PROGESTINS

Interest in the effects of gonadal hormones on plasma lipoprotein metabolism has initiated extensive reviews (15, 41). To avoid repetition, we intend to concentrate on recent developments in this field, including the use of less androgenic progestins, of transdermal routes of administration, and of lower doses of gonadal steroids.

Effects of Unopposed Estrogens

Recognition of the potent hepatic effects of synthetic estrogens, such as ethinyl estradiol and mestranol, has led to the discontinuation of their use for the relief of postmenopausal symptoms. Although the synthetic estrogens have been superseded by "natural" estrogens, such as 17β-estradiol and conjugated equine estrogens, their effects on plasma lipoprotein levels are of historical significance and will be briefly discussed.

The first convincing demonstration of the effects of estrogens on plasma lipoproteins came from Barr et al. (42). These authors showed that ethinyl estradiol given to male myocardial infarction survivors induced an increase in HDLs (measured then as α-lipoproteins) and a decrease in LDLs (measured as β-lipoproteins). Following this, Robinson et al. (43) reported on 108 women given 0.01 mg/day ethinyl estradiol or 0.625 to 10.0 mg/day conjugated equine estrogens (CEE) (Premarin: Wyeth-Ayerst). A fall in the α/β ratio, clearly related to estrogen dose, developed within 1 month and was maintained over the 1-year duration of the study.

Subsequent investigation of a wide range of estrogens (reviewed by Godsland et al.) (15) has confirmed the general impression that they lower LDLs, raise HDLs, and increase triglycerides. These changes are dose related, and their extent varies according to the type of estrogen. Importantly, the effects of estrogens on plasma lipoproteins depends on the route of administration, and it is appropriate to distinguish between studies using oral and non-oral routes.

Because gonadal steroids induce reciprocal changes in LDLs and HDLs, a finding of "no change" in total cholesterol is of little value, as it may hide substantial changes in the lipoprotein profile. Because of this, it is necessary to exclude studies that have only measured total lipids and not the lipoprotein fractions.

EFFECTS OF ORAL ESTROGENS

Although various reports of the effects of postmenopausal estrogens were published in the late 1960s, the first detailed evaluation of the effects of oral estrogen on plasma lipoproteins was performed by Wallentin and Larsson-Cohn (44). They compared the effects of 50 μg/day ethinyl estradiol and 2 mg/day estradiol valerate (Progynova; Schering Corporation, Kenilworth, NJ) over 6 months in postmenopausal women.

With the synthetic estrogen, LDLs fell by 30%, triglycerides and HDLs both increased by 30 to 40% (Fig. 7.5). Lesser falls in LDLs (6 to 8%) were seen with the natural estrogen; triglycerides were not significantly changed but HDL levels increased by 4 to 14%. Based on these data, the authors speculated that estrogen replacement therapy might reduce the incidence of CHD, although they were concerned by the increases in triglycerides seen with ethinyl estradiol.

The dose of ethinyl estradiol used in this study was high. Subsequent comparisons (45, 46) have shown that the extent of these changes is reduced when the dose of ethinyl estradiol is lowered, although the differences between "synthetic" and "natural" estrogens, especially in terms of triglyceride levels, are generally maintained.

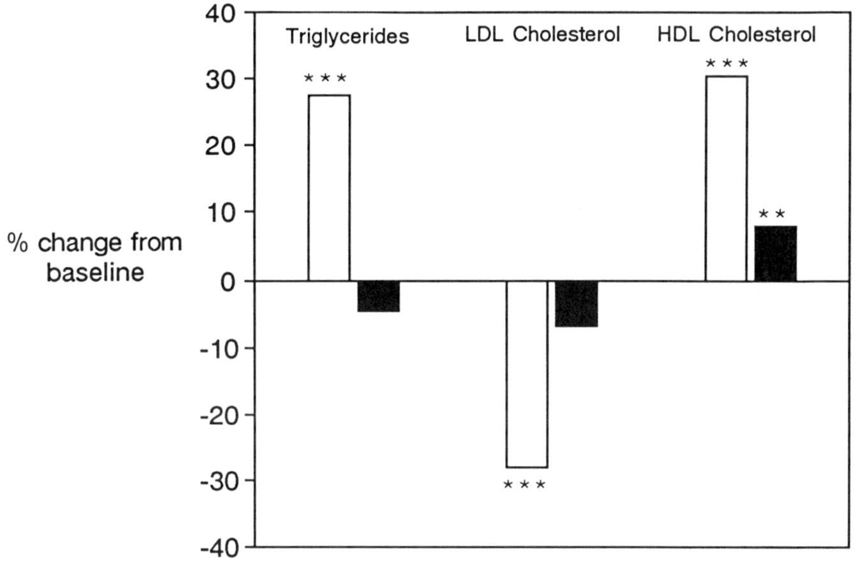

Figure 7.5. Comparison of the effects of synthetic versus natural estrogen on plasma triglycerides, LDL cholesterol, and HDL cholesterol. 39 women were randomized to receive either 50 μg/day ethinyl estradiol (*open bars*) or 2 mg/day estradiol valerate (*closed bars*). Mean changes over 6 months of treatment are plotted; significant differences from baseline are coded as ** $P<0.01$, *** $P<0.001$. (Adapted from Wallentin L, Larsson-Cohn U. Metabolic and hormonal effects of post-menopausal oestrogen replacement therapy. II. Plasma lipids. Acta Endocrinol 1977;86:597–607.)

These observations with oral estradiol valerate were extended by Tikkanen et al. (47, 48). When a mixed group of normo- and hypercholesterolemic postmenopausal women were given 2 mg/day estradiol valerate, HDL cholesterol levels increased significantly (but only after 6 months of treatment), whereas LDL cholesterol levels fell within 3 months. It is of interest that the extent of the LDL-lowering effect depends on the initial level (Fig. 7.6). Thus, LDL levels were not lowered if the pretreatment LDL level was normal or low.

This important observation may explain some of the differences in response to estrogens reported by various studies: the effect of an estrogen formulation on LDL cholesterol will depend on the baseline LDL levels in that particular study group. This must be borne in mind when data on LDLs are reported and interpreted, and especially when the effects of different estrogens are compared. Presentation of absolute values is mandatory if meaningful

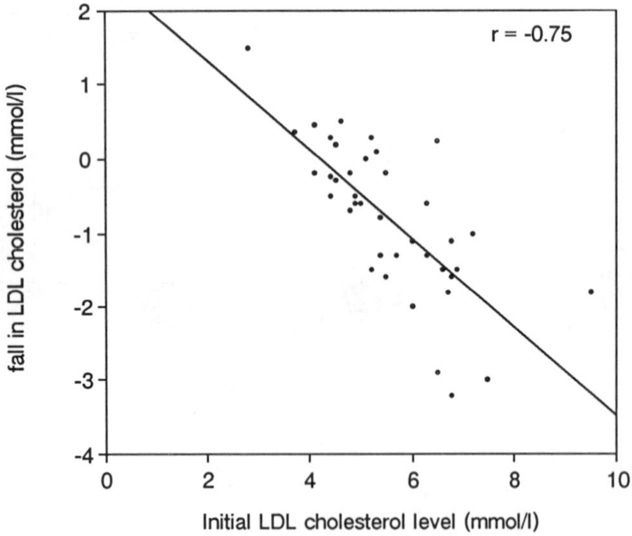

Figure 7.6. Relation between initial LDL cholesterol levels and subsequent changes in LDL cholesterol levels. Thirty-nine women were treated with estradiol valerate 2 mg/day for 3 months. The effects of this therapy on LDL cholesterol are plotted relative to the pretreatment level. (Adapted from Tikkanen MJ, Nikkila EA, Vartiainen E. Natural oestrogen as an effective treatment for Type II hyperlipoproteinaemia in postmenopausal women. Lancet 1978;2:490–491.)

comparisons of different therapies are to be made; presentation as "percentage changes" may mask significant differences in pretreatment values between the various treatment groups.

In the United States, the most widely prescribed preparation used for replacement therapy is CEE, a mixture of various steroids, predominantly estrone sulfate. The first large study of the effects of CEE came from the Lipid Research Clinics program. Using a cross-sectional multicenter study design, Wahl et al. (49) compared 239 women taking various regimens of CEE with 370 controls closely matched for age, body mass, smoking habits, and alcohol use. Women using various doses of CEE had 25% higher triglyceride levels, 13% higher HDL cholesterol levels, and 14% lower LDL cholesterol levels compared to nonusers.

Subsequent studies with different estrogen preparations and doses have shown that the increase in HDLs seen in estrogen users is predominantly due to an increase in the HDL_2 fraction (50, 51), the fraction most closely correlated with cardioprotection. Increasing the dose of estradiol valerate from 2 to 4 mg/day did not increase the effects on the plasma lipoprotein profile (52), suggesting that it may not be possible to increase HDLs above a certain level. The ability of high doses of natural estrogens to increase triglycerides has been confirmed by Fahreus et al. (53) using oral micronized 17β-estradiol 4 mg/day.

In some studies, the doses of estrogen prescribed were higher than those in current use. With the more commonly used dose of CEE (0.625 mg/day), not all of the expected changes have been seen. With this dose, Barnes et al. (54) reported increases of 13% in HDL cholesterol and decreases of 16% in LDL cholesterol at 1 year, but no change in triglycerides. In contrast, Farish et al. (51) studied 21 women every 2 months for 6 months of therapy with the same dose of CEE and reported that triglycerides were increased by 15% and HDL cholesterol by 15% (with the HDL_2 fraction increasing by 36%), while LDL cholesterol levels decreased by 9%. However, not all of these changes were statistically significant at all visits.

Many subsequent studies of unopposed CEE 0.625 mg/day support this overall pattern (55, 56) but the changes have not always achieved statistical significance. Some studies have tended to involve relatively small numbers of subjects and are unlikely to have had sufficient statistical power to detect small changes. This is particularly relevant with triglycerides, where a large intra-and inter-patient variability exists.

What are the effects of estrone? Lagrelius et al. (57) showed that 2.5 mg/day piperazine estrone sulfate (Ogen; Abbott Laboratories, Chicago, IL) for 3 weeks out of 4 increased HDL cholesterol. Recently, Colvin et al. (58) compared the effects of graduated doses of 17β-estradiol and piperazine estrone sulfate on plasma lipoprotein metabolism in six postmenopausal women. Identical plasma estrone and estradiol levels were observed with the two preparations due to interconversion of estradiol and estrone. Surprisingly, estrone induced greater falls in LDLs and increases in HDLs than did estradiol. The authors suggested that these differences were due to different hepatic effects. Further investigation of this phenomenon is needed.

EFFECTS OF NON-ORAL ESTROGENS

Oral estrogens are partially absorbed as a bolus, which may exaggerate hepatic effects. This "first-pass" effect on clotting factors and lipoprotein metabolism may induce unwanted metabolic disturbances, such as increased secretion of triglyceride-rich lipoproteins. Various non-oral routes of administration have been developed (Table 7.2). The rationale behind their use derives not only from avoidance of the inconvenience of pill-taking, but from a reduction of the effect of these steroids on the liver.

Table 7.2.
Non-Oral Estrogens

Patches
Gels
Pellets
Others (buccal, injectables, etc.)

Percutaneous administration of estradiol from gels (Oestrogel; Laboratoires Besins-Iscovesco) induces less change in plasma lipoproteins than oral administration. Fahreus et al. (53) randomized 38 postmenopausal women to either oral or percutaneous administration of 17β-estradiol 2 to 4 mg/day. Oral, but not percutaneous, estradiol increased HDL cholesterol. The percutaneous preparation reduced LDLs after 6 months, but to a lesser extent than was seen with oral administration. These authors subsequently reported that the increase in HDL cholesterol seen with oral administration was restricted to the HDL_2 fraction (50). Using the same percutaneous therapy, Basdevant et al. (59) observed no effect on LDLs or HDLs, but a fall in triglycerides.

There are conflicting reports on the effects of subcutaneous estradiol pellets (implants) on plasma lipoproteins (60). Using a 25-mg estradiol pellet, Lobo et al. (61) found no effect on LDLs but a striking increase (nearly 50%) in HDL cholesterol. Subsequent studies, including one from the same group (62) have failed to detect such a large effect. In the most comprehensive evaluation of estradiol pellets (63), 14 women given 50-mg pellets of 17β-estradiol were studied for 6 months. Small but significant falls in LDL cholesterol (3 to 9%) and increase in HDLs (5 to 8%) were seen. The increase in HDLs appeared to be due to increases in both HDL_2 and HDL_3, although these measurements were not made in all subjects. Plasma triglyceride levels fell by 4 to 8%, but this fall was not statistically significant.

The most recent development in estrogen administration has been transdermal delivery systems or "patches." Preliminary reports conflict as to whether transdermal estradiol (Estraderm; Ciba Pharmaceutical Co., Summit, NJ) affects plasma lipoprotein metabolism. Chetkowksi et al. (55) found no effect of estradiol patches given at a range of doses up to 200 μg/day. However, the patches were used for only 21 days, which may have been insufficient time for effects on plasma lipoproteins to become evident. Stanzyk et al. (62) randomized 20 women to receive estradiol pellets or patches. Both therapies increased HDLs, whereas neither regimen had a significant effect on LDL cholesterol levels.

Our own studies with a group of 30 women receiving transdermal estradiol show that this regimen will lower triglycerides and LDL cholesterol but has little effect on HDL cholesterol (Crook, Stevenson and Whitehead, unpublished observations).

Effects of Unopposed Progestins

An evaluation of the effects of unopposed progestins on plasma lipoprotein levels is of interest not only because these agents have been used as postmenopausal monotherapy, but because an understanding of the effects of combined therapies demands appreciation of the metabolic effects on both components.

When given orally, natural progesterone is poorly absorbed and is also rapidly metabolized, and so various synthetic progestins have been developed. These can be divided into two groups: *pregnanes* (C-21 progestins derived from 17α-hydroxyprogesterone), such as medroxyprogesterone acetate (MPA) (Provera; Upjohn, Kalamazoo, MI) and dydrogesterone (Duphaston: Duphar), and *estranes* (C-19 progestins derived from 19-nor-testosterone), such as norethindrone (Micronor; Ortho Pharmaceutical Corp., Raritan, NJ) and levonorgestrel (Neogest; Schering Corporation, Kenilworth NJ) (Fig. 7.7).

There is a further division of C-19 progestins into those derived from norethindrone, such as norethindrone acetate, and those derived from levonorgestrel, such as desogestrel (Fig. 7.7). This latter group result from molecular manipulations in which the androgenic characteristics of the parent compound have been minimized, leaving the progestational properties unchanged.

In addition to binding to progesterone receptors, synthetic progestins may also demonstrate other hormonal and anti-hormonal activities, such as estrogenicity, anti-estrogenicity, androgenicity, and anti-androgenicity. If given in sufficiently high doses, virtually all progestins can display such characteristics in bioassay systems.

Progesterone and the C-21 derivatives have a high affinity for progesterone receptors and minimal, but definite, estrogenic and androgenic activities, whereas progestins derived from testosterone can be divided into two distinct groups: those such as levonorgestrel that retain some of the androgenic activities of the parent compounds, and the "third-generation" progestins such as desogestrel (Organon, Teknika Corp., Durham, NC), gestodene (Schering) and norgestimate (Ortho), which have minimal androgenic activity.

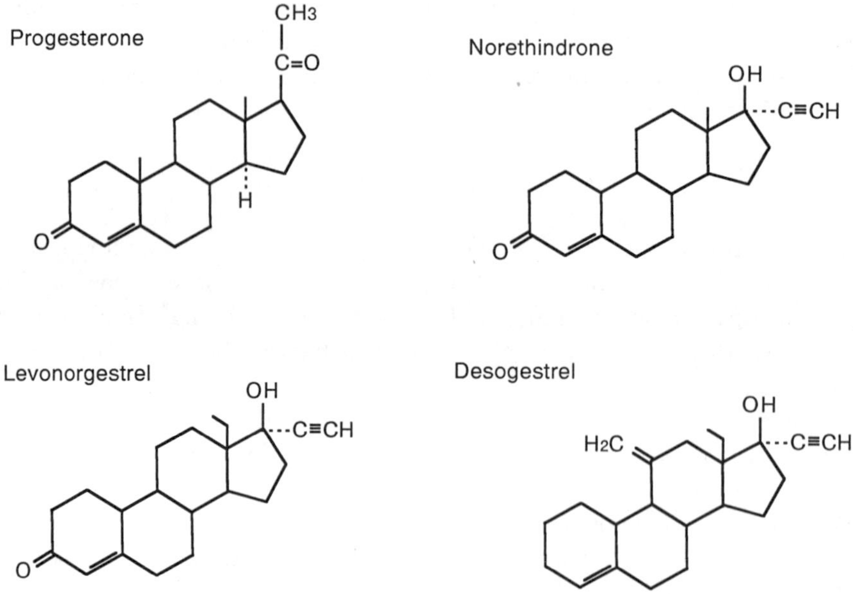

Figure 7.7. Structure of selected progestogens used for hormone replacement therapy.

Natural progesterone is usually given as a micronized preparation and has virtually no effect on plasma lipoproteins (64, 65), although the number of subjects in these studies was small. Cyproterone acetate (Schering), a steroid with anti-androgenic properties, has been reported to have no effect on LDLs or HDLs when given at a dose of 2 mg/day (66). MPA has been held to be similarly inert, although the data from which this conclusion was reached (67–69) have been challenged on statistical grounds (41). When given at high doses (100 mg/day) to women with endometrial cancer, MPA reduces HDLs in a dose-dependent manner, consistent with the residual androgenic properties of this steroid (70). Intramuscular MPA injections, 150 mg every 3 months, had no effects on HDLs, but LDLs fell by 20% (54). In contrast, when the same dose was given every second week, large falls in HDLs (especially a 60% fall in HDL_2) were reported (71). These authors concluded that MPA lowers HDL levels in accord with its identity as a progestin, but has no effect on LDL, conflicting with the observations of Barnes et al. (54).

When given on their own, both levonorgestrel and norethindrone have potentially adverse effects on CHD risk markers. Work by Silfverstolpe et al. (68), Hirvonen et al. (67), and Tikkanen et al. (69) has conclusively shown that these progestins increase LDL levels and reduce HDL levels. In the long-term study of Farish et al. (72), postmenopausal women were treated with norethindrone (5 mg/day) for 1 year. LDL cholesterol levels increased by 14% and triglyceride levels were decreased by 17 to 30%. HDL cholesterol levels fell by 40%, and this was due principally to a reduction in HDL_2.

Less information is available concerning third-generation progestins. Kuusi et al. (73) treated postmenopausal women with desogestrel 125 μg/day. This progestin had no effect on HDL cholesterol, whereas levonorgestrel, given at the same dose, lowered HDL cholesterol, especially HDL_2.

Effects of Combined Estrogen/Progestin Therapy

Interest in the safety of ERT has led to a large and often contradictory series of publications that have compared the metabolic effects of various estrogen/progestin combinations (15, 41, 74). In many studies, the doses of steroids were excessively high. It must also be emphasized that the effects of a given dose of progestin will depend on the estrogen with which it is combined. Most of our understanding of the effects of estrogen/progestin combinations arises from studies in Europe and Scandinavia that use 17β-estradiol or estradiol valerate. Comparable data relating to combinations using CEE, the most commonly used estrogen in the United States, are limited. Thus, the applicability of the existing data to current U.S. prescribing habits is questionable. For example, a given dose of a progestin may result in an overall reduction in HDL cholesterol levels when combined with estrogen administered percutaneously, but this may not apply when the same dose of progestin is combined with an oral estrogen.

The major problem in the interpretation of studies of combined therapies lies in the conventional choice of blood sampling during the estrogen plus progestin phase of the treatment cycle. With very few exceptions (e.g., Jensen et al. [75]), investigators do not study their patients during both estrogen-alone and combined phases. Thus, we cannot assess net risk because we do not know if the changes seen during the combined phases would be ameliorated by those seen during the estrogen-only phase.

Logically, the net effect of an estrogen/progestin combination will depend on the relative potencies of the two steroids, and it should be possible to formulate a combined regimen that maintains the potentially cardioprotective pattern of low LDL and high HDL levels seen in users of unopposed estrogen. Evidence that this is possible comes from the cross-sectional study of Barrett-Connor et al. (76). These authors found no difference in plasma lipoprotein levels between users of estrogen-only formulations and of combined formulations containing MPA, although the number of users of combined therapy was relatively small (69 women). Prospective data confirming these findings are urgently needed.

COMBINED FORMULATIONS CONTAINING PROGESTERONE AND PROGESTERONE DERIVATIVES

Natural progesterone (Utrogestan; Laboratoires Besins-Iscovesco) 200 to 300 mg/day for 10 days each cycle has been reported to have no significant effect on levels of LDLs, HDLs, and HDL subfractions when combined with percutaneous estradiol or oral estradiol valerate (77, 78). However, in the former study a statistically significant fall of 10% in HDL cholesterol was evident.

In a pilot study, Hargrove et al. (79) treated 10 women with a continuous regimen of 0.35 mg/day micronized estradiol and 200 to 300 mg/day micronized progesterone. Although this regimen induced amenorrhea without endometrial proliferation or hyperplasia, the lipoprotein data are difficult to interpret. The authors claim to have obtained a 50% increase in mean HDL cholesterol levels. The pretreatment HDL cholesterol levels in these subjects were well below the lower limits of normality for U.S. women, and in one subject, levels of HDL cholesterol increased by 300% after 12 months of therapy. Such large changes in HDLs have not previously been reported using any form of drug therapy, and may reflect methodological problems such as artifactual losses during storage of frozen samples.

Cyproterone acetate has been evaluated as a progestin for combined ERT. A combination of cyproterone acetate, 2 mg/day and ethinyl estradiol, 35 to 50 μg/day or estradiol valerate, 2 mg/day, lowered LDL cholesterol (66, 80), presumably reflecting an inability of the progestin to oppose the effects of the estrogen. In contrast, the progestin appeared to oppose the action of estrogen on HDLs, with no overall changes being seen with the combined formulation.

Sporrong et al. (81) used a continuous regimen of 2 mg/day 17β-estradiol and either 5 or 2.5 mg/day megestrol acetate (Megace; Bristol-Myers, Evansville, IN). After 1 year, LDL was lowered by the formulation containing the higher dose of megestrol but, paradoxically, not by the formulation containing the lower dose of progestin. Although both regimens reduced HDL cholesterol after 4 months, there were no significant changes from baseline after 1 year. We have previously suggested that these inconsistencies may reflect withdrawal of subjects from the study (82).

Recently, Sonnendecker et al. (56) have presented a double-blind crossover study of 22 postmenopausal women given CEE 0.625 mg/day with or without medrogestone (Colprone; Wyeth-Ayerst, Philadelphia, PA) 5 mg/day for 10 days each cycle. The reductions in LDL cholesterol levels induced by CEE were not opposed by the progestin, and, unlike the previous studies concerning cyproterone acetate, the increase in HDL cholesterol was maintained. Similar results have been obtained in a pilot study (83) of dydrogesterone 10 to 20 mg/day for 12 days/cycle combined with CEE 1.25 mg/day.

Some studies have reported that when added to estradiol valerate 2 mg/day, MPA 10 mg/day for 10 days each cycle will lower HDL and HDL_2 (e.g., Ottosson et al. [78]); others (e.g., Hirvonen et al. [84]) using the same formulation reported no significant effect of MPA on HDL cholesterol. One possible explanation for this discrepancy is that the bioavailability of the MPA preparations differed between the studies.

One of the more interesting studies of MPA in combined therapy is that of Sherwin and Gelfand (85). This was a double-blind study of 95 women randomly assigned to either CEE 0.625 or 1.25 mg/day, combined with a 10-day course of either MPA 5 mg/day or placebo. In the groups given unopposed estrogen, only the higher estrogen dose lowered LDL cholesterol, but both estrogen doses increased HDL cholesterol and triglycerides (Table 7.3). When MPA was added, the progestin countered the increase in HDLs seen with the low estrogen dose formulation, although HDLs remained elevated with the higher estrogen dose.

Many of the studies that have evaluated continuous combined estrogen/progestin regimens are flawed because only small numbers of patients were recruited; few have included a control group. Weinstein (86) evaluated a range of formulations containing CEE and various doses of MPA, including

Table 7.3.
Effects of Conjugated Equine Estrogens (CEE) with and without Medroxyprogesterone Acetate (MPA) on Serum Lipids and Lipoproteins[a]

Treatment Group	% Change in LDL[b]	% Change in HDL[b]
0.625 mg/day CEE	−0.6 (ns)	+13.2 (P<0.01)
0.625 mg/day CEE + 5 mg/day MPA	−3.8 (ns)	+4.6 (ns)
1.25 mg/day CEE	−17.6 (P<0.01)	+18.8 (P<0.01)
1.25 mg/day CEE + 5 mg/day MPA	−8.7 (P<0.01)	+14.1 (P<0.01)

[a]Adapted from Sherwin BB, Gelfand MM. A prospective one-year study of estrogen and progestin in postmenopausal women: effects on clinical symptoms and lipoprotein lipids. Obstet Gynecol 1989; 73:759–766.
[b]Over 1 year of therapy.

both sequential and continuous progestin administration. No statistically significant changes in HDL cholesterol were seen. LDL cholesterol levels fell with the sequential and lower MPA dose continuous regimens, but not with the higher-dose continuous MPA formulation.

Prough et al. (87) investigated 16 women given continuous CEE 0.625 mg/day and MPA either 2.5 mg or 10 mg/day, both continuously. After 9 months of treatment, no significant changes in HDL cholesterol, LDL cholesterol, or triglycerides were seen, indicating that the progestin had countered the abilities of CEE to lower LDL and increase HDL and triglycerides. Similar results were obtained by Luciano et al. (88) using 10 mg/day MPA.

COMBINED FORMULATIONS CONTAINING NORETHINDRONE AND NORETHINDRONE DERIVATIVES

Combinations of estradiol and norethindrone reduce LDL cholesterol (89, 90). Additionally, very high doses of this progestin (10 mg/day) can overwhelm the ability of estradiol to increase HDL cholesterol (67): indeed, a fall of 20% from pretreatment values was observed. Subsequent studies using lower doses (e.g., 1 mg/day) have reported similar falls in HDL cholesterol (90). Although Jensen et al. (89) measured HDL cholesterol in women treated with low-dose norethindrone, the results of this study are difficult to interpret due to large changes in HDL cholesterol seen in the placebo group.

Continuous regimens containing 17β-estradiol 2 mg/day and norethindrone acetate 0.5 or 1 mg/day have been evaluated by Sporrong et al. (81). After 1 year, LDL was consistently lowered in users of the formulation containing norethindrone 1 mg/day, but paradoxically, not by the formulation containing 0.5 mg/day. The higher norethindrone dose formulation lowered HDL cholesterol by 15% after 1 year, whereas the lower-dose formulation lowered HDL cholesterol by 15% after 4 months, with levels returning to baseline over the following 8 months. We have previously voiced our concerns over the changing study population seen in this trial.

Farish et al. (91) studied 38 women given a continuous regimen containing estradiol valerate 2 mg/day (with or without estriol 1 mg/day) and norethindrone (1 mg/day) for 48 weeks. Decreases of 10% in both LDL and HDL cholesterol were reported. The fall in HDL appeared to be due to a decrease in the HDL_3 subfraction.

The importance of estrogen dose on the net effect of combined HRT was elegantly demonstrated by the work of Christiansen and colleagues (75).

These authors gave 30 healthy postmenopausal women one of three different combinations of micronized 17β-estradiol and norethindrone acetate. The progestin was always given for 10 days of the cycle at a dose of 1 mg/day, but the estrogen was prescribed for 28 days at doses of 1, 2, or 4 mg/day. This study is one of the few to question how the overall exposure to combined ERT affects the plasma lipoprotein risk profile: fasting blood samples were taken at frequent intervals over two cycles of therapy. During the estrogen-alone phase, HDL cholesterol increased in a dose-dependent manner, returning toward baseline when the progestin was added (Fig. 7.8). Mirroring these changes, levels of LDL cholesterol fell, again in a dose-dependent manner, but returned toward baseline during the combined phase of treatment. However, even during the times of maximal progestational impact, HDL remained high and LDL low with the higher estrogen dose. This study both emphasizes the importance of the timing of blood sampling when performing metabolic studies and demonstrates that minimizing the dose of estrogen will reduce the effects on plasma lipoproteins.

Transdermal administration of norethindrone in combined HRT is cur-

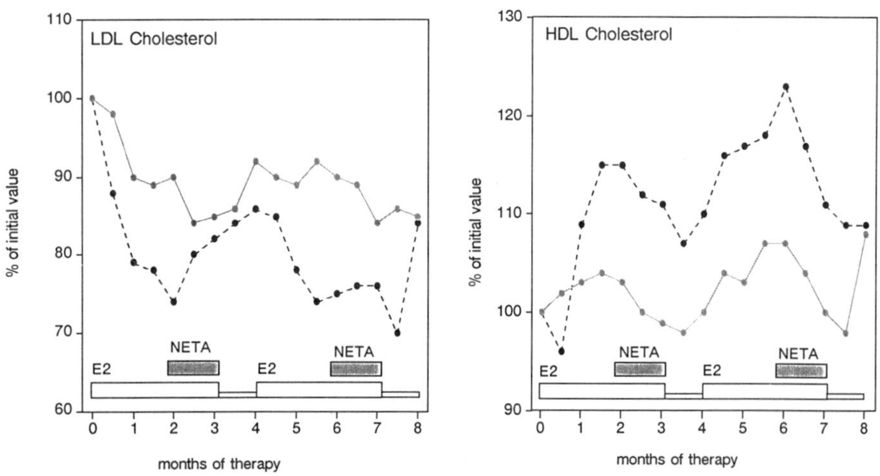

Figure 7.8. Cyclical changes in LDL and HDL cholesterol in women treated with ERT. Twenty women were treated with 17β-estradiol (E2) at doses of 1 mg/day (*solid line*) or 4 mg/day (*broken line*) together with sequential norethindrone acetate (NETA) 1 mg/day for 10 days per cycle. (Adapted from Jensen J, Nilas L, Christiansen C. Cyclic changes in serum cholesterol and lipoproteins following different dose of combined postmenopausal hormone replacement therapy. Br J Obstet Gynaecol 1986;93:613–618.)

rently under development. Non-oral administration of norethindrone and 17β-estradiol does not avoid the falls in HDL cholesterol seen with the oral combined HRT, but these are mainly in the HDL_3 subfraction with no consistent changes in HDL_2 (Crook, Stevenson and Whitehead, unpublished observations). Falls in LDL are still evident with nonoral norethindrone.

COMBINED FORMULATIONS CONTAINING LEVONORGESTREL

Comparative studies (67, 68, 84) have shown that levonorgestrel is able to counter the increase in HDL seen with estrogens, and result in lowered HDL levels (Fig. 7.9). These findings have been supported by others (77, 78). However, the dose of levonorgestrel used in these studies (120 to 250 μg/day) was greatly in excess of that required for endometrial protection. When a more reasonable dose of 75 μg/day is used, which still affords endometrial protection, no overall effects on HDL or LDL were seen (92).

One of the most detailed metabolic studies of the effects of combined

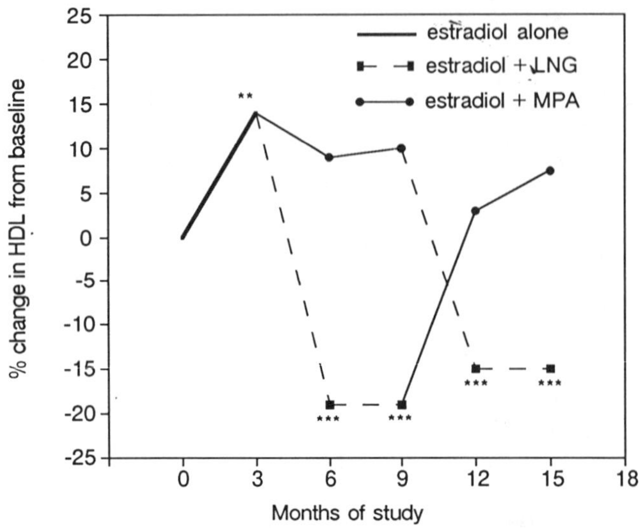

Figure 7.9. Effects of different progestins on HDL cholesterol. After 3 months of unopposed therapy, 24 women were randomized to receive estradiol plus 12-day monthly courses of medroxyprogesterone (MPA) 10 mg/day or levonorgestrel (LNG) 0.25 mg/day. After a further 6 months of combined therapy, the treatment groups were crossed over for a further 6-month period. Mean changes from baseline are coded as ** $P<0.01$; *** $P<0.001$. (Adapted from Hirvonen E, Lipasti A, Malkonen M, et al. Clinical and lipid metabolic effects of unopposed oestrogen and two oestrogen-progestogen regimens in post-menopausal women. Maturitas 1987;9:69–79.)

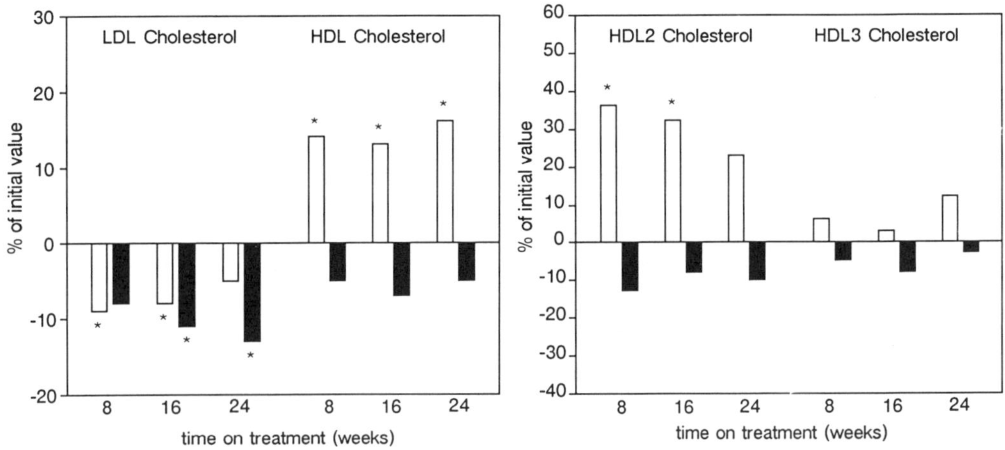

Figure 7.10. Effects of conjugated equine estrogens with and without progestin on plasma lipoprotein levels. Forty-two women received either unopposed CEE 0.625 mg/day (*open bars*) or CEE 0.625 mg/day plus levonorgestrel 75 μg/day for 12 days per cycle (*closed bars*). Mean changes from baseline are coded as * $P<0.05$. (Adapted from Farish E, Fletcher CD, Hart DM, et al. The effects of conjugated equine oestrogens with and without a cyclical progestogen on lipoproteins and HDL subfractions in postmenopausal women. Acta Endocrinol (Copenh) 1986;113:123–127.)

formulations containing levonorgestrel is that of Farish et al. (51). In this careful 24-week study, women were treated with unopposed CEE 0.625 mg/day or with CEE 0.625 mg/day plus levonorgestrel 75 μg/day for 12 days each cycle. Levonorgestrel opposed the increase in triglycerides seen in users of unopposed CEE (Fig. 7.10). This progestin did not oppose the LDL-lowering ability of unopposed estrogen, and LDL cholesterol levels with combined therapy remained low. In contrast, levonorgestrel opposed the action of estrogen on HDL, and HDL levels fell although this was not statistically significant.

SUMMARY AND CONCLUSIONS

The past 2 decades have been seen a sequence of comparative studies that have evaluated the effect of postmenopausal estrogens and progestins on plasma lipoproteins. The effects of these hormones on plasma lipoproteins are dose dependent, and many of these studies are difficult to reconcile because the doses of different steroids used were not strictly comparable. In particular, studies in which the doses of progestins used were the minimum needed for endometrial protection are rare. Allowing for the substantial differences in study design and methodologies, the following statements are, we believe, valid.

Effects of Unopposed Estrogens

Oral estrogens increase plasma triglycerides, whereas non-oral estrogens have no effect or may even lower triglycerides. "Synthetic" estrogens such as ethinyl estradiol have the greatest effect on triglyceride levels. Both oral and non-oral estrogens decrease LDL levels, and greater decreases have been seen with the oral route compared to estradiol creams and pellets. Scant data on patches is available. Oral estrogens, and some non-oral estrogens such as estradiol pellets, increase HDL levels. The increase in HDL seen with currently used doses of CEE has not been demonstrated in all studies. This has major implications if the cardioprotective effect of unopposed estrogen therapy is held to operate through HDL metabolism.

Effects of Combined Therapy

Where unopposed ERT is inadvisable, a progestin must be added, either cyclically or continuously. In general, progestins oppose the actions of estrogen on plasma lipoproteins. The overall effect on the plasma lipoprotein profile will depend on the dose and type (specifically, the androgenicity) of the progestin and on the dose and type of the estrogen. The progestin may oppose the estrogen poorly, giving rise to a formulation that retains some (or even all) of the potentially favorable effects on plasma lipoproteins, or it may overwhelm the estrogen, giving rise to a formulation with a potentially detrimental lipoprotein pattern. Between these two extremes are a wide range of options. Reducing the progestin dose in continuous combined therapy has not been conclusively shown to improve the lipoprotein profile seen with equivalent cyclical combined therapies.

A series of recommendations for studies into the risk profile of combined ERT can be made. Because the metabolic effects of progestins are so clearly dose related, it is essential that doses that confer similar degrees of endometrial protection are compared. In this context, the published literature often appears to refer to excessive doses of levonorgestrel and norethindrone, but inadequate doses of C-21 progestins. Furthermore, plasma lipoprotein levels may change with age and declining ovarian function, and studies that do not control for these factors by including an untreated referent group may be of limited interest. The issue of statistical power must be addressed; the loss to follow-up of subjects during a prospective trial may be so high as to confound the conclusions of the study.

Progestins lower triglyceride levels and can therefore oppose the potentially undesirable action of unopposed oral estrogen. Combined therapy results in no change in triglycerides, or perhaps an overall reduction in this lipid. Progestins tend to increase LDL cholesterol. However, they appear unable to match the ability of estrogens to lower LDL cholesterol, and the net result of most combinations is a fall in LDL cholesterol. Progestins decrease HDL cholesterol according to their androgenic characteristics. Progesterone derivatives with minimal androgenicity are weak in their opposition to the effects of estrogen. Progestins with established androgenic characteristics, such as norethindrone and levonorgestrel, are able to overwhelm the action of estrogen on HDL, particularly at high doses, leading to a net fall in this potentially cardioprotective lipoprotein. MPA comes somewhat in between the two categories, and the net effect will depend on the dose of MPA used.

Preliminary studies of progesterone derivatives such as megestrol and dydrogesterone offer the possibility of an oral combined regimen that increases HDL levels and decreases those of LDL. "Third-generation" progestins may also achieve this profile.

Overall, this research shows that the judicious balancing of estrogen and progestin in combined ERT will lead to a formulation that will maintain the potentially favorable lipoprotein profile and, hopefully, the cardiovascular protection associated with the use of unopposed estrogen.

Key Points

- The major public health benefit of estrogen replacement therapy (ERT) is a 50% reduction in the incidence of cardiovascular disease. Although this protection may be due in part to the effects of estrogen on arterial tone, changes in plasma lipoprotein risk markers have been held responsible for much of the protection enjoyed by users of unopposed ERT.

- Estrogens reduce plasma levels of low-density lipoprotein (LDL) and increase those of high-density lipoprotein (HDL). Both of these changes would be expected to reduce the incidence of arterial disease. The role of plasma triglycerides in atherogenesis is controversial. When given orally, estrogens raise plasma triglyceride levels, which may be undesirable. Such increases may offset some of the benefit accrued from lowering LDL and raising HDL levels.

- In non-hysterectomized women, most ERT is now prescribed as a combination of estrogen and a 10- to 14-day course of progestin. Progestins may oppose the potentially beneficial effects of estrogens. To retain the low-risk plasma lipoprotein profile associated with the use of unopposed ERT, there has been a concerted effort to develop combined regimens in which levels of LDL are lowered and those of HDL increased.

- The effects of estrogen/progestin combinations depend on the doses of the steroids, their type (synthetic versus natural), the route of administration (oral versus non-oral) and above all on the balance between the estrogen and the progestin.
- Non-oral estrogens have less influence on the plasma lipoprotein profile, but may still be beneficial. Progestins vary widely in their ability to oppose estrogen-induced changes in plasma lipoproteins. The ability of progestins to lower plasma triglyceride levels may be beneficial. Progesterone derivatives such as megestrol and dydrogesterone offer the possibility of an oral combined regimen that increases HDL levels and decreases those of LDL. "Third-generation" progestins such as desogestrel and gestodene may also achieve this profile.
- Overall, research suggests that judicious balancing of estrogen and progestin will give a formulation that will maintain a favorable lipoprotein profile and, hopefully, the cardiovascular protection associated with the use of unopposed estrogen.

References

1. Bush TL, Barrett-Connor E, Cowan LD, et al. Cardiovascular mortality and noncontraceptive use of estrogem in women: results from the Lipid Research Clinics Program Follow-up Study. Circulation 1987;75:1102–1109.
2. Henderson BE, Paganini-Hull A, Ross RK. Estrogen replacement therapy and protection from acute myocardial infarction. Am J Obstet Gynecol 1988;159:312–317.
3. Stampfer MJ, Willett WC, Colditz JA, et al. A prospective study of postmenopausal estrogen therapy and coronary heart disease. N Engl J Med 1985;313:1044–1049.
4. Bourne T, Hillard TC, Whitehead MI, Crook D, Campbell S. Oestrogens, arterial status, and postmenopausal women. Lancet 1990;335:1470–1471.
5. Sarrel P. Effects of ovarian steroids on the cardiovascular system. In: Ginsburg J, ed. The circulation in the female from the cradle to the grave pp117–141. Carnforth, Lancs, England: Parthenon, 1989.
6. Gordon T, Castelli WP, Mjortland MC, Kannel WB, Dawber TR. High density lipoprotein as a protective factor against coronary heart disease: The Framingham Study. Am J Med 1977;62:707–714.
7. Kannel WB, Castelli WP, Gordon T, McNamara PM. Serum cholesterol lipoproteins, and risk of coronary heart disease. The Framingham Study. Ann Intern Med 1971;24:1–12.
8. Perrson I, Adami HO, Bergkvist L, et al. Risk of endometrial cancer after treatment with oestrogen alone or in conjunction with progestogens: results of a prospective study. Br Med J 1989;298:147–151.
9. Whitehead MI, Townsend PT, Pryse-Davies J, et al. Effects of estrogens and progestins on

the biochemistry and morphology of the postmenopausal endometrium. N Engl J Med 1981;305:1599–1607.
10. Montgomery JC, Crook D. Progestagens: symptomatic and metabolic side-effects. In: Drife JO, Studd JWW, eds. MRT and Osteoporosis. London: Springer-Verlag, 1990;197–208.
11. Steinberg D. Lipoproteins and the pathogenesis of atherosclerosis. Circulation 1987;76: 508–514.
12. Assmann G. Lipid metabolism and atherosclerosis. New York: Schattauer, 1982.
13. Eisenberg S. High density lipoprotein metabolism. J Lipid Res 1984;25:1017–1058.
14. Havel RJ. Lipid transport function of lipoproteins in blood plasma. Am J Physiol 1987;253:E1–E5.
15. Godsland IF, Wynn V, Crook D, Miller NE. Sex, plasma lipoproteins and atherosclerosis: prevailing assumptions and outstanding questions. Am Heart J 1987;114:1467–1503.
16. Crook D, Seed M. Endocrine control of plasma lipoprotein metabolism: effects of gonadal steroids. Baillière's Clin Endocrinol Metab: Lipid and Lipoprotein Disorders. 1990; 175(4):851–876.
17. Letterie GS, Klein TA, Winkel CA. Modulation of hepatic cholesterol metabolism by ethinyl estradiol and norgestrel. Contraception 1988;37:405–413.
18. Gordon DJ, Rifkind BM. High-density lipoprotein—the clinical implications of recent studies. N Engl J Med 1989;321:1311–1316.
19. Miller NE. Associations of high-density lipoprotein subclasses and apolipoproteins with ischaemic heart disease and coronary atherosclerosis. Am Heart J 1987;113:589–597.
20. Frick MH, Elo MO, Haapa K, et al. Helsinki Heart Study: primary prevention trial with gemfibrozil in middle-aged men with dyslipidemia: safety of treatment, changes in risk factors, and incidence of coronary heart disease. N Engl J Med 1987;317:1237–1245.
21. Manninen V, Elo MO, Frick MH, et al. Lipid alterations and decline in the incidence of coronary heart disease in the Helsinki Heart Study. JAMA 1988;260:641–651.
22. Zilversmit DB. Atherogenesis: a postprandial phenomenon. Circulation 1970;60:473–485.
23. Austin MA. Plasma triglycerides as a risk factor for coronary heart disease. The epidemiological evidence and beyond. Am J Epidemiol 1989;129:249–259.
24. Avins AL, Haber J, Hulley SB. The status of hypertriglyceridemia as a risk factor for coronary heart disease. Clin Lab Med 1989;9:153–168.
25. Bush TL, Fried LP, Barrett-Connor E. Cholesterol, lipoproteins, and coronary heart disease in women. Clin Chem 1988;34(suppl B):60–70.
26. Jacobs DR Jr, Mebane IL, Bangdiwala SI, et al. High density lipoprotein cholesterol as a predictor of cardiovascular disease mortality in men and women: the Follow-up Study of the Lipid Research Clinics Prevalence Study. Am J Epidemiol 1990;131:32–47.
27. Wilson PWF, Abbott RD, Castelli WP. High density lipoprotein cholesterol and mortality. The Framingham Heart Study. Arteriosclerosis 1988;8:737–741.
28. Castelli WP. The triglyceride issue: a view from Framingham. Am Heart J 1986;112:432–437.
29. Muuronen A, Kaste M, Nikkila EA, Tolppanen E-M. Mortality from ischaemic heart disease among patients using anti-convulsant drugs: a case-control study. Br Med J 1985;291: 1481–1483.
30. U.S. Department of Health and Human Services, National Institutes of Health. Lipid Research Clinics Population Studies Data Book, vol 1: The Prevalence Study. (Publication No 80-1527). Washington, DC: U.S. Government Printing Office, 1980.
31. Kannel WB, Hjortland MC, McNamara PM, Gordon T. Menopause and risk of cardiovascular disease: The Framingham Study. Ann Intern Med 1976;85:447–452.
32. Campos H, McNamara JR, Wilson PWF, Ordovas JM, Schaefer EJ. Differences in low density lipoprotein subfractions and apolipoproteins in premenopausal and postmenopausal women. J Clin Endocrinol Metab 1988;67:30–35.

33. Crouse JR, Parks JS, Schey HM, Kahl FR. Studies of low density lipoprotein molecular weight in human beings with coronary artery disease. J Lipid Res 1985;26:566–574.
34. Matthews KA, Meilahn E, Kuller LH, et al. Menopause and risk factors for coronary heart disease. N Engl J Med 1989;321:641–646.
35. Sznajderman M, Oliver MF. Spontaneous premature menopause, ischaemic heart-disease, and serum-lipids. Lancet 1963;1:962–965.
36. Montgomery JC, Crook D, Godsland IF, Wynn V, Studd JWW. Plasma lipid risk factors in oophorectomised women. Br J Obstet Gynaecol 1989;96:1236–1238.
37. Punnonen R, Rauramo L. Effect of bilateral oophorectomy and peroral estradiol valerate therapy on serum lipids. Int J Gynecol Obstet 1976;14:13–16.
38. Crook D, Gardner R, Worthington M, et al. Zoladex versus danazol in the treatment of pelvic endometriosis: effects on plasma lipid risk factors. Horm Res 1989;32(suppl 1): 157–160.
39. Henzl MR, Corson SL, Moghissi K, et al. Administration of nasal nafarelin as compared with oral danazol for endometriosis. N Engl J Med 1988;318:484–489.
40. Beaglehole R, Trost DC, Tamir I, et al. Plasma high-density lipoprotein cholesterol in children and young adults. The Lipid Research Clinics Program Prevalence Study. Circulation 1980;62(suppl IV):83–92.
41. Bush TL, Miller VT. Effects of pharmacological agents used during menopause: impact on lipids and lipoproteins. In: Mishell DR Jr, ed. Menopause: physiology and pharmacology. Chicago: Year Book, 1986:187–208.
42. Barr DP, Russ EM, Eder HA. Influence of estrogens on lipoproteins in atherosclerosis. Trans Assoc Am Physicians 1952;65:102–111.
43. Robinson RW, Higano N, Cohen WD. Effects of long-term administration of estrogens on serum lipids of postmenopausal women. N Engl J Med 1960;263:828–831.
44. Wallentin L, Larsson-Cohn U. Metabolic and hormonal effects of post-menopausal oestrogen replacement therapy. II. Plasma lipids. Acta Endocrinol 1977;86:597–607.
45. Lindberg U-B, Enk L, Crona N, Silfverstolpe G. A comparison of the effects of ethinyl estradiol and estradiol valerate on serum and lipoprotein lipids. Maturitas 1988;10:343–352.
46. Silfverstolpe G, Gustafson A, Samsioe G, Svanborg A. Lipid metabolic studies in oophorectomized women: effects induced by two different estrogens on serum lipids and lipoproteins. Gynecol Obstet Invest 1980;11:161–169.
47. Tikkanen MJ, Kuusi T, Vartiainen E, Nikkila EA. Treatment of postmenopausal hypercholesterolaemia with estradiol. Acta Obstet Gynceol Scand (Suppl) 1979;88:83–88.
48. Tikkanen MJ, Nikkila EA, Vartiainen E. Natural oestrogen as an effective treatment for Type II hyperlipoproteinaemia in postmenopausal women. Lancet 1978;2:490–491.
49. Wahl P, Walden C, Knopp R, et al. Effect of estrogen/progestin potency on lipid/lipoprotein cholesterol. N Engl J Med 1983;308:862–867.
50. Fahreus L, Wallentin L. High density lipoprotein subfractions during oral and cutaneous administration of 17β-estradiol to menopausal women. J Clin Endocrinol Metab 1983;56: 797–801.
51. Farish E, Fletcher CD, Hart DM, et al. The effects of conjugated equine oestrogens with and without a cyclical progestogen on lipoproteins and HDL subfractions in postmenopausal women. Acta Endocrinol (Copenh) 1986;113:123–127.
52. Enk L, Crona N, Samsioe G, Silfverstolpe G. Dose and duration effects of oestradiol valerate on serum and lipoprotein lipids. Horm Metab Res 1986;18:551–554.
53. Fahreus L, Larsson-Cohn U, Wallentin L. Lipoproteins during oral and cutaneous administration of oestradiol 17-β to menopausal women. Acta Endocrinol (Copenhagen) 1982;101:597–602.
54. Barnes RB, Roy S, Lobo RA. Comparison of lipid and androgen levels after conjugated

estrogen of depo-medroxyprogesterone acetate treatment in postmenopausal women. Obstet Gynecol 1985;66:216–219.
55. Chetkowski RJ, Meldrum DR, Steingold KA, et al. Biologic effects of transdermal estradiol. N Engl J Med 1986;314:1615–1620.
56. Sonnendecker EWW, Polakow ES, Benadé AJS, Simchowitz E. Serum lipoprotein effects of conjugated estrogen and a sequential conjugated estrogen-medrogestone regimen in hysterectomized postmenopausal women. Am J Obstet Gynecol 1989;160:1128–1134.
57. Lagrelius A, Johnson P, Lunell N-O, Samsoie G. Treatment with oral estrone sulphate in the female climacteric. 1. Influence on lipids. Acta Obstet Gynecol Scand 1981;60:27–31.
58. Colvin PL, Auerbach BJ, Korotnik DR, Hazzard WR, Applebaum-Bowden D. Differential effects of oral estrone versus 17β-estradiol on lipoproteins in postmenopausal women. J Clin Endocrinol Metab 1990;70:1568–1573.
59. Basdevant A, De Lignieres B, Guy-Grand B. Differential lipemic and hormonal responses to oral and parenteral 17β-estradiol in postmenopausal women. Am J Obstet Gynecol 1983; 147:77–81.
60. Whitehead MI, Fraser D. Controversies over the safety of estrogen replacement therapy. Am J Obstet Gynecol 1987;156:1313–1322.
61. Lobo RA, March CM, Goebelsmann U, Krauss RM, Mishell DR Jr. Subdermal estradiol pellets following hysterectomy and oophorectomy. Am J Obstet Gynecol 1980;138:714–719.
62. Stanczyk FZ, Shoupe D, Nunez V, et al. A randomized comparison of nonoral estradiol delivery in postmenopausal women. Am J Obstet Gynecol 1988;159:1540–1546.
63. Farish E, Fletcher CD, Hart DM, et al. The effects of hormone implants on serum lipoproteins and steroid hormones in bilaterally oophorectomised women. Acta Endocrinol (Copenh) 1984;106:116–120.
64. Engleberg H, Glass SJ. Influence of physiological doses of sex steroid hormones on serum lipids and lipoproteins in humans. Metabolism 1955;4:298–312.
65. Svanborg A, Vikrot O. The effect of estradiol and progesterone on plasma lipids in oophorectomized women. Acta Med Scand 1966;179:615–622.
66. Lindberg U-B, Crona N, Enk L, Samsioe G, Silfverstolpe G. Effects of cyproterone acetate (CPA) on serum lipoproteins when administered alone and in combination with ethinyl estradiol (EE). Horm Metab Res 1987;19:222–225.
67. Hirvonen E, Malkonen M, Manninen V. Effects of different progestagens on lipoproteins during postmenopausal replacement therapy. N Engl J Med 1981;304:560–563.
68. Silfverstolpe G, Gustafson A, Samsioe G, Svanborg A. Lipid metabolic studies in oophorectomized women. Effects of three different progestogens. Acta Obstet Gynecol Scand (Suppl) 1979;88:89–95.
69. Tikkanen MJ, Nikkila EA, Kuusi T, et al. Different effects of two progestins on plasma high density lipoprotein (HDL_2) and postheparin plasma hepatic lipase activity. Atherosclerosis 1981;40:365–369.
70. Lehtonen A, Ronroos M, Marniemi J, et al. Effect of high dose progestin on serum lipids and lipid metabolizing enzymes in patients with endometrial cancer. Horm Metab Res 1985;17:32–34.
71. Fahreus L, Sydsjo A & Wallentin L. Lipoprotein changes during treatment of pelvic endometriosis with medroxyprogesterone acetate. Fertil Steril 1986;45:503–506.
72. Farish E, Fletcher CD, Hart DM, Kitchener H, Sharpe GLM. A long-term study of the effects of norethisterone on lipoprotein metabolism in menopausal women. Clin Chim Acta 1983;132:193–198.
73. Kuusi T, Nikkila EA, Tikkanen MJ, Sipenen S. Effects of two progestins with different androgenic properties on hepatic endothelial lipase and high density $lipoprotein_2$. Atherosclerosis 1985;54:251–262.

74. Krauss RM. Effects of progestational agents on serum lipids and lipoproteins. J Reprod Med 1982;27(suppl):502–510.
75. Jensen J, Nilas L, Christiansen C. Cyclic changes in serum cholesterol and lipoproteins following different dose of combined postmenopausal hormone replacement therapy. Br J Obstet Gynaecol 1986;93:613–618.
76. Barrett-Connor E, Wingard DL, Criqui MH. Postmenopausal estrogen use and heart disease risk factors in the 1980s. Rancho Bernardo, Calif, revisited. JAMA 1989;261:2095–2100.
77. Fahreus L, Larsson-Cohn U, Wallentin L. L-norgestrel and progesterone have different influences on plasma lipoproteins. Eur J Clin Invest 1983;13:447–453.
78. Ottoson UB, Johansson BG, von Schoultz B. Subfractions of high-density lipoprotein cholesterol during estrogen replacement therapy: a comparison between progestogens and natural progesterone. Am J Obstet Gynecol 1985;151:746–750.
79. Hargrove JT, Maxson WS, Wentz AC, Burnett LS. Menopausal hormone replacement therapy with continuous daily oral micronized estradiol and progesterone. Obstet Gynecol 1989;73:606–612.
80. Jensen J, Riis B, Christiansen C. Cyproterone acetate, an alternative progestogen in postmenopausal hormone replacement therapy? Effects on serum lipids and lipoproteins. Br J Obstet Gynaecol 1987;94:136–141.
81. Sporrong T, Hellgren M, Samsioe G, Mattsson L-A. Metabolic effects of continuous estradiol-protestin therapy in postmenopausal women. Obstet Gynecol 1989;73:754–758.
82. Whitehead MI, Hillard TC, Crook D. The role and use of progestogens. Obstet Gynecol 1990;75(suppl):59–76.
83. Siddle NC, Jesinger DK, Whitehead MI, et al. Effect on plasma lipids and lipoproteins of postmenopausal oestrogen therapy with added dydrogesterone. Br J Obstet Gynaecol 1990;97:1093–1100.
84. Hirvonen E, Lipasti A, Malkonen M, et al. Clinical and lipid metabolic effects of unopposed oestrogen and two oestrogen-progestagen regimens in post-menopausal women. Maturitas 1987;9:69–79.
85. Sherwin BB, Gelfand MM. A prospective one-year study of estrogen and progestin in postmenopausal women: effects on clinical symptoms and lipoprotein lipids. Obstet Gynecol 1989;73:759–766.
86. Weinstein L. Efficacy of a continuous estrogen-progestin regimen in the menopausal patient. Obstet Gynecol 1987;69:929–932.
87. Prough SG, Aksel A, Wiebe RH, Shepherd J. Continuous estrogen/progestin therapy in menopause. Am J Obstet Gynecol 1987;157:1449–1453.
88. Luciano AA, Turksoy RN, Carleo J, Hendrix JW. Clinical and metabolic responses of menopausal women to sequential versus continuous estrogen and progestin replacement therapy. Obstet Gynceol 1988;71:39–43.
89. Jensen J, Riis BJ, Strøm V, Christiansen C. Continuous oestrogen-progestogen treatment and serum lipoproteins in postmenopausal women. Br J Obstet Gynaecol 1987;94:130–135.
90. Mattsson L-A, Cullberg G, Samsioe G. A continuous estrogen-protestagen regimen for climacteric complaints. Acta Obstet Gynecol Scand 1984;63:673–677.
91. Farish E, Fletcher CD, Dagen MM, et al. Lipoprotein and apolipoprotein levels in postmenopausal women on continuous oestrogen/progestogen therapy. Br J Obstet Gynaecol 1989;96:358–364.
92. Garnett TJ, Crook D, Worthington M, et al. Prospective study of a novel hormone replacement therapy combining continuous oestradiol valerate (2mg/day) with sequential levonorgestrel (75μg/day for 12/28 days): effects on plasma lipoprotein risk markers. In: Christiansen C, ed. Osteoporosis. Copenhagen, Osteopress, 1990:1829–1831.

8

Estrogen Replacement Therapy: Current Regimens

Paul Stumpf

RATIONALE

It is helpful to consider the irreversible ovarian failure associated with menopause to represent an endocrine deficiency state or endocrinopathy, at least for women who are at risk for the pathologic consequences of estrogen deficiency. This basic premise can then be used as a framework for designing a rational approach to many aspects of postmenopausal hormone replacement therapy, including the selection of specific treatment regimens (1).

The term "endocrinopathy" can be defined as a disorder in the function of an endocrine gland and the consequences of that dysfunction (2). As discussed in more detail elsewhere in this book, a specific endocrine gland, namely the ovary, discontinues its normal functions at the time of menopause. Indeed, it is possible to artificially produce a pathologic condition resembling natural menopause by prematurely removing the ovaries or by destroying their function with radiation or chemotherapy. Specific endocrine products become deficient after ovarian failure, most importantly 17β-estradiol (E_2) and progesterone. A variety of specific pathologic consequences develop subsequent to this well-defined endocrine deficiency; for example, vasomotor instability, urogenital atrophy, and postmenopausal osteoporosis, among others. Finally, the application of hormone therapy to replace the endocrine deficiency has been proved to prevent, delay, or ameliorate many of these pathologic consequences of ovarian failure. Thus, menopause fulfills the criteria for an endocrinopathy, at least for postmenopausal women who experience, or are at risk to experience, the pathologic consequences of ovarian failure.

For endocrinopathies in general, several principles of properly designed replacement can be proposed (1). It is generally desirable to replace the specific hormones that are deficient, if possible. Replacement of the specific hormones should be accomplished at a dose, pattern of administration, and portal of entry that approximates the characteristics of production from the functioning endocrine gland, as closely as possible. The replacement therapy should aim to relieve or prevent as many as possible of the pathologic consequences of the endocrine deficiency state being considered. Finally, replacement therapy should seek to avoid unphysiologic consequences that may result from the exogenous administration of the hormone. I propose that it is possible to apply these principles to regimens used for treatment of the menopausal state.

Prior to menopause, ovarian follicles produce 17β-estradiol (E_2), which is the principal naturally occurring endogenous human estrogen, at a controlled rate that is between approximately 60 and 600 μg/day, resulting in levels of E_2 in the general circulation ranging from approximately 40 to 400 pg/ml. At the age of menopause, irreversible ovarian failure marks the cessation of ovarian follicle development, and therefore a dramatic reduction in E_2 production and circulating levels. After menopause, ovarian production of E_2 drops to less than 20 μg/day, and circulating levels of E_2 are generally less than 30 pg/ml. Relatively small amounts of circulating E_2 are derived from the metabolism of estrone (E_1), the second major naturally occurring human estrogen (3–5).

E_1 binds to the estrogen receptor with a lower affinity than does E_2. Since all activities of sex steroids are thought to be mediated through binding and activation of steroid receptors, E_1 may be considered less potent than E_2. The E_1 in circulation comes either from the metabolism of E_2 or from aromatization of androstenedione. Since levels of E_2 fluctuate during the ovarian cycle, the levels of E_1 fluctuate as well, and range from approximately 40 to 200 pg/ml. Androstenedione levels, on the other hand, are fairly constant, since androstenedione is produced rather constantly from the adrenal gland and to some extent by the ovary itself. Production of androstenedione by the adrenal gland continues after menopause, of course, and therefore E_1 becomes an important endogenous estrogen after ovarian failure. Serum levels of E_1 after menopause remain above 40 pg/ml, and thus there is no significant deficiency of E_1 in post-menopausal women. The estradiol to estrone ratio is a mechanism used to express which one of these two estrogens is predominant at any given time. Prior to menopause the E_2 to E_1 ratio is generally greater than 1.0, indicating that estradiol is the predominant estrogen in circulation. After menopause, the E_2 to E_1 ratio is reversed, becoming less than 1.0, indicating that estrone is predominant following ovarian failure (3, 5). (For completeness, it should be mentioned that the third principal human estrogen is estriol, a compound characterized by a hydroxyl group at the 16 position on the D ring. Estriol is only produced in any clinically significant amount during pregnancy. In the non-pregnant state, estriol has little importance, and it is therefore extraneous to the present discussion.)

The selection of a particular type of hormone administration is strongly influenced by the side effects, patient tolerability, and pharmacologic effects of the method being considered. Because sex steroids exert their effect through intracellular receptor binding, any estrogen administered in appropriate dosages through any feasible portal of administration should be able to diminish the pathology associated with estrogen deficiency, as long as that estrogen is cable of binding effectively to an estrogen receptor. It may be possible to distinguish *physiologic* effects of replacement therapy, which depend on the ambient levels of circulating estrogen, from the *pharmacologic* effects of administration, which are related to either supraphysiologic levels of estrogen in circulation or specific effects that are peculiar to the route of administration, such as "first-pass" through the liver.

In describing and comparing the possible regimens to be used for hormone replacement therapy, the following variables must be considered: the type of estrogen to be used, the route of administration, the addition of progestins, the schedules of hormone administration, the duration of therapy, and the various factors affecting patient compliance. The following discussion examines each of these considerations.

TYPES OF ESTROGEN

Conjugated Equine Estrogens

In animals, as well as in humans, estrogens are excreted in the urine, principally as estrogen conjugates. Over 60 years ago, estrogenic compounds were identified in the urine of animals, and were found in large quantities during pregnancy because of the large amount of estrogen being produced and excreted. One of the earliest forms of estrogen replacement therapy was the oral administration of estrogens that had been purified from the urine of pregnant mares, and this form of estrogen is still in clinical use today. These urinary estrogens are actually a mixture of estrogenic compounds, principally estrone sulfate (about 50%), equilin sulfates (about 40%), and other conjugated and unconjugated estrogens (6). Some of these compounds, such as equilin, are not naturally produced in humans at all. The fact that several different types of estrogenic compounds are being administered simultaneously and may undergo additional metabolic conversion during absorption through the gastrointestinal tract, and the fact that separation and identification of these compounds from blood samples are tedious, using assays that are not readily available, make studying the pharmacokinetics of orally administered conjugated equine estrogens (CEE) difficult and complicated. Nevertheless, oral CEE has a long history of clinical study and experience.

Doses of oral CEE used today, such as 0.625 and 1.25 mg/day, are associated with levels of E_2 and E_1 in circulation that are similar to the lower levels produced endogenously in a normal ovarian cycle. However, levels of equilin associated with these same doses of oral CEE are reported to be much higher than the levels of E_2 or E_1. These equine estrogens in circulation appear to have relatively little biological activity in humans, but represent a large steroid load to be metabolized, cleared, and excreted.

Estradiol

E_2 was purified from sow ovaries in 1935. However, oral administration of this principal product of the normally functioning ovary was limited because of problems with poor absorption and deactivation of E_2 in the gastrointestinal tract. In 1972, it was reported that micronization allows effective oral administration of E_2 (7). Nevertheless, during absorption, there is significant conversion of the administered E_2 to E_1 and other estrogens before passage into the general circulation. Micronized E_2 has been reported to be effective in relieving menopausal symptoms. As expected, oral micronized E_2 also appears to be effective in preventing the loss of bone density associated with postmenopausal osteoporosis. The most commonly used dosages of micronized E_2 appear to be 1.0 or 2.0 mg/day.

Estrone

Pure E_1 is not available for oral administration today. However, a water-soluble estrone conjugate is available, specifically estropipate or piperazine estrone sulfate. The piperazine moiety is apparently necessary to enhance solubility and to stabilize the molecule. Orally administered E_1 has been shown to produce clinical relief for menopausal symptoms and is said to be extensively used in Europe. At one time it was believed that E_1 might be less likely to produce endometrial hyperplasia or carcinoma. E_1 binds less avidly to the intracellular estrogen receptor. However, it seems likely that a given dose of E_1 sufficient to produce clinical relief of symptoms would also have an equivalent effect on the endometrium. Therefore, there seems to be little objective evidence that oral E_1 is an inherently safer form of estrogen administration. Furthermore, as outlined above, the hormone deficiency associated with ovarian failure is a loss of E_2 production but not of E_1 production, so there seems little reason to supplement E_1 levels specifically.

Estradiol Derivatives

Combination oral contraceptives contain either 17-ethinyl-estradiol or 17-ethinyl-estradiol-3-methyl-ether (mestranol). Both of these synthetic estrogens appear to have a dramatic pharmacologic effect on liver metabolism, and in the United States, they are not currently recommended for postmenopausal estrogen replacement. Another estradiol derivative, 17-ethinyl-estradiol-3-cyclopentoether (quinestrol) is also available. Quinestrol appears to be stored in adipose tissue after oral administration, and is then slowly released back into the general circulation to produce clinical effects. This particular form of estrogen administration has gained little popularity because of concerns about the difficulty in stopping therapy quickly if it becomes necessary or desirable.

Nonsteroidal Estrogens

Diethylstilbestrol (DES) is approved in the United States for palliative treatment of prostatic cancer. DES is a potent estrogen that has profound effects on several markers of liver function. At the present time, it is not recommended for postmenopausal estrogen replacement.

ROUTE OF ADMINISTRATION

On the practical level, estrogen administration can be divided into two major groups: oral and parenteral. Oral administration of estrogen has a long history and is still currently used. As mentioned above, estradiol, estrone, and conjugated estrogens can all be administered orally in tablets. Oral estrogens are subject to intestinal absorption and metabolism before their entry into the circulation and their subsequent access to target tissues. Parenteral administration, on the other hand, has been accomplished by a variety of different mechanisms, including intravenous or intramuscular injections; subcutaneous pellet administration; transvaginal administration using creams, solutions, tablets, or silastic vaginal rings; and percutaneous and transdermal administration through the skin (1). Parenteral administration is characterized by predictable levels of absorption without significant intermediate metabolism directly into the systemic blood stream. The parenteral route allows specifically the administration of 17β-estradiol, which is the major active estrogen produced by a normally functioning ovary. (Progestins can also be administered through either the oral or the parenteral route. Progesterone, progesterone derivatives, and 19-nor testosterone derivatives are all available for oral administration. Progesterone can be administered also by vaginal or rectal suppositories, by vaginal rings, or by injection. Other progestins can be administered by intramuscular injection, subcutaneous rods, or vaginal rings. Most recently, the transdermal administration of progestins has also been reported.)

The features of absorption and metabolism, and the pharmacologic characteristics of these major forms of hormone administration are examined below.

Oral Estrogens

One of the most commonly used mechanisms to deliver estrogens clinically is oral administration. Estrogens taken orally are subject to the vagaries of intestinal absorption and may have an exaggerated pharmacologic impact on the liver. The liver is an important organ in determining the status of sex steroids. Metabolic conversion, conjugation, and bile excretion of estrogens occur primarily in the liver. The liver is also the principal site for the conjugation of estrogens into water-soluble estrogen sulfates and estrogen glucuronides to prepare for their subsequent extraction and excretion through the kidney. Estrogens are also excreted directly through the liver into the bile. Estrogens in the gastrointestinal tract are absorbed into the portal blood stream and carried directly to the liver, which establishes enterohepatic recirculation of estrogens. In addition to metabolic conversion, conjugation, excretion, and reabsorption of estrogens, the liver also influences the activity of estrogens in the circulation by modulating the production of sex hormone–binding globulin. (SHBG). SHBG is the major serum protein that specifically binds estrogens, and therefore the levels of circulating SHBG determines, in part, the bioavailability of sex steroids in the circulation (6, 8). SHBG production is in turn influenced by the levels of sex steroids in the circulation and by the exposure of the liver to sex steroids absorbed through the gastrointestinal tract, via the first-pass effect. In addition, liver production of other proteins, including other binding proteins and clotting factors, is influenced by the exposure of the liver to estrogen and other sex steroids. Carbohydrate metabolism, lipid metabolism, bile production, and other metabolic functions of the liver are also influenced by sex steroid exposure. Therefore, the metabolism and activity of estrogen and other sex steroids is influenced by liver functions by interactions that are sensitive and complex. Clearly, the influence of liver metabolism is an important consideration in analyzing the current regimens for postmenopausal hormone replacement therapy.

(More recently, attention has been directed toward the hepatic interactions with progestin administration as well (8). Progestins appear to affect many of the metabolic functions of the liver as described above. In addition, the activity of progestins may also be determined, in part, by liver activity, through metabolic conversion, binding, and excretion.)

Parenteral Administration

Several different approaches to administering estrogens non-orally have been studied as alternatives to the oral route described above. Some possible advantages of non-oral administration of estrogen include the ability to use types of estrogen that are normal products of the functioning ovary and to deliver those estrogens directly into the systemic circulation, which more closely resembles the normal ovarian delivery of estrogen.

Intravenous and Intramuscular Injection

Extracts of ovarian tissue were demonstrated to produce estrus characteristics when injected into animals in the early 1900s. Aqueous suspensions of estrogen were found to be impractical, because of the poor water solubility of unconjugated estrogens. Intravenous injection of aqueous suspensions of conjugated estrogens has been recommended for the control of acute uterine bleeding in certain circumstances. For intramuscular injection, estrogen suspensions in oil can be used. Lipid solutions of simple estrogens are rapidly absorbed and quickly metabolized when injected intramuscularly. Because esters of estradiol are less polar than 17β-estradiol itself, estradiol esters in oil have a slower rate of absorption after intramuscular injection, and therefore the clinical effects may be prolonged (6). Estradiol valerate and estradiol cypionate show clinical response for several weeks after intramuscular injection of lipid solutions with concentrations ranging from 1 to 40 mg/ml. Polyestradiol phosphate can be used for intramuscular injection because estradiol is released from the parent molecule; however, in the United States, polyestradiol phosphate is approved only as treatment for prostatic cancer, and is not recommended for postmenopausal hormone replacement. Solutions of estrone, sometimes called natural estrogenic substance, can also be used for intramuscular injection (9).

Pellets for Subcutaneous Injection

Crystalline 17β-estradiol has been prepared as pellets intended for implantation under the skin (10, 11). E_2 appears to be spared from metabolism in the subcutaneous tissue, so these E_2 pellets enable systemic administration of E_2 without intermediate metabolism to E_1 or other compounds. The absorption rates are relatively constant, and therefore the E_2 levels in serum are highly predictable. Pellets containing 25 mg of E_2 are associated with circulating levels of E_2 in serum of about 50 to 70 pg/ml. Pellets containing 50 mg of E_2 produce serum levels of E_2 of about 100 to 120 pg/ml. These E_2 levels in serum can be maintained for several months following implantation of one or more E_2 pellets (10). Therefore, pellet insertion may have certain advantages for compliance in selected patients. However, this form of administration has several disadvantages. Perhaps most important is the difficulty of stopping estrogen therapy if necessary, since these pellets are difficult or impossible to remove following the insertion. The insertion itself and any attempted removal require local anesthesia and a minor surgical procedure, to which some patients may object. Subcutaneous pellets of E_2 may continue to play a role, albeit minor, in postmenopausal hormone replacement therapy.

Vaginal Estrogen Solutions and Tablets

Most estrogens are readily absorbed across the vaginal epithelium. For example, an aqueous solution containing 0.5 mg of E_2, when placed in the vagina, produced preferential increases in E_2 levels in the systemic circulation without significant intermediate metabolism. By about 6 hours after application, serum levels of E_2 returned to baseline. A similar application of 0.5 mg of E_1 in solution results in a preferential increase in circulating levels of E_1, no significant change in E_2 levels, and a return to pretreatment levels within about 6 hours (12). Tablets containing E_2, placed in the vagina, also demonstrate absorption with little intermediate metabolism. These E_2 tablets achieve serum levels approaching 1000 pg/ml, and return to baseline by about 24 hours. In the United States, there are no clinically approved preparations available to administer estrogen in solution or tablet through the vaginal epithelium.

Vaginal Estrogen Creams

Estrogen-containing vaginal creams are available in the United States. At one time, it was believed that these creams could achieve clinical relief of urogenital symptoms in women by local effect, without systemic absorption. However, it has been recognized that estrogen is readily absorbed through the vaginal epithelium from vaginal creams, establishing this route as an alternative for parenteral administration of estrogen. Many patients find such creams rather messy to use. In clinical use, it is rather difficult to control the specific dosage being administered. Nevertheless, preparations containing CEE, E_2, estropipate, and dienestrol are clinically available. They represent only a relatively small proportion of estrogens prescribed for postmenopausal hormone replacement.

Vaginal Estrogen Rings

From the above discussion, it is clear that the vaginal epithelium is an available route for the absorption of estrogen systemically. In an attempt to avoid the patterns of bolus absorption described above, sustained release systems have been stuided for possible long-term administration of estradiol through the vagina. Several polymers are capable of releasing estrogen in a predictable fashion, if the estrogen has been incorporated into the structure prior to polymerization. The characteristics of absorption from these rings depend in part on the surface area of the ring, and the duration of effectiveness depends in part on the amount of estrogen that is incorporated into each ring structure (8). The author has studied polydimethylsiloxane vaginal rings containing 100, 200, and 400 mg of pure 17β-estradiol per ring. Vaginal rings containing 100 mg of E_2 produce levels of E_2 in serum of about 40 to 50 pg/ml, while rings containing 200 mg of E_2 achieve levels of E_2 in serum of about 70 to 80 pg/ml, and 400-mg E_2 rings produced levels of about 140 pg/ml (13). It is possible to design vaginal rings containing sufficient estrogen to maintain fairly constant circulating levels of estradiol for up to 3 months per ring. There appears to be little intermediate metabolism in the vaginal epithelium, as expected, and therefore 17β-estradiol itself can be administered through this route. Study subjects have reported good comfort and compliance with this system, since the vaginal rings may be removed periodically for short periods of time for rinsing and for vaginal hygiene. While the rings are in place, the levels are maintained fairly constantly, and the different dosages are capable of achieving rather precise levels in serum. In this way, it is possible to design a system wherein several different vaginal rings are used to produce serum levels of sex steroids, including progesterone, that resemble the levels seen in a normal ovarian cycle. Serum E_2 levels rise rapidly when the ring is first placed in the vagina, remain fairly constant while the ring is in place, and then are cleared rapidly when the system is removed. These characteristics have been advantageous for certain investigational purposes to administer pure 17β-estradiol and/or pure progesterone. Other investigators have also demonstrated the possibility of delivering E_1 from similar vaginal rings for estrogen replacement, and ethinyl estradiol and progestins for contraceptive purposes. None of these vaginal ring systems are currently clinically approved for use in the United States.

Percutaneous Estrogen Creams or Gels

In Europe, E_2 gel has been studied as a form of parenteral administration (14, 15). The E_2 suspension is applied, usually to the anterior abdominal wall, and the E_2 is absorbed through the skin. Circulating serum levels of E_2 are increased preferentially, with little evidence of significant intermediate metabolism. Both clinical relief of symptoms, and evidence of clinical effectiveness, have been reported. For at least some patients, percutaneous creams or gel may be messy. A practical consideration may be the relative difficulty of achieving precise control of the dosage being self-administered by the patient.

Transdermal Estrogen

To avoid the potential problems of messiness and difficulties in controlling dosage, an alternative system has been developed to take advantage of the absorption of estrogen through the skin (16–18). Transdermal patches have been approved for clinical use in the United States, designed to deliver 0.05 mg or 0.1 mg of estradiol per day. Each patch is constructed with five layers: (*a*) an outer occlusive membrane, (*b*) a reservoir containing an alcohol solution of 17β-estradiol, (*c*) a control membrane that determines the release rate, (*d*) a layer of adhesive that enables the patch to adhere to the skin, and (*e*) a plastic film that protects the adhesive and is designed to be removed before the patch is applied. Each patch provides rather constant serum levels of E_2 for approximately 84 hours. Clinically, patches are changed twice per week, being applied to the skin, usually on the lower trunk. E_2 is absorbed rapidly through the skin when the patch is first applied, remains fairly constant while the patch is in place, and then falls rapidly when the patch is removed. Serum E_2 levels are preferentially increased, with little evidence of significant intermediate metabolism through the skin. Relief of menopausal symptoms, suppression of gonadotropins, reduction in urinary excretion of calcium, and maintenance of bone density have all been reported in subjects using transdermal E_2 administration. Patient compliance is generally good, and the system is relatively easy to prescribe. This system appears to represent a further refinement of available regimens for parenteral administration of hormone replacement therapy.

TYPE OF PROGESTIN

Progestins or progestogens are compounds that have been found to have activity resembling the effects of natural progesterone, such as secretory changes in the endometrium and delay of menses. It is possible to divide the clinically useful progestogens into three major groups: (*a*) the naturally occurring 21-carbon compounds, specifically progesterone itself and 17-hydroxyprogesterone, its derivative; (*b*) the 21-carbon synthetic progesterone derivatives, specifically medroxyprogesterone acetate and megestrol acetate; and (*c*) the synthetic 19-nortestosterone derivatives, such as norethindrone, norethindrone acetate, and norgestrel. Although all these compounds have progestational effects, they differ considerably in their absorption, activity, potency, and side effects.

The Naturally Occurring 21-Carbon Progestins

The two naturally occurring human progestogens are progesterone itself and its 17-hydroxy derivative. Of these two compounds, pure progesterone is the more active.

When administered orally, pure progesterone is only poorly absorbed, and is subject to rapid deactivation by the liver through hydroxylation and conjugation (19). As described above for estradiol, micronization of progesterone improves the results of oral administration. Nevertheless, relatively large doses and frequent administration, such as 100 or 200 mg twice daily, are necessary to achieve satisfactory progesterone levels in circulation. For this and other reasons, oral administration of pure progesterone has received relatively little use in the United States.

Pure progesterone may also be administered parenterally from vaginal or rectal suppositories, vaginal rings, nasal administration, and intramuscular injection. Vaginal and rectal suppositories require rather large doses, such as 25 or 50 mg, with frequent administration, once or twice per day. Some clinicians have prepared aqueous suspensions of progesterone for rectal administration, but this is also relatively inconvenient and unpleasant for patients, and there has been little scientific evaluation describing this technique. Similarly, a progesterone ointment designed to be administered nasally has been described, but there is very little experience. Vaginal rings and vaginal cylinders containing pure progesterone, with or without concomitant estradiol, have been shown to effectively administer progesterone through the vaginal epithilium but are not available clinically (20, 21). Intramuscular injections of progesterone in oil result in adequate systemic levels of circulating progesterone and have been used for the "progesterone challenge test" but are generally not used for long-term therapy in postmenopausal women.

The 21-Carbon Synthetic Progesterone Derivatives

The most important example of this group, medroxyprogesterone acetate (MPA), appears to be the most popular progestin used for postmenopausal therapy. MPA is a synthetic compound in which one methyl group has been added to the 6 position and one acetoxy group has been added to the 17α position of the progesterone molecule. These additional side chains appear to increase the progestational activity of the compound and delay its metabolism. MPA is usually administered orally at dosages ranging from 2.5 to 10 mg/day in most instances. The absorption appears to be rapid, with peak levels achieved by 4 hours and a return to near baseline by 24 hours. Serum levels of about 3 or 4 mg/ml have been reported after a 10-mg dose of MPA given orally. However, it has been reported that the absorption characteristics are quite variable.

Megestrol acetate is similar to MPA in structure, except for an additional double bond in the B ring. It is approved in the United States primarily for oncologic purposes.

Parenteral administration of MPA is also possible. A depot form of MPA is available clinically for contraceptive and oncologic purposes, but there is little published information regarding its usefulness in postmenopausal women. The synthetic derivatives of 17-hydroxyprogesterone, namely the valerate and caproate derivatives, have been described as long-acting injectable forms of progestogens.

The Synthetic 19-Nortestosterone Derivatives

These so-called 19-norprogestogens are actually derivatives of the testosterone molecule in which the C-19 carbon has been removed from its attachment to the C-10 carbon position. The loss of the 19th carbon reduces, but does not entirely eliminate, the androgenic activity of the molecule. An acetyl group is added at the 17th position to enhance potency when the compound is administered orally. These 19-norprogestogens were primarily developed for use as contraceptives, but have recently attracted increasing attention for possible usefulness in postmenopausal women. It appears that the largest experience has been accumulated for norethindrone for this purpose, although there is some information about norgestrel and levonorgestrel as well. These progestogens appear to provide adequate protection to the endometrium at low doses, which appear to have minimal side effects. Recently, the parenteral administration of 19-norprogestogens by means of a transdermal patch has been reported in an attempt to decrease still further the side effects and metabolic impact of these compounds when given to postmenopausal women.

SCHEDULES OF ADMINISTRATION

Given the several different types of estrogen which are available, at the various approved dosages, with or without the addition of progestogens, the various types and dosages of progestogen available, the possible routes of administration and the various possible patterns of dosing, there are, theoretically, hundreds of possible regimens which could be used for post menopausal hormone replacement therapy. Indeed, one survey among gynecologists in the Los Angeles area described 84 different patterns of use among only 283 physicians. In order to make any possible order out of such variety, one might conveniently group the various possible patterns into: (1) cyclic estrogen alone; (2) continuous estrogen alone; (3) cyclic estrogen plus cyclic progestin; (4) continuous estrogen plus cyclic progestin; (5) continuous estrogen plus continuous progestogen; (6) cyclic or continuous progestin alone.

Cyclic Estrogen Alone

Prior to the 1970s, it was popular to administer estrogens without progestins in a cyclic pattern, whether or not the patient had an intact uterus. A common regimen was CEE given orally at a dose of 1.25 mg or 2.5 mg per day for 21 of every 28 days, or 25 days of each calendar month. A less common regimen was to administer the estrogen for 5 days each week. It is said that the cyclic administration of estrogen alone is well tolerated and produces little withdrawal bleeding if the patient has a uterus, but there is little published information to support this clinical contention. Furthermore, there is no evidence that the cyclic (as opposed to continuous) administration of estrogen alone provides any real protection against endometrial hyperplasia or adenocarcinoma. For this reason, the use of unopposed estrogen, even given cyclically, is discouraged for patients who have an intact uterus. In patients without a uterus, cyclic estrogen alone can be used but may not provide any real advantage over a simpler regimen of continuous unopposed estrogen, described below. However, if cyclic unopposed estrogen is to be used in a woman without a uterus, some reasonable treatment patterns would include estrogen administration for 25 days each calendar month, using oral CEE at 0.625 mg/day, or oral micronized estradiol at 1 mg/day, or oral estropipate at 1.25 mg/day, or transdermal estradiol at 0.05 or 0.1 mg patch dose.

Continuous Estrogen Alone

Because of the concern about endometrial hyperplasia or adenocarcinoma, continuous unopposed estrogens are not recommended for patients with an intact uterus. However, at the present time, unopposed estrogens may be used in postmenopausal patients without a uterus. (It should be noted that it is possible that progestins may help to decrease the risk of breast cancer. Although this has not been conclusively demonstrated at the present time, this possibility may represent a reason to use progestins, even in patients without a uterus.) The continuous administration of estrogen has the following advantages: it may resemble the normal pattern of estrogen production by the ovary more closely, since the ovary produces estrogen at all times during the ovulatory cycle, although at varying levels; this regimen may be easier for patients to remember, and therefore may enhance compliance; the regimen may eliminate estrogen withdrawal symptoms experienced by some patients using cyclic estrogen therapy; and it increases the number of days of estrogen exposure, which may enhance some of the benefits associated with estrogen administration. If continuous unopposed estrogen is used, the same dosages described above could be selected except that there would be no days off estrogen. Clinically, it appears that women using transdermal estradiol administration may be more comfortable when the patches are used continuously, because estradiol is cleared so rapidly from the system that estrogen withdrawal side effects may be uncomfortable for patients during the days when they are not wearing a patch.

Cyclic Estrogen plus Cyclic Progestin

The addition of progestins to estrogen replacement therapy has been advocated to reduce the risk of endometrial hyperplasia and adenocarcinoma, to increase the possibility of new bone formation, and perhaps to reduce the risk of breast cancer. When estrogens are administered, as described above, for the first 25 days of each calendar month, progestins are usually added beginning on the 14th or 16th day of the month, for a total progestin exposure of 10 or 12 days. After the 25th of the month, the patient is receiving no medication and will usually experience vaginal bleeding at this time. Some commonly used progestin regimens include MPA at 5 or 10 mg/day or norethindrone acetate at 2.5 or 5 mg/day orally.

Continuous Estrogen plus Cyclic Progestin

For reasons described above, continuous estrogen may provide some advantages in postmenopausal hormone replacement therapy, especially when accompanied by a progestin. On these regimens, the patient takes estrogen every day, and therefore she may use the calendar date simply to dictate the timing of her progestin dosage. Some clinically useful regimens in this category would include continuous estrogen given either orally (CEE at 0.625 mg/day or micronized estradiol at 1 mg/day, or estropipate at 1.25 mg/day) or transdermally (with 0.05-mg or 0.1-mg patches worn continuously, changing each patch every 3½ days) plus progestin (either MPA at 5 or 10 mg/day or norethindrone acetate at 2.5 or 5 mg/day) taken from the first to the 12th of each calendar month. Vaginal bleeding after the 10th day of progestin administration may be considered normal withdrawal bleeding, according to some investigators. This treatment plan appears to be easier for patients to remember, and clinically seems to be well tolerated.

Continuous Estrogen plus Continuous Progestin

Some older patients object to the experience of monthly withdrawal bleeding, which is usually induced when progestins are added to estrogen replacement therapy. To eliminate this problem, it has been suggested that estrogens and progestins could both be given every day, sometimes called the continuous-combined regimen. Because the duration of progestin administration is increased, the daily dose of progestin may be reduced. At the present time in the United States, an apparently common regimen for continuous-combined therapy is to use both an estrogen (such as CEE at 0.625 mg, or oral micronized estradiol at 1 mg, or oral estropipate at 1.25 mg, or transdermal estradiol at 0.05 or 1.0 mg) plus a progestin (such as MPA at 2.5 mg, or norethindrone acetate at 2.5 mg, or norethindrone at 0.35 or 0.7 mg) taken every day, without any pill-free interval. Based on limited published data, it appears that this regimen produces amenorrhea in most patients after 6 months of therapy, with minimal adverse affects on lipid metabolism. However, many patients will experience unpredictable breakthrough bleeding during the first 6 months, which may cause them to stop therapy. Furthermore, for patients who experience adverse side effects while using progestin, the continuous exposure to progestin may be more uncomfortable than cyclic exposure. Nevertheless, this regimen appears to be gaining increasing popularity, and may become a favored method in the future if the preliminary safety data are confirmed.

Cyclic or Continuous Progestin Alone

Some investigators have advocated the use of a so-called progesterone challenge test to determine estrogen deficiency. To perform this clinical test, a short course of a progestin is administered, usually MPA 10 mg/day for 5 or 7 days. If bleeding occurs, usually within 7 to 10 days after the last MPA tablet, it has been suggested that this demonstrates that the patient's circulating estrogen levels are high enough that replacement therapy is not necessary. It has been recommended that such patients should receive progestin periodically, usually every 3 to 6 months, both to determine their estrogen status and to induce shedding of the endometrium to decrease the risk of endometrial hyperplasia or adenocarcinoma. Unfortunately, there is no published information that correlates the results of a progesterone challenge test with the relative risks of postmenopausal osteoporosis, cardiovascular disease, vasomotor symptoms, urogenital atrophy, or other menopausal complications. Nevertheless, in patients who are reluctant to use estrogen or are not candidates for estrogen therapy, the periodic administration of progestins may be desirable. Furthermore, there is some evidence that progestins, particularly MPA, may provide some relief of vasomotor symptoms and may have some beneficial effect on calcium metabolism. For patients who cannot or will not use estrogen, therefore, continuous progestin therapy may offer some possible alternative. To my knowledge, a scientific study of the appropriate dosage has not yet been performed, but presumably, MPA at 10 mg/day might be considered. It is possible that other progestins, or the depot form of MPA might also be useful for this purpose.

DURATION OF THERAPY

If menopause is truly an endocrine deficiency state, then presumably one would need to continue replacement therapy indefinitely. Indeed, at least for bone metabolism, it has been demonstrated that stopping estrogen therapy, even after a number of years, will result in an acceleration of bone loss. Furthermore, it has not been demonstrated that the protective effect of estrogen replacement therapy in preventing cardiovascular disease diminishes with the length of time of exposure to estrogen. If estrogen has been prescribed to treat or prevent urogenital atrophy or dyspareunia, then therapy needs to be continued for as long as those beneficial effects are desired. For these reasons, at the present time, it does not appear possible to define a specific duration of therapy, after which estrogen will no longer be useful. Since therapy may need to be continued indefinitely, it is highly desirable to select a pattern of administration that provides maximum safety for that particular patient over long periods of administration.

While hormone replacement therapy is being prescribed, it seems reasonable to have the patient visit the physician every 6 months. At these visits, the patient is interviewed carefully regarding compliance, symptomatology, complications, and side effects. Height, weight, and blood pressure are measured and breast and pelvic examinations are performed at each visit. A more complete physical examination, including a Papanicolaou smear with a maturation index, is performed annually. Consistent with the recommendations of the American Cancer Society, women over age 50 should receive annual mammograms, whether or not they are receiving hormone therapy. At the present time, there is some disagreement about the timing, and even the necessity, for routine endometrial biopsy. Because the incidence of endometrial cancer in asymptomatic patients is so low, random screening endometrial biopsies do not appear to be cost effective. In a patient who has been estrogen deficient for some time, performing an endometrial biopsy can be quite difficult and can be painful for the patient. Therefore, in such patients, if a screening biopsy is to be performed, it may be done after several months of estrogen exposure, which appears to make the biopsy easier to perform. Although *any* abnormal or unpredicted vaginal bleeding after menopause requires further evaluation with some form of endometrial sampling, it may not be necessary to perform biopsies on asymptomatic patients who are having regular, predictable withdrawal bleeding on hormone replacement therapy. Nevertheless, with newer equipment that makes the biopsy less uncomfortable, it has been suggested that periodic endometrial biopsies be performed, presumably annually.

COMPLIANCE

As mentioned above, hormone replacement therapy may need to be continued indefinitely. For this reason, it is extremely important that the patient be comfortable, and committed to her treatment regimen. Clearly, some patients feel more comfortable taking tablets by mouth, and some patients will feel more comfortable using a transdermal patch. As long as there are no obvious contraindications or complications, every attempt should be made to comply with the individual patient's preference. The type of estrogen, the dosage, the type and dose of progestin, and the schedule of administration may all be modified to help make the treatment as comfortable as possible for each individual patient. Clinicians are encouraged to gain experience with each of the possible alternatives so that a customized treatment plan can be proposed when necessary. Books, pamphlets, and written instructions are often helpful to allow the patient to fully understand the rationale and details of her treatment, so that she can make a well-informed decision and commitment to therapy, if indicated. The twice-annual visits are good opportunities to review the details of menopause and hormone therapy, to discuss the information that appears in the media, and to answer the patient's questions and concerns.

SUMMARY

Menopause is an endocrine deficiency state that results in pathology for at least some women. Postmenopausal hormone replacement therapy can be designed using the principles that are applied to other endocrine deficiency states. It appears that any form of estrogen therapy that results in adequate levels of estrogen in circulation should be acceptable for therapy. A pattern of hormone replacement can be customized for each patient by using a type and dose of estrogen, a type and dose of progestin, a route of administration, and a treatment schedule that provides maximum safety, comfort, and effectiveness. The selected regimen can be modified, within certain bounds, to accommodate the needs of each individual patient. The ultimate goal is to design a treatment plan that is able to minimize as much as possible any potential risks of hormone replacement therapy while at the same time maximizing patient comfort and the documented benefits of hormone replacement therapy in appropriately selected patients.

Key Points

- Menopause is an endocrine deficiency state, with pathologic consequences in at least some women.
- Postmenopausal hormone replacement therapy can be designed based on general principles applied to other endocrine deficiencies.
- The specific hormones that are deficient after menopause are 17β-estradiol and progesterone. Testosterone is also reduced but to a greater degree after surgical menopause (bilateral oophorectomy).

- The *physiologic* effects of hormone replacement appear to be related to the ambient, circulating levels of hormone achieved. The *pharmacologic* effects of hormone replacement are related to the route of administration as well as to the type, dosage, and schedule used.
- Postmenopausal hormone replacement may be administered using a variety of different compounds. The dosage and schedule must be adjusted for the type of hormone used.
- Both oral and parenteral routes of administration are possible; each route has its own individual advantages and disadvantages.
- Every attempt should be made to select a form of therapy that provides maximal comfort, safety, effectiveness, and convenience for each individual patient.

References

1. Stumpf PG. Pharmacokinetics of estrogen. Obstet Gynecol 1990;75:9S–14S.
2. Stedman's medical dictionary. 25th ed. Baltimore: Williams & Wilkins, 1990:510.
3. Sherman BM. Endocrinologic and menstrual alterations. In: Mishell DR, ed. Menopause: physiology and pharmacology. Chicago: Year Book, 1987:41–51.
4. Powers MS, Schenkel L, Darley PE, Good WR, Balestra JC, Place VA. Pharmacokinetics and pharmacodynamics of transdermal dosage forms of 17β-estradiol: comparison with conventional oral estrogens used for hormone replacement. Am J Obstet Gynecol 1985;152:1099–1106.
5. Casey ML, MacDonald PC. Origin of estrogen and regulation of its formation in postmenopausal women. In: Buchssbaum HJ, ed. The menopause. New York: Springer-Verlag, 1983:1–8.
6. Quirk JG, Wendel GD. Biologic effects of natural and synthetic estrogens. In: Buchsbaum HJ, ed. The menopause. New York: Springer-Verlag, 1983:55–75.
7. Martin PL, Burnier AM, Greaney MO: Oral menopausal therapy using 17-β micronized estradiol: a preliminary study of effectiveness, tolerance and patient preference. Obstet Gynecol 1972;39:771.
8. Stumpf PG, Nakamura RM, Mishell DR. Changes in physiologically-free circulating estradiol and testosterone during exposure to levonorgestrel. J Clin Endocrinol Metab 1981;52:138–143.
9. Haynes RC, Murad F. Estrogens and progestins. In: Gilman AG, Goodman LS, Rall TW, Murad F, eds. Goodman and Gilman's the pharmacologic basis of therapeutics. 7th ed. New York: Macmillan, 1985:1412–1439.
10. Lobo RA, March CM, Goebelswann U, et al. Subdermal estradiol pellets following hysterectomy and oophorectomy: effect upon serum estrone, estradiol, luteinizing hormone, follicle-stimulating hormone, cortisol binding globulin-binding capacity, testosterone-estradiol binding globulin-binding capacity, lipids and hot flushes. Am J Obstet Gynecol 1980;138:714–719.
11. Notelovitz M, Johnston M, Smith S, Kitchens C. Metabolic and hormonal effects of 25 mg and 50 mg 17β-estradiol implants in surgically menopausal women. Obstet Gynecol 1987;70:749–754.

12. Schiff I, Tulchinsky D, Ryan KJ. Vaginal absorption of estrone and 17β-estradiol. Fertil Steril 1977;28:1063–1066.
13. Stumpf PG. Selecting constant serum estradiol levels achieved by vaginal rings. Obstet Gynecol 1986;67:91–94.
14. Riis BJ, Thomsen K, Strom V, Christiansen C. The effect of percutaneous estradiol and natural progesterone on postmenopausal bone loss. Am J Obstet Gynecol 1987;156:61–65.
15. Jensen J, Riis BJ, Strom V, Nilas L, Christiansen C. Long-term effects of percutaneous estrogen and oral progesterone on serum lipoproteins in postmenopausal women. Am J Obstet Gynecol 1987;156:66–71.
16. Laufer LR, DeFazio JL, Lu JKH, et al. Estrogen replacement therapy by transdermal estradiol administration. Am J Obstet Gynecol 1983;146:533–540.
17. Selby PL, Peacock M. Dose dependent response of symptoms, pituitary, and bone to transdermal estrogen in postmenopausal women. Br Med J 1986;293:1337–1339.
18. Judd H. Efficacy of transdermal estradiol. Am J Obstet Gynecol 1987;156:1326–1331.
19. Lobo RA. Absorption and metabolic effects of different types of estrogens and progestogens. Obstet Gynecol Clin North Am 1987;14(1):143–167.
20. Simon JA, Rodi IA, Stumpf PG, et al. Polysiloxane vaginal rings and cylinders for physiologic endometrial priming in functionally agonadal women. Fertil Steril 1986; 46:619–625.
21. Steingold K, Stumpf PG, Kreiner D, Liu H-C, Vanot D, Rosenwaks Z. Estradiol and progesterone replacement regimens for induction of endometrial receptivity. Fertil Steril 1989;52:756–760.

9

Complications of Estrogen Replacement Therapy

R. Don Gambrell Jr.

While the many benefits of estrogen replacement therapy were being increasingly recognized, some of the complications became emphasized in the mid-1970s. Several reports indicated that unopposed estrogens increased the risk for endometrial cancer. Concern had also been expressed for many years that estrogen replacement therapy might also increase the risk for breast cancer. However, numerous published studies have failed to incriminate exogenous estrogen use as a cause of breast cancer in postmenopausal women. Questions have also been raised about estrogen use and hypertension, thromboembolic and gallbladder diseases, and possible adverse effects of progestogens upon lipids. Many contraindications are listed in the product literature, including breast cancer, estrogen-dependent neoplasia, pregnancy, undiagnosed genital bleeding, and thromboembolic disorders. These are all discussed in detail in this chapter.

ENDOMETRIAL HYPERPLASIA

Hyperplasia of the endometrium has been established as a precancerous lesion in some women. In a prospective study of 562 women with adenomatous hyperplasia, 18.5% developed adenocarcinoma of the endometrium after a few years, but by the 10th year the incidence of cancer rose to 30% (1). In another study, 115 patients with hyperplasia or carcinoma-in-situ were observed for 2 to 8 years without any therapy, either hysterectomy or hormonal manipulation (2). A significant number developed invasive adenocarcinoma, including 26.7% of those with atypical hyperplasia and all of those with adenocarcinoma-in-situ. Shanklin suggested that cancer tendencies are set as early as age 30 and that the risk of focal hyperplasia, hyperplasia, adenomatous hyperplasia, atypical hyperplasia, carcinoma-in-situ, and carcinoma are a function of increasing age (3).

Of the 31 patients with endometrial cancer in the Wilford Hall USAF Medical Center studies, 11 (39.3%) had a previous diagnosis of hyperplasia from 4 months to 8 years before the detection of cancer (4). Although earlier studies contend that adenomatous hyperplasia may be precancerous, any degree of hyperplasia may be a significant lesion since six of these 11 patients had only benign or cystic hyperplasia, yet all developed adenocarcinoma of the endometrium within a relatively short period of time. Unopposed estrogens have a role in the development of endometrial hyperplasia and neoplasia, primarily because of incomplete shedding of the endometrium (Fig. 9.1) (6). Progestogen therapy ensures more complete sloughing of the endometrium, leaving behind fewer glands and cells for continued proliferation and growth.

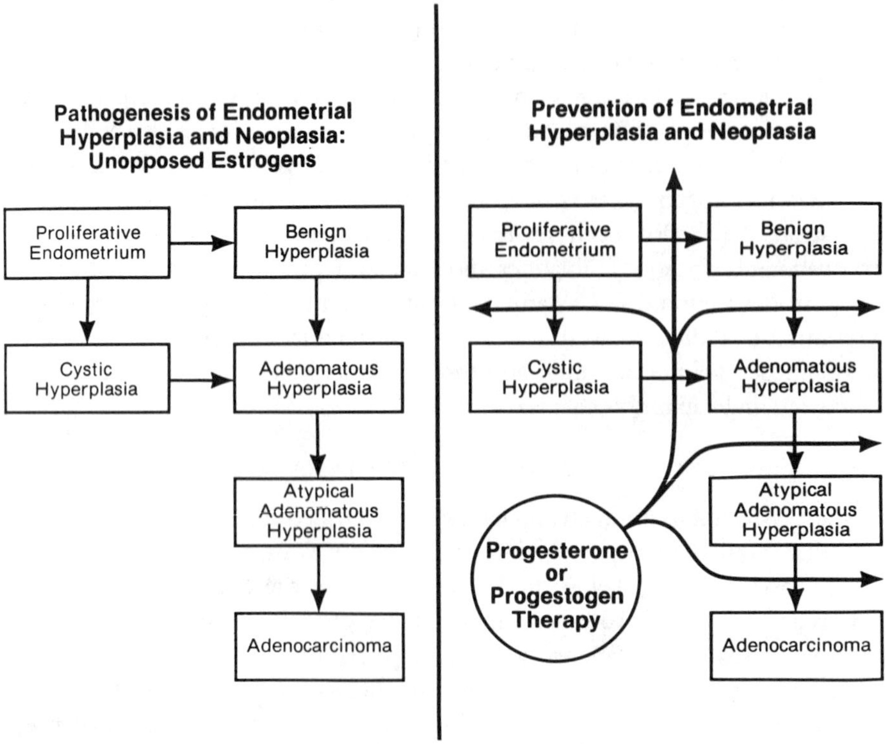

Figure 9.1. Schematic representation of the role of unopposed estrogens in the development of endometrial hyperplasia and cancer and the effect of progesterone or progestogens on these pathologic changes. (Reproduced from Gambrell RD Jr. The menopause: benefits and risks of estrogen-progestogen replacement therapy. Fertil Steril 1982;37:457.)

The protective action of progesterone is primarily physical. However, there are additional actions of both natural progesterone and synthetic progestogens that may be important (5). Progestogens decrease estrogen receptors in endometrial cells and induce estradiol dehydrogenase and isocitrate activity, which is the enzyme mechanism by which endometrial cells metabolize and excrete estrogens.

Treatment of Endometrial Hyperplasia

In our 5-year prospective study, 325 women were found to have varying degrees of endometrial hyperplasia (Table 9.1). They were treated with progestogens for 7 to 10 days each month for 3 to 6 months and the curettage was repeated after therapy. Hyperplasia reversed to normal endometrium in 307 (94.5%). Of the 18 patients with persistent hyperplasia after therapy, 14 had been given progestogens for only 7 days each month, while four patients with persistent hyperplasia had been treated with progestogens for 10 days monthly. During the past 8 years at the Medical College of Georgia, the duration of progestogens has been increased to 13 days. To date, all 55 patients with endometrial hyperplasia have reversed to normal endometrium. During the reproductive years, the human corpus luteum produces progesterone for 12 to 14 days during the normal 28-day ovulatory cycle. Therefore it is only logical that progestogens should be given to estrogen-treated women for at least 13 days during a 30-day or 31-day month.

The preferred method of treatment for endometrial hyperplasia is an initial curettage followed by a 6-month course of progestogen therapy. Norethindrone acetate 2.5 to 5 mg or medroxyprogesterone acetate 10 mg should be prescribed for 13 days each month. After 6 months of progestogen therapy,

Table 9.1.
Effects of Progestogens on Endometrial Hyperplasia

Pathology before Therapy	Number of Patients	Endometrium after Therapy	Number of Patients
Benign hyperplasia	196	Proliferative	156
Cystic hyperplasia	34	Secretory	98
Adenomatous hyperplasia	28	Atrophic	53
Atypical adenomatous hyperplasia	67	Benign hyperplasia	12
		Adenomatous hyperplasia	4
		Atypical adenomatous hyperplasia	2
Total patients	325	Total patients	325

the curettage should be repeated to ensure that the hyperplasia has reversed to normal endometrium. Should the hyperplasia persist after 6 months of progestogen therapy, hysterectomy should be considered. If the patient is on estrogen therapy, discontinuance is not necessary during the 6 months of progestogen therapy. The hyperplasia will reverse equally well on combined estrogen-progestogen therapy.

ENDOMETRIAL CANCER

Since the mid-1970s, numerous reports have implicated estrogen replacement therapy as a possible cause of endometrial cancer (7–16). These retrospective epidemiologic case-control studies indicate that postmenopausal estrogen users have a 1.7-fold to 20-fold increased relative risk for the development of endometrial carcinoma. Although the incidence of endometrial cancer was rising in the 1970s, mortality from this malignancy was decreasing, in part because of early detection and a high cure rate. Of all gynecologic cancers, adenocarcinoma of the endometrium is associated with the lowest mortality. In fact, the 5-year survival rate from endometrial cancer at Wilford Hall USAF Medical Center was in excess of 96.7% (17), and most institutions report a 5-year survival of 90% or greater.

Since simple hysterectomy without irradiation therapy is usually curative in these early diagnosed, well-differentiated lesions, some physicians are suggesting that annual endometrial biopsies be performed and progestogens not given. However, patients just cannot accept the fact that unopposed estrogens may cause endometrial cancer even though they have a 90% or better chance of being cured by hysterectomy. A recent report suggests that long-term use of estrogens increase the risk for both localized and widespread adenocarcinoma of the endometrium (for Stages III and IV combined, the relative risk (RR) was 3.1) (15). Although this study is probably flawed by methodology, their data also suggested that women who have taken estrogens for 1 year or longer remain at increased risk for endometrial carcinoma for at least 10 years after they discontinue use.

In another obviously flawed study, Swedish investigators claimed to have conducted a prospective study in which estrogen use increased the risk for both endometrial and breast cancer (16, 18). This study was not a cohort, long-term study of 23,244 women studied for 133,375 person-years, as they claimed. What this study represents is a case-control analysis of 74 cases of endometrial carcinoma and 33 cases of premalignant lesions of the endometrium. Only 90 of their 107 women answered their questionnaire to provide detailed information for proper assessment. The duration and dosages of added progestogens were inadequate in that they used 7- to 10-day combinations with levonorgestrel 25 to 150 μg or medroxyprogesterone acetate 5 to 10 mg. This group neither found the same magnitude of endometrial cancer with unopposed estrogens (relative risk of 1.8) nor the same protection from added progestogens (relative risk of 0.9) that has been universally observed (4, 5, 17, 19–20).

USE OF THE PROGESTOGEN CHALLENGE TEST TO PREVENT ENDOMETRIAL CANCER

The concept of adding cyclic progestogens to shed the endometrium of estrogen-treated postmenopausal women was introduced at Wilford Hall USAF Medical Center in 1971. Progestogen therapy was initially prescribed at this institution for 5 to 7 days each month. However, soon after our prospective study began in 1975, it was recognized that administration of progestogens for 5 to 7 days monthly was insufficient to reverse all endometrial hyperplasias and consequently prevent all endometrial cancers, so the duration of progestogens was increased to 10 days each month (17). Continuing studies demonstrated that even 10 days of progestogens each month may not be enough, since this duration will reverse only 98.4% of endometrial hyperplasias (4). There are now four cases of endometrial cancer among our estrogen-progestogen users in whom progestogens were used for 10 days each month. We concur with the recommendations of our British colleagues (19–21) that the minimal duration of cyclic progestogens should be for 12 to 14 days each month.

The progestogen challenge test (PCT) is another concept that evolved at our institution when it was recognized that the second highest incidence of endometrial cancer was consistently observed in our untreated women (Table 9.2). Not all postmenopausal women need estrogen replacement, since many

Table 9.2.
Incidence of Endometrial Cancer at Wilford Hall USAF Medical Center: 1975–1983

Therapy Group	Patient-Years of Observation	Patients with Cancer	Incidence (per 100,000)
Estrogen-progestogen users	16,327	8	49.0
Unopposed estrogen users	2,560	10	390.6
Estrogen vaginal cream users	2,716	2[a]	73.6
Progestogen or androgen users	1,160	0	—
Non-users	4,480	11	245.5
TOTAL	27,243	31	113.8

[a]Includes past estrogen vaginal cream users.

produce sufficient endogenous estrogens to remain asymptomatic and prevent the metabolic changes of long-term estrogen deprivation. However, within this group may be those in need of progestogen therapy to prevent hyperplasia of the endometrium, which may lead to adenocarcinoma. The PCT should be administered to all postmenopausal women with an intact uterus, including estrogen-treated patients, women being evaluated for estrogen therapy, and asymptomatic postmenopausal women at their annual examination. If there is a positive response, as manifested by withdrawal bleeding, then the progestogen should be continued for 13 days each month for as long as withdrawal bleeding follows. If there is no response, it is recommended that the PCT be repeated in the asymptomatic non-estrogen users each year.

Our original work on the PCT has been confirmed by a prospective study utilizing 100 mg of progesterone in oil given intramuscularly (23). In this study of 30 asymptomatic postmenopausal women, five had withdrawal bleeding to the PCT, and three of these five (60%) had either adenomatous or atypical adenomatous hyperplasia. In the 25 subjects with no withdrawal bleeding, the endometrial histology was entirely normal, mostly atrophic or inactive endometrium. There were no adenocarcinomas in either group, and although the number of subjects was small, the difference between these two groups was statistically significant ($P \leq 0.001$). In the second phase of this study, in which the authors tested this concept in 10 patients with known adenomatous hyperplasia, the PCT resulted in withdrawal bleeding in nine, confirming the effectiveness of this test in detecting abnormal endometrial pathology.

During the 5 years of prospective study and 4 years of follow-up from 1975 through 1983, 5563 postmenopausal women were registered in the hormone use survey (22). However, approximately 40% had a previous hysterectomy and so were not at risk for endometrial cancer and were not included in the study. Adenocarcinoma of the endometrium was diagnosed in 31 patients during 27,243 patient-years of observation, for an overall incidence of 113.8 per 100,000 women per year (Table 9.2). The largest group of patients, the estrogen-progestogen users, had the lowest incidence of cancer, with eight cases for an annual incidence of 49.0 per 100,000 women. The highest incidence of endometrial carcinoma was observed in the unopposed estrogen users, in whom 10 cases were detected during 2,560 patient-years of observation, for an incidence of 390.6 per 100,000. The difference between these two groups was highly statistically significant, with $P \leq 0.0006$. Eleven untreated women were found to have adenocarcinoma during 4,480 patient-years, for an incidence of 245.4 per 100,000. The estrogen-progestogen users also had a significantly lower incidence of cancer than the untreated women with $P \leq 0.004$. No cancers were detected in the progestogen or androgen users. This group consisted primarily of progestogen users, women who had been identified as being at increased risk for adenocarcinoma by the PCT and who were being treated with cyclic progestogens only.

Figure 9.2 illustrates the incidence of endometrial cancer in the various groups on a yearly basis from 1975 through 1983. The estrogen-progestogen users had a consistently lower incidence of endometrial malignancy than either the unopposed estrogen users or the untreated women. All of the 10 adenocarcinomas of the endometrium observed in the unopposed estrogen

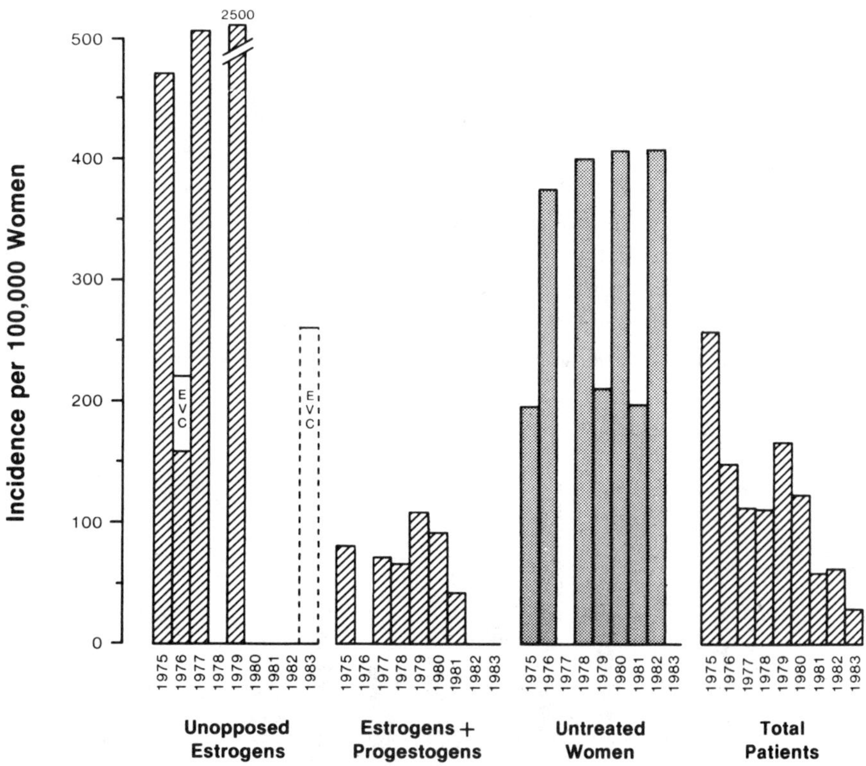

Figure 9.2. Incidence of endometrial cancer in the various treatment groups compared with that in the untreated women. *Solid lines,* current users: *broken lines,* past users. (Reproduced from Gambrell RD Jr. Prevention of endometrial cancer with progestogens. Maturitas 1986;8:159.)

users occurred during the first 5 years of study. Of the two cases in the estrogen vaginal cream (EVC) users, one was diagnosed during 1976 following 7 months of EVC use (1 g three times weekly). The other case occurred in 1983 in a former EVC user who had used this unopposed estrogen for two years but who had ceased therapy 4½ years before the cancer was diagnosed. Since the duration of progestogen was increased to 13 days in 1982 and 1983, there have been no additional cases in the estrogen-progestogen users. Ever-increasing use of the PCT has decreased the overall incidence of this malignancy from 257.3 per 100,000 in 1975 to 29.1 per 100,000 during 1983.

Figure 9.3 compares the number of estrogen users and the number of estrogen-progestogen users to the number of cancer cases each year for the 12 years from 1972 through 1983. Three years of retrospective data were added to the prospective and follow-up study for 1972–1974, by obtaining cases of endometrial malignancy from the tumor registry and estimating hormone use from computerized pharmacy records. With ever-increasing estrogen use from approximately 1000 postmenopausal women in 1972 to 2300 by 1975, there was no increase in the cases of endometrial cancer: six in 1972, five in 1973, and seven each during 1974 and 1975. However, with ever-increasing progestogen addition, from approximately 10% of the estrogen users in 1972 to 98.7% of the estrogen users by 1983, the number of cancers decreased from seven in 1975 to three or four each over the next 5 years, to two cases each in 1981 and 1982, and finally down to a single case during 1983.

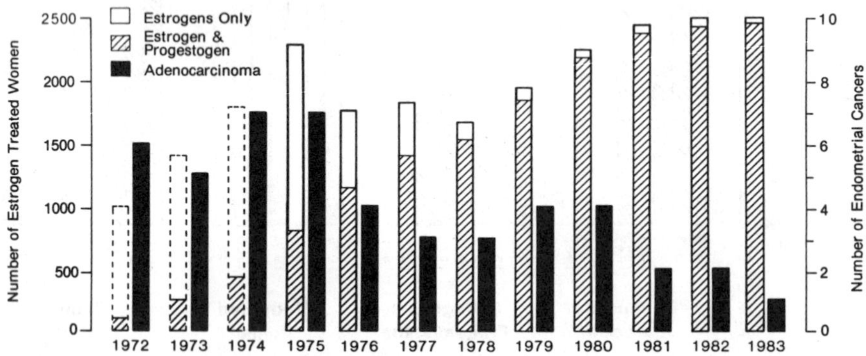

Figure 9.3. Number of cases of adenocarcinoma of the endometrium in hormone users compared to number of estrogen and estrogen-progestogen users from 1972 to 1983. *Solid lines,* data from prospective and follow-up study; *broken lines,* estimated data from computerized pharmacy records. (Reproduced from Gambrell RD Jr. Prevention of endometrial cancer with progestogens. Maturitas 1986;8:159.)

BENIGN BREAST DISEASE

Whether benign breast disease is related to carcinoma of the breast is still uncertain. According to most studies, women with fibrocystic disease of the breast have a two-fold to four-fold increased risk of developing breast cancer (24–26). It may be that women with fibrocystic disease are at increased risk, while those with fibroadenoma are not at any increased risk. The actual etiology of benign breast disease is unknown but is believed to result from an exaggerated or inappropriate tissue response induced by the ebb and flow of ovarian hormones (27). Most women with symptomatic benign breast disease have some relief after menopause, which may be exacerbated with estrogen replacement therapy. Both nodularity and mastodynia may decrease at menopause, only to return when estrogen therapy is begun.

When there is an increase in breast tenderness with estrogen use, it was clinically recognized that progestogens, particularly medroxyprogesterone acetate, may afford relief; however, it may take months to accomplish and ironically there may be an increase in mastodynia during the first few months of use. In some patients the nodularity of fibrocystic disease may decrease as evidenced by mammography after 12 to 18 months of progestogen use. Certainly, review of the studies regarding oral contraceptives and benign breast disease, have consistently shown a reduction in the risk with increasing duration of use (24). About one-third of women with fibrocystic breast disease will have intraductal epithelial hyperplasia (28). Women with hyperplasia have a threefold, and women with atypical hyperplasia have a sixfold increased risk of breast cancer.

Long-term treatment with either a progestogen or a low-estrogen/high-progestogen oral contraceptive effectively reduces intraductal epithelial hyperplasia and atypical hyperplasia (29). The relative risk of ductal carcinoma-in-situ in 1080 patients treated for 6 years was 0.2 from that expected (29). Other hormones that may reduce benign breast disease, and consequently the subsequent development of carcinoma, include androgens such as methyl testosterone 5 mg daily or fluoxymesterone 2 to 5 mg daily, tamoxifen 10 mg daily, bromocriptine 2.5 mg b.i.d., and danazol 100 to 400 mg daily (24).

BREAST CANCER

Women fear breast cancer as much as, if not more than, any other malignancy. Rightfully so, since carcinoma of the breast will strike one in nine women in the United States. It is the most frequent malignancy in females, accounting for 32% of all cancers (30). The American Cancer Society estimated that

180,000 new cases of breast carcinoma would be diagnosed in the United States in 1992 and that 46,000 women would die from this tumor that year. The good news is that the mortality from breast cancer is leveling off in that the percent increase in mortality from breast cancer has steadily declined during the past 5 years: from 3.8% between 1985 and 1986, to 2.7% in 1987, 2.4% in 1988, 2.3% in 1989, 2.1% in 1990, and down to 1.1% during 1991.

The frequency of breast cancer increases throughout the female life span (Fig. 9.4). In this respect, the incidence of this malignancy differs from cervical, endometrial, and ovarian cancer, which peak in the fourth, fifth, and sixth decades of life, respectively, and then either decline or plateau. The sharpest increase in the frequency of breast cancer occurs between the mid-30s and early 50s, or just prior to menopause. Then the incidence continues to rise steeply throughout the postmenopausal years, when estrogen levels are lower but not completely absent.

There are at least 28 published studies of exogenous estrogen use and breast cancer in postmenopausal women (Table 9.3) (4, 18, 31–56). None have been able to assess all the risk factors for mammary malignancy, and there is wide variance in the design and quality of these studies. What is quite obvious is that all of the relative risks hover around 1.0, or no increased risk at all. There are also five meta-analyses of estrogen therapy and breast cancer that confirm that there is no increased risk (relative risk 1.01 to 1.3; 95% confidence interval 0.87 to 1.6) (56a–56e). That estrogen replacement therapy may be causally related to carcinoma of the breast has been debated for many years. Yet none of these studies have incriminated exogenous estrogen use as a cause of mammary malignancy in postmenopausal women. There are four studies—including the recent Swedish study (18) that received such wide press coverage—that have observed a significantly increased risk for breast cancer in small subgroups of estrogen users, but not in their overall patient population. The publication of this Swedish study linking estrogen therapy to an increased risk of breast cancer was premature, to say the least (18). Their mean duration of follow-up (5.7 years) is too short, since most breast cancers have been developing for 7 to 8 years before being clinically detectable. Only 29 of their 253 patients with breast cancer used estrogens for 9 years or longer (relative risk 1.7; 95% confidence interval, 1.1 to 2.7). Yet the 45 women who never used estrogens had a similar relative risk of 1.6 (95% confidence interval, 1.1 to 2.1).

Their conclusions that breast cancer is not prevented and may even be increased by added progestogens is invalid, not only because of the short follow-up (6 years) but also because it is based on only 10 patients with breast

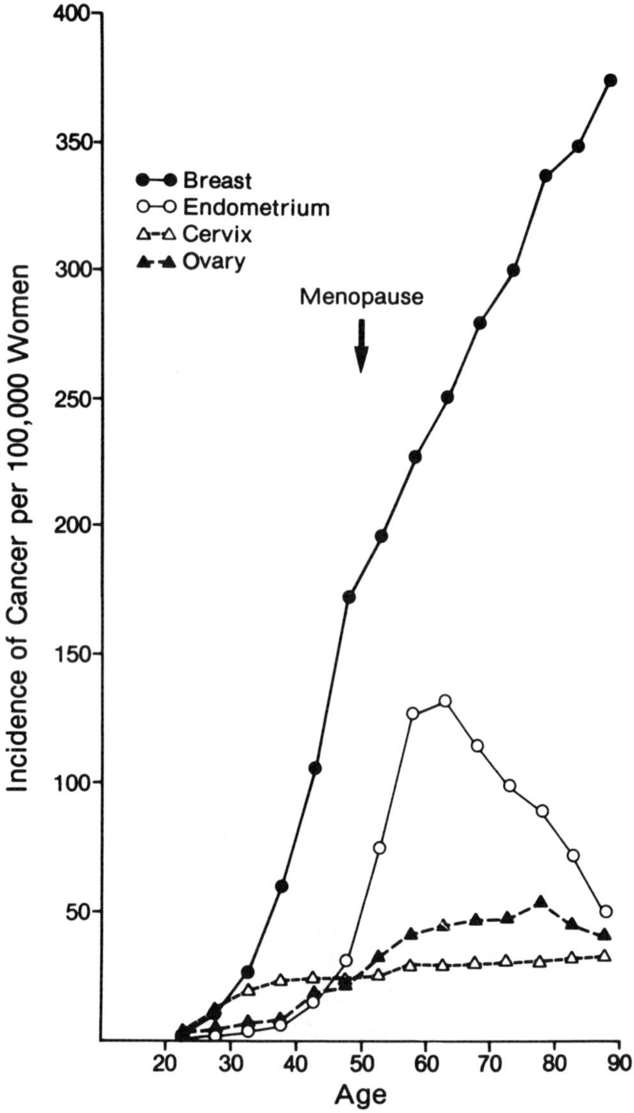

Figure 9.4. Incidence of breast, endometrial, cervical, and ovarian cancer in women according to age. (Reproduced from Gambrell RD Jr. Breast disease in the postmenopausal years. Semin Reprod Endocrinol 1983;1:27.)

Table 9.3.
Studies of Exogenous Estrogens and Breast Cancer

Authors	Number of Cases	Relative Risk		
		Intact Ovaries		Ovaries Removed
Bergkvist et al., 1989 (18)	253		1.7	
Bland et al., 1980 (31)	25		0.4	
Boston Drug Surveillance, 1974 (32)	51		1.0	
Brinton et al., 1981 (33)	881	1.2		1.5
Brinton et al., 1986 (34)	1,960	1.05	1.0	1.14
Brinton et al., 1986 (35)	320		1.5	
Burch et al., 1976 (36)	33		1.4	
Casagrande et al., 1976 (37)	47		3.1	
Craig et al., 1974 (38)	134		1.0	
Gambrell, 1987 (4)	69		0.7	
Hammond et al., 1979 (39)	8		1.1	
Henderson et al., 1974 (40)	308		0.8	
Hoover et al., 1976 (41)	49		1.3	
Hoover et al., 1981 (42)	345	1.3		1.5
Hulka et al., 1982 (43)	199	1.7		1.2
Hunt et al., 1987 (44)	50		1.59	
Jick et al., 1980 (45)	97	3.4		1.1
Kaufman et al., 1984 (46)	1,610	0.7–1.3	0.9	0.5–1.1
Kelsey et al., 1981 (47)	332	0.8–1.1		0.9–1.5
Lauritzen and Meier, 1984 (48)	10		0.9	
Nachtigall et al., 1979 (49)	4		0.0	
Rohan & McMichael, 1988 (50)	281		1.03	
Ross et al., 1980 (51)	138	0.9–2.5		0.7–0.9
Sartwell et al., 1983 (52)	284		0.8	
Sherman et al., 1983 (53)	113		0.6	
Volker, 1980 (54)	120		0.9	
Wingo et al., 1987 (55)	1,369	0.8	1.1	1.3
Wynder et al., 1978 (56)	785		1.1	

cancer (relative risk 4.4; 95% confidence interval, 0.9 to 22.4). As shown in their companion report on endometrial cancer (16), the duration and dosage of the added progestogens were inadequate, using as little as 7 days of medroxyprogesterone 5 mg each month. In our studies of breast cancer in estrogen users, with and without added progestogens, we observed a slight but insignificant increase in the incidence of breast cancer during the first 5 years of prospective study (4). A significant decrease in the incidence of breast cancer was not observed until the ninth and tenth years of ever-increasing addition of progestogens to estrogen replacement.

Also in August 1989, this same Swedish group published another paper in a different journal, utilizing the same data base of 253 breast cancer patients, where they observed a significantly higher survival rate in estrogen users (57). It is a shame that this information was not included in the press release, for if it had been, the terrible impact on hormone replacement would have been lessened. The authors stated that this had not been previously studied; however, their report confirmed several earlier studies, with none to the contrary, indicating an improved prognosis of breast cancer developing in estrogen users (36, 44, 58). Now with 8 to 18 years' follow-up of the 256 postmenopausal women with breast cancer at Wilford Hall USAF Medical Center, life-table analysis reveals median survival times of 77.7 months for never users and greater than 192 months for the hormone users ($P \leq 0.001$). In the study from England of 4544 hormone users, the mortality from breast cancer was significantly reduced to a relative risk of 0.55 (95% confidence interval, 0.28 to 0.96) (44).

PROTECTION FROM BREAST CANCER WITH ADDED PROGESTOGEN

During the 9 years of prospective study at Wilford Hall USAF Medical Center from 1975 to 1983, 69 postmenopausal women were diagnosed with breast cancer during 48,669 patient-years of observation for an overall incidence of 141.9:100,000 women per year (Table 9.4). The lowest incidence of mammary malignancy was in the estrogen-progestogen users, with 11 patients diagnosed with cancer during 16,466 patient-years of observation for an annual incidence of 66.8:100,000 women. During 19,676 patient-years of unopposed estrogen use, there were 28 cancers for an incidence of 142.3:100,000. With 22 carcinomas of the breast during 6,404 patient-years of observation, the incidence in the non-users was 343.6:100,000. The incidence of mammary malignancy in the estrogen-progestogen users

Table 9.4.
Incidence of Breast Cancer at Wilford Hall USAF Medical Center: 1975–1983

Therapy Group	Patient-Years of Observation	Patients with Cancer	Incidence (per 100,000)
Estrogen-progestogen users	16,466	11[a]	66.8
Unopposed estrogen users	19,676	28[a]	142.3
Estrogen vaginal cream users	4,298	5[a]	116.3
Progestogen users	1,825	3[a]	164.4
Non-users	6,404	22	343.5
Total Patients	48,669	69	141.8

[a]Includes past users.

(66.8:100,000) was significantly lower than that in the non-users (343.6:100,000) with $P \leq 0.01$. The difference between the estrogen-progestogen users (66.8:100,000) and unopposed estrogen users (142.3:100,000) was not significant but does indicate a trend in that direction ($P \leq 0.08$). The expected incidence of breast carcinoma in this age group, according to the Third National Cancer Survey (59), is 188.3:100,000 and for ages 55 to 59, according to the National Cancer Institute Surveillance, Epidemiology, and End Results (SEER) data (60), would be 229.2:100,000. The risk for breast cancer in the estrogen-progestogen users was significantly lower than expected when compared to the NCI SEER data (relative risk 0.3; 95% confidence interval, 0.1 to 0.8). The risk was also lower than expected in the unopposed estrogen users; however, this was not statistically significant (relative risk 0.7; 95% confidence interval, 0.5 to 1.1).

The concept of adding progestogens to estrogen replacement therapy for postmenopausal women was introduced at Wilford Hall USAF Medical Center in 1971. Figure 9.5 compares the number of estrogen and estrogen-progestogen treated women with the incidence of breast cancer for the 12 years from 1972 through 1983, including 3 years of retrospective data from

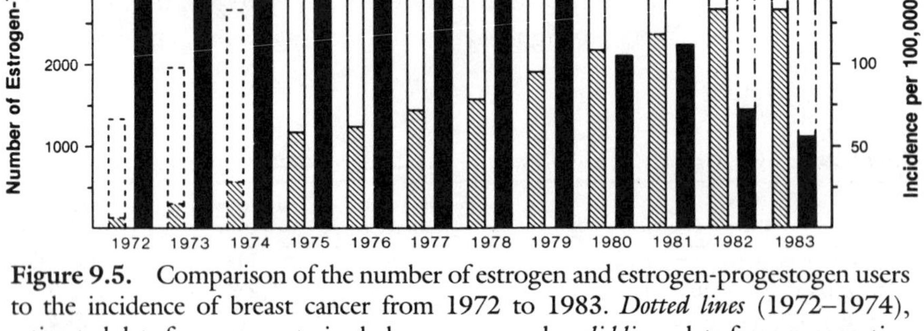

Figure 9.5. Comparison of the number of estrogen and estrogen-progestogen users to the incidence of breast cancer from 1972 to 1983. *Dotted lines* (1972–1974), estimated data from computerized pharmacy records; *solid lines,* data from prospective and follow-up study; *broken lines* (1982 and 1983), former users. (Reproduced from Gambrell RD Jr. Role of progestogens in the prevention of breast cancer. Maturitas 1986;8:169.)

1972 to 1974. With increased estrogen use, from approximately 1320 patients in 1972 to 3940 estrogen-treated women during 1975, there was no increase in the incidence of mammary malignancy. The apparent decline in the incidence of breast carcinoma from 189.4:100,000 in 1972 to 143.4:100,000 during 1975 was not statistically significant. However, with ever-increasing progestogen addition from approximately 9.1% of the estrogen users in 1972 to 61.1% of the estrogen users by 1983, a significant decrease in the incidence of breast carcinoma occurred in the ninth and tenth years of study, from 183.8:100,000 in 1978 to 104.3:100,000 in 1980 and 110.4:100,000 during 1981, and finally down to 53.9:100,000 in the continuing users during 1983.

There are two other studies in addition to ours indicating that adding progestogens to estrogen therapy may decrease the risk for carcinoma of the breast (48, 49). A study from West Germany also observed a lower incidence of breast carcinoma in the unopposed estrogen users (123:100,000) compared to non-users (154:100,000); however, this was not significant (48). The incidence of mammary malignancy in the estrogen-progestogen users (109:100,000) was significantly lower ($P \leq 0.05$) compared to either the estrogen users or non-users. The New York group studied 84 estrogen users for 10 years in a carefully controlled double-blind study and compared these to 84 placebo users (49). No carcinomas of the breast were found in the 84 estrogen-progestogen users, while four were observed in the placebo users, which was significant with $P \leq 0.05$. In no way does the Swedish study (18) detract from these other studies with their higher relative risk of breast cancer in estrogen-progestogen users. It was not statistically significant (relative risk 4.4; 95% confidence interval, 0.9 to 22.4) and was based on only 10 patients with more than 6 years of use. Very convincing evidence will be published in 1992 confirming that added progestogen reduces the risk for breast cancer in long-term estrogen users.

There is other evidence that progesterone deficiency may increase the risk for breast cancer. In a long-term follow-up of a group of infertility patients, those with progesterone deficiency had 5.4 times the risk of premenopausal carcinoma of the breast when compared to women in the non-hormone group, those whose infertility was caused by other factors (61). The incidence of postmenopausal breast cancer did not differ significantly between the two groups; however, these patients were just reaching menopause. Another study of progesterone deficiency did observe an increased risk of postmenopausal breast cancer (62). Chronic anovulation increased the risk of endometrial cancer 5-fold, and the risk of breast carcinoma after age 55 was increased

3.6-fold. These studies in both premenopausal and postmenopausal women indicate that progestogens should be added to estrogen replacement therapy, even after hysterectomy, to reduce the risk for carcinoma of the breast.

HYPERTENSION

Because the original high-dosage oral contraceptives were associated with transient hypertension in some young women, estrogen replacement therapy had been expected to have a similar effect. However, numerous studies have indicated that estrogen therapy has a beneficial effect on hypertension. In the study from Duke University, the incidence of new hypertensive cardiovascular disease was 16.3% in estrogen-treated women compared to 31.7% in non-users ($P \leq 0.001$) (63). A study of 1496 women from southern California, after adjusting for the effects of obesity, observed that estrogen users tended to have lower blood pressure and blood glucose than controls (64). In our Wilford Hall USAF Medical Center studies, the estrogen users had a significantly lower diastolic blood pressure while non-users were more obese (65). Australian studies observed a lowered systolic blood pressure with one natural estrogen (estropipate) and a lowered diastolic blood pressure with another (conjugated estrogens) (66). An English study observed that both systolic and diastolic blood pressure are significantly reduced in women on various regimens of hormone replacement (67).

Hypertension increases in the age group of postmenopausal women; cases will therefore be found among estrogen users (68, 69). However, these do not establish the role of estrogens in hypertension. Elevations in blood pressure can coexist with hormone replacement, so blood pressure should be routinely monitored. Other studies have reported the effect of estrogen use on the renin-angiotensin system. One study showed no activation of the renin-aldosterone system in patients using estradiol valerate therapy (70). Another study reported an increased plasma renin activity in users of conjugated estrogens, but no effect on the renin concentration itself (71). Neither study observed any adverse effect of estrogens on blood pressure when hormone users were matched to controls and corrected for age and weight.

If hypertension does occur in estrogen users, estrogen replacement does not have to stop (72). Instead, as a first step, salt intake should be restricted to 3000 mg daily. If salt restriction alone does not control the hypertension, a mild antihypertensive such as hydrochlorothiazide (25 to 50 mg daily) can be added. Only if these two measures fail to improve blood pressure levels should there be consideration of ending estrogen replacement. Most hypertensive patients require less medication after hormone replacement.

THROMBOEMBOLIC DISEASE

Estrogen replacement therapy has been thought to increase thromboembolic phenomena, which are listed as contraindications. This concept is based largely on observations suggesting an association between oral contraceptives and vascular thrombosis. Despite a positive association between aging and thrombotic complications, clinical studies have failed to observe any increased risk of these disorders (36, 49, 63, 73). The concentrations of coagulation factors V and VII, and possibly VIII, increase with aging (73). Antithrombin III activity does not change after menopause. Prothombin time and partial thromboplastin time are not affected by estrogen replacement therapy. Fibrinogen concentration increases with estrogen use; however, the magnitude of the rise varies with the type of estrogen. With conjugated estrogens, fibrinogen values increase but remain within the normal range. Mestranol significantly increases fibrinogen levels and may provide a thrombogenic hazard. Coagulation factor V decreases during estrogen therapy, but factors VII and X do not change. Antithrombin III activity is probably the most sensitive and clinically reliable test of hypercoagulability. It is significantly decreased in pregnant women and oral contraceptive users but is only slightly decreased with conjugated estrogens, remaining within the normal range. In postmenopausal women treated with mestranol, antithrombin III activity decreases significantly, suggesting that synthetic estrogens, such as mestranol, produce greater changes in certain coagulation factors than do natural estrogens.

In a long-term clinical study, deaths from cerebral vascular accidents (CVAs) declined from an expected 15 to eight during estrogen replacement in 1000 women studied for 15 years (36). It was concluded that estrogens delay aging of the arteries. Although another more recent study observed an increase in CVAs, the only significant increase was in women who smoked, and there were some problems with the methodology in this study (74). The Duke University study observed a significantly lower incidence of stroke syndromes in long-term estrogen users compared with a similar group who had never used estrogens (63). No significant difference in the incidence of either thrombophlebitis or embolism was observed between estrogen-treated women and patients who had never received estrogens. In a double-blind study, thrombophlebitis occurred in 13 of 84 estrogen-progestogen users and 17 of 84 placebo users (49). Only one incidence of pulmonary embolism was encountered during the 10 years of this study and it occurred in a placebo user. In the most recent report, 20 of 4962 estrogen users died from stroke compared with 43 of 3845 non-users (relative risk 0.53, 95% confidence interval 0.31 to 0.91) (75). Protection was found in all age groups except the youngest and was unaffected by adjustment for possible confounding factors such as hypertension, smoking, alcohol consumption, body mass, and exercise.

Estrogen labeling has recently been changed so that no longer are all thromboembolic events a contraindication. Active thrombophlebitis or thromboembolic disorders remain a contraindication as does a past history of thrombophlebitis, thrombosis, or thromboembolic disorders associated with previous estrogen use. No longer are postpartum, postoperative, or traumatic blood clots a contraindication. However, in patients with any history of thromboembolic disease, it would seem prudent to obtain coagulation studies, including antithrombin III activity, and repeat these after 3 to 6 months of estrogen use.

GALLBLADDER DISEASE

Some studies have indicated that estrogen replacement therapy increases the risk for gallbladder disease, especially cholelithiasis. The liver responds to oral estrogens by an increase in sex hormone–binding globulin (SHBG), so non-oral routes of administration may be safer. It has been suggested that oral estrogens may affect the liver's excretory functions and may increase the incidence of gallstones. Gallstones seem to occur more frequently in the silent form. In one study, oral cholecystography showed that 5.1% of those tested had gallstones present (76). Silent cases occurred twice as often, and the diet was not significantly different in those with or without gallstones.

One evaluative study reported that the risk of surgically confirmed gallbladder disease increased 2.5 times with estrogen therapy (32). In another study, the risk of cholesterol cholelithiasis was increased by both estrogens and obesity (77). Both factors operated independently, with estrogen increasing the risk of gallstones at all weight levels. However, in the Duke University study, new occurrences of gallbladder disease were significantly lower ($P \leq 0.05$) in the estrogen users when compared to never-users (63). At the end of the 10-year study from New York, the estrogen-progestogen group had a higher, although statistically insignificant, incidence of cholelithiasis (49). The most recent study found no increased risk for gallstones among estrogen users (relative risk 1.18; 95% confidence interval, 0.65 to 2.13) (78). Among estrogen users, the duration of use was similar in cases and controls.

Since it is not feasible to screen all postmenopausal women for occult gallbladder disease prior to the initiation of estrogen therapy, it has been suggested that patients should be instructed about the early signs of cholelithiasis (77). These include right upper quadrant pain, indigestion, eructation, and nausea.

POTENTIAL ADVERSE EFFECTS OF PROGESTOGENS ON LIPIDS

Concern has been expressed that adding progestogens to estrogen replacement therapy may adversely affect the estrogen-induced beneficial effects on lipids, thus negating the benefit of hormone replacement on heart disease. In our prospective study, a standard dosage of estrogen was used (50 mg of estradiol by subcutaneous implantation of pellets every 6 months) and was combined with three different progestogens for 10 days each month (79). Lipoproteins were drawn at baseline and repeated at 6-, 12-, and 18-month intervals. With this dosage of estrogen combined with medroxyprogesterone acetate 10 mg, there was a significant increase in HDL cholesterol with a significant decrease of LDL cholesterol and an insignificant decrease in VLDL cholesterol (Fig. 9.6). It was not the medroxyprogesterone acetate that increased the HDL cholesterol and decreased the LDL cholesterol, but this C-21 progestogen did not adversely affect the estrogen-induced improvement in the LDL/HDL ratio over the long term. With norgestrel 0.075 mg, HDL increased only slightly with no change in LDL but a significant decrease

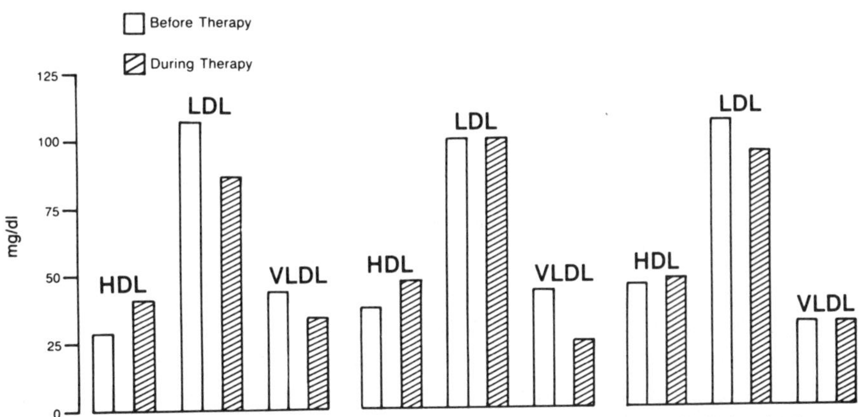

Figure 9.6. Changes in various fractions of lipoproteins with estrogen therapy combined with three different progestogens. (Reproduced from Gambrell RD Jr. The menopause: benefits and risks of estrogen-progestogen replacement therapy. Intern Med Specialists 1985;6:135.)

in VLDL. Using norethindrone acetate 5 mg, there was still a slight increase in HDL, a moderate decrease in LDL, and no change in VLDL. Lower dosages of this 19-norsteroid progestogen are fully protective of the endometrium, so 2.5 mg of this progestogen and especially 2.5 mg of norethindrone may produce just as favorable a lipid pattern as the C-21 progestogens. Although only medroxyprogesterone acetate left the significantly improved estrogen-induced lipid pattern, neither of the 19-nortestosterone progestogens fully negated the estrogen effects in that LDL/HDL ratios were improved from baseline.

In a cross-sectional study of the long-term effects of estrogens and progestogens on lipids and lipoproteins, no adverse effects of progestogens were observed in postmenopausal women receiving therapy for up to 44 years (79a). In this study of 556 women aged between 44 and 85 years (mean age 57.14 ± 10.56 years) receiving hormone replacement for 1 to 44 years (mean duration of therapy 11.97 ± 8.11 years), there were no significant differences in mean HDL cholesterol levels: 67.0 ± 3.94 mg/dl in those receiving unopposed estrogen; 64.5 ± 4.16 mg/dl in those receiving estrogen plus C-21 progestogen; and 61.9 ± 3.84 mg/dl in those receiving estrogen plus C-19 progestogen. Triglyceride levels were related to weight and were significantly different only between non-hormone users of normal weight (128.3 ± 7.80 mg/dl) and hormone users weighing more than 200 pounds (252.9 ± 9.44 mg/dl). Smoking significantly depressed HDL cholesterol in both the hormone users (56.3 ± 4.26 mg/dl) and non-users (48.8 ± 3.69 mg/dl).

Other studies with postmenopausal hormone replacement also indicate that it may take several months to reach the beneficial improvement in lipids, so short-term studies should be discounted. In a study from Denmark using percutaneous estrogens combined with micronized oral progesterone in the second year, HDL cholesterol did not change until 12 months, when it increased (80). After oral progesterone was added in the second year, there was an initial decrease in HDL, followed by a rise at 18 and 24 months. Total cholesterol and LDL cholesterol decreased significantly throughout the first 12 months of unopposed estrogen use. There was a further decrease in both total cholesterol and LDL throughout the second year when oral micronized progesterone was added to the estrogen therapy. It may be the dosage of estrogen that is most important in improving the lipid pattern to decrease the risk for cardiovascular disease. In a study comparing different dosages of micronized estradiol, 1, 2, and 4 mg, combined with a standard dosage of progestogen, norethindrone acetate 1 mg for 11 days, HDL cholesterol increased significantly only with the 2 mg and 4 mg of estradiol (81). Total cholesterol decreased significantly only with the 4 mg of estradiol combined with 1 mg of norethindrone acetate, but there were significant decreases in LDL cholesterol with all three dosages of estradiol.

CONTRAINDICATIONS

There are several contraindications listed in the product literature for both estrogens and progestogens that are strikingly similar (Table 9.5). There is no evidence that estrogen replacement therapy increases the risk for breast cancer. However, estrogens are the growth hormones of mammary tissue and these contraindications must be observed until further data are accumulated. Theoretically, estrogen receptors would allow selection of some patients for estrogen therapy, yet only 50% of estrogen receptor–positive tumors will respond to either endocrine ablative surgery or anti-estrogen or progestogen therapy. When progesterone receptors in mammary cancer are also positive, this predictive response increases to 70%. However, it has not yet been determined which patients could be treated safely.

Endometrial cancer may not have to remain a strict contraindication. Gynecologic oncologists at Wilford Hall USAF Medical Center provided estrogen replacement in women with Stage I well-differentiated adenocarcinoma of the endometrium since there was little likelihood of metastases. The 5-year survival was in excess of 96.7%. A recent study from Duke University indicated that the prognosis was actually improved in endometrial cancer patients treated with estrogens after definitive therapy for the malignancy (82). Any abnormal postmenopausal bleeding should be thoroughly evalu-

Table 9.5.
Contraindications for Estrogens and Progestogens

Estrogens	Progestogens
Known or suspected cancer of the breast	A past or present history of:
Known or suspected estrogen-dependent neoplasia	Thrombophlebitis
	Thromboembolic disorders
Known or suspected pregnancy	Cerebral apoplexy
Undiagnosed abnormal genital bleeding	Liver dysfunction or disease
Active thrombophlebitis or thromboembolic disorders	Known or suspected carcinoma of the breast
A past history of problems associated with previous estrogen use:	Undiagnosed vaginal bleeding
	Missed abortion
Thrombophlebitis	As a diagnostic test for pregnancy
Thrombosis	
Thromboembolic disorders	

ated. Once malignancy is excluded and endometrial hyperplasia has been adequately treated with progestogens, estrogen-progestogen replacement therapy can be safely administered (83). Although there is no evidence that low dosages of natural estrogens have any adverse effect on coagulation factors or thromboembolic disease, estrogen replacement should be withheld in women who had blood clots previously while using estrogens. Thromboembolic events not related to a previous history of hormone use are no longer contraindications for replacement therapy.

Almost identical contraindications are listed for progestogens as for estrogens, although there is no evidence that progestogens have any adverse effect on coagulation factors or thromboembolic disorders. This labeling should not preclude the physician from using his or her best judgment in the interest of the patient. If liver function studies are normal, a patient with a history of liver dysfunction or disease can safely be given progestogens; however, liver function studies should be repeated after 3 to 6 months of progestogen therapy.

There is no evidence that progestogens increase the risk for breast cancer. In fact, there is increasing evidence that adding progestogens to estrogen replacement may decrease the risk for carcinoma of the breast in some women. Long-term progesterone deficiency can increase the risk of breast cancer (61, 62). For medicolegal reasons, however, the only progestogen that can be used in patients who have had breast cancer is megestrol acetate, which is used to treat metastatic breast cancer. Although medroxyprogesterone acetate is used in Europe and Canada to treat metastatic breast carcinoma, it has not yet been approved for this use in the United States. Undiagnosed genital bleeding becomes diagnosed in the course of proper evaluation of postmenopausal women. Endometrial hyperplasia should be treated with progestogens to prevent adenocarcinoma of the endometrium.

Key Points

Endometrial Hyperplasia

- Untreated adenomatous hyperplasia may lead to endometrial cancer in 30% of cases over 8 to 10 years.
- Cyclic 13-day progestogen treatment of hyperplasia with follow-up endometrial biopsy appears to be curative in most cases. Cyclic progestogen therapy is recommended for 13 days monthly.

Endometrial Cancer

- The progestogen challenge test (e.g., 13 days of 10 mg of medroxyprogesterone acetate daily) is useful in asymptomatic postmenopausal women not employing sequential replacement and should be used at each annual examination.
- Multiple studies indicate that estrogen-only users experience a 1.7- to 20-fold increased relative risk for endometrial carcinoma.
- In a prospective study of 16,327 patient-years of observation of the use of sequential estrogen-progestogen replacement therapy, endometrial cancer incidence was significantly lower (49 per 100,000 women) than in unopposed estrogen users 390.6 per 100,000, or in women using no hormonal replacement (245.4 per 100,000 women).
- When the duration of progestogen was increased to 13 days in this large study, no additional cases of endometrial cancer occurred to date.

Benign Breast Disease

- One-third of women with fibrocystic breast disease will have intraductal epithelial hyperplasia.
- Ductal hyperplasia increases breast cancer risk threefold.
- Long-term treatment of ductal hyperplasia with either a progestogen or a high-progestin oral contraceptive reduces ductal hyperplasia and atypical hyperplasia.

Breast Cancer

- The American Cancer Society estimates there will be 180,000 new cases and 46,000 deaths of women in the United States in 1992 from breast cancer.
- Breast cancer increases throughout the entire female life span.
- 28 published studies of exogenous estrogen therapy and breast cancer failed to prove convincingly that exogenous estrogen use was a cause in postmenopausal women.
- Most breast cancers have been present for 7 to 8 years before being clinically detectable.

- In 16,466 woman patient-years of sequential estrogen-progestogen hormonal replacement, the incidence of breast cancer was 66.8 per 100,000; in 19,676 woman patient-years of unopposed estrogen use the incidence was 142.3 per 100,000; and in 6,404 woman patient-years of observation in non-hormone users the observed incidence was 343.5 per 100,000.
- Progestogens should be added to estrogen replacement therapy even in post-hysterectomy women to reduce the incidence of carcinoma of the breast.

Hypertension

- Numerous studies indicate that estrogen therapy has a beneficial effect on hypertension.
- Although hypertension occurs in the postmenopausal age group, this observation does not establish estrogens as etiologic in that hypertension.
- Only if salt restriction and mild antihypertensive therapy fails to control hypertension in a patient employing estrogen replacement should consideration be given to discontinuing the estrogen use.

Thromboembolic Disease

- Antithrombin 3 activity is probably the most sensitive test of hypercoagulability. It is significantly decreased in pregnant women and in users of oral contraceptives but remains within the normal range (slightly decreased) with conjugated estrogen therapy.
- Mestranol significantly increases fibrinogen levels and may be a thrombogenic hazard.
- Postpartum, postoperative, or traumatic thrombophlebitis or embolic episodes are no longer regarded as contraindications to estrogen therapy.
- Only thrombosis or thromboembolic disorders associated with prior estrogen use are now regarded as contraindications to renewed use.
- It may be prudent to measure antithrombin 3 activity in patients with any prior history of thromboembolic disease and to repeat the study 3 to 6 months after commencing estrogen therapy.

Gallbladder Disease

- Oral estrogen therapy is reported by some to increase cholelithiasis; other reports find a decrease.
- Transdermal estrogen may obviate increased risk, if present.

Potential Adverse Effects of Progestogens on Lipids

- In a study using subcutaneous implantations of estradiol combined with one of three progestogens for 10 days monthly, medroxyprogesterone acetate permitted a significant increase in HDL cholesterol and a significant decrease of LDL cholesterol. Norgestrel 0.075 mg allowed only a slight increase in HDL, no change in LDL, but a significant decrease in VLDL; Norethindrone acetate 5 mg allowed only a slight increase in HDL, a moderate decrease in LDL, and no change in VLDL.
- With transdermal estrogen alone, HDL cholesterol did rise but it required 12 months to observe the increase. The addition of micronized oral progesterone in a second year not only did not result in any long-term decrease in HDL, but the HDL rose further after 6 and 12 months of the added oral progesterone. LDL cholesterol and total cholesterol decreased throughout the first 12 months of percutaneous estrogen use.

References

1. Gusberg SB. The individual at high risk for endometrial carcinoma. Am J Obstet Gynecol 1988;115:954.
2. Wentz WB. Progestin therapy in endometrial hyperplasia. Gynecol Oncol 1974;2:362.
3. Shanklin DR. Endometrial carcinoma, diagnostic criteria, pathogenesis, natural history, and associations. Pathol Annu 1978;13:233.
4. Gambrell RD Jr. Use of progestogen therapy. Am J Obstet Gynecol 1987;156:1304.
5. Whitehead MI, Fraser D. The effects of estrogens and progestogens on the endometrium. Obstet Gynecol Clin North Am 1987;14:299.
6. Gambrell RD Jr. The menopause: benefits and risks of estrogen-progestogen replacement therapy. Fertil Steril 1982;37:457.
7. Smith DC, Prentice R, Thompson DC, et al. Association of exogenous estrogen and endometrial carcinoma. N Engl J Med 1975;293:1164.
8. Ziel HK, Finkle WD. Increased risk of endometrial carcinoma among users of conjugated estrogens. N Engl J Med 1975;293:1167.
9. Mack TM, Pike MC, Henderson BE, et al. Estrogens and endometrial cancer in a retirement community. N Engl J Med 1976;294:1262.
10. McDonald TW, Annegers JF, O'Fallon WM, et al. Exogenous estrogen and endometrial carcinoma: case-control and incidence study. Am J Obstet Gynecol 1977;127:572.

11. Gray LA Sr, Christopherson WM, Hoover RN. Estrogens and endometrial carcinoma. Obstet Gynecol 1977;49:385.
12. Antunes CMF, Stolley PD, Rosensheim NB, et al. Endometrial cancer and estrogen use. Report of a large case-control study. N Engl J Med 1979;300:9.
13. Jick H, Watkins RN, Hunter JR, et al. Replacement estrogens and endometrial cancer. N Engl J Med 1979;300:218.
14. Horwitz RI, Feinstein AR. Alternative analytic methods for case-control studies of estrogens and endometrial cancer. N Engl J Med 1978;299:1089.
15. Shapiro S, Kelly JP, Rosenberg L, et al. Risk of localized and widespread endometrial cancer in relation to recent and discontinued use of conjugated estrogens. N Engl J Med 1985;313:969.
16. Persson I, Adami H-O, Bergkwist L, et al. Risk of endometrial cancer after treatment with oestrogens alone or in conjunction with progestogens: results of a prospective study. Br Med J 1989;298:147.
17. Gambrell RD Jr, Massey FM, Castaneda TA, et al. Use of the progestogen challenge test to reduce the risk of endometrial cancer. Obstet Gynecol 1980;55:732.
18. Bergkvist L, Adami H-O, Persson I, et al. The risk of breast cancer after estrogen and estrogen-progestin replacement. N Engl J Med 1989;321:293.
19. Sturdee DW, Wade-Evans T, Paterson MEL, et al. Relationship between bleeding pattern, endometrial histology and oestrogen treatment in menopausal women. Br Med J 1978:1:1575.
20. Thom MH, White PJ, Williams RM, et al. Prevention and treatment of endometrial disease in climacteric women receiving oestrogen therapy. Lancet 1979;2:445.
21. Whitehead MI, Townsend PT, Pryse-Davies J, et al. Effects of estrogens and progestins on the biochemistry and morphology of the postmenopausal endometrium. N Engl J Med 1981;305:1599.
22. Gambrell RD Jr. Prevention of endometrial cancer with progestogens. Maturitas 1986;8:159.
23. Hanna JH, Brady WK, Hill JM, et al. Detection of post-menopausal women at risk for endometrial carcinoma by a progesterone challenge test. Am J Obstet Gynecol 1983; 147:872.
24. Gambrell RD Jr. Breast disease in the postmenopausal years. Semin Reprod Endocrinol 1983;1:27.
25. Berkowitz GS. Risk factors. *In:* Marchant DJ, ed. Breast disease. New York, Churchill Livingstone, 1986:13–43.
26. Roberts MM, Jones V, Elton RA, et al. Risk of breast cancer in women with history of benign disease of the breast. Br Med J 1984;228:275.
27. Greenblatt RB, Vasquez J, Samaras C. Fibrocystic breast disease. Postgrad Med 1982;71:159.
28. Voherr H. Fibrocystic breast disease: pathophysiology, pathomorphology, clinical picture and management. Am J Obstet Gynecol 1986;154:161.
29. Voherr H. Oral contraception and hormone replacement: are progestogens and progestins breast mitogens? Am J Obstet Gynecol 1986;155:1140.
30. American Cancer Society. Cancer statistics, 1992. CA 1992;42:21.
31. Bland KI, Buchannan JB, Weisberg BF, et al. The effects of exogenous estrogen replacement therapy on the breast: breast cancer risk and mammographic parenchymal patterns. Cancer 1980;45:3027.
32. Boston Collaborative Drug Surveillance Program. Surgically confirmed gallbladder disease, venous thrombosis, and breast tumors in relation to postmenopausal estrogen replacement therapy. N Engl J Med 1974;290:15.

33. Brinton LA, Hoover RN, Szklo M, et al. Menopausal estrogen use and the risk of breast cancer. Cancer 1981;47:2517.
34. Brinton LA, Hoover R, Fraumeni JF. Menopausal oestrogens and breast cancer risk: an expanded case-control study. Br J Cancer 1986;54:825.
35. Brinton LA, Schairer C, Stanford JL, et al. Cigarette smoking and breast cancer. Am J Epidemiol 1986;123:614.
36. Burch JC, Byrd BF, Vaughn WK. Results of estrogen treatment in one thousand hysterectomized women for 14,318 years. In: van Keep PA, Greenblatt RB, Albeaux-Fernet M, eds. Consensus on menopause research. Lancaster, England: MTP Press Ltd, 1976:164.
37. Casagrande J, Gerkins V, Henderson BE, et al. Exogenous estrogens and breast cancer in women with natural menopause. J Natl Cancer Inst 1976;56:839.
38. Craig TJ, Comstock GW, Geiser PB. Epidemiologic comparison of breast cancer patients with early and late onset of malignancy and general population controls. J Natl Cancer Inst 1974;53:1577.
39. Hammond CB, Jelovsek FR, Lee KI, et al. Effects of long term estrogen replacement therapy: II. Neoplasia. Am J Obstet Gynecol 1979;133:537.
40. Henderson BE, Powell D, Rosario I, et al. An epidemiologic study of breast cancer. J Natl Cancer Inst 1974;53:609.
41. Hoover R, Gray LA Sr, Cole P, et al. Menopausal estrogens and breast cancer. N Engl J Med 1976;295:401.
42. Hoover R, Glass A, Finkle WD, et al. Conjugated estrogens and breast cancer risk in women. J Natl Cancer Inst 1981;67:815.
43. Hulka BS, Chambless LE, Deubner DC, et al. Breast cancer and estrogen replacement therapy. Am J Obstet Gynecol 1982;143:163.
44. Hunt K, Vessey M, McPherson K, et al. Long-term surveillance of mortality and cancer incidence in women receiving hormone replacement therapy. Br J Obstet Gynaecol 1987;94:620.
45. Jick H, Walker AM, Watkins RN, et al. Replacement estrogens and breast cancer. Am J Epidemiol 1980;112:586.
46. Kaufman DW, Miller DR, Rosenberg L, et al. Noncontraceptive estrogen use and the risk of breast cancer. JAMA 1984;252:63.
47. Kelsey JL, Fischer DB, Holford TR, et al. Exogenous estrogens and other factors in the epidemiology of breast cancer. J Natl Cancer Inst 1981;67:327.
48. Lauritzen C, Meier F. Risks of endometrial and mammary cancer morbidity and mortality in long-term oestrogen treatment. In: van Herendael H, van Herendael B, Riphagen FE, Goessens L, van der Pas H, eds. The climacteric—an update. Lancaster, England: MTP Press Ltd, 1984:207.
49. Nachtigall LE, Nachtigall RH, Nachtigall RB, et al. Estrogen replacement: II. A prospective study in the relationship to carcinoma and cardiovascular and metabolic problems. Obstet Gynecol 1979;54:74.
50. Rohan TE, McMichael AJ. Noncontraceptive exogenous oestrogen therapy and breast cancer. Med J Aust 1988;148:221.
51. Ross RK, Paganni-Hill A, Gerkins VR, et al. A case-control study of menopausal estrogen therapy and breast cancer. JAMA 1980;243:1635.
52. Sartwell PE, Arthes FG, Tonascia JA. Exogenous hormones, reproductive history, and breast cancer. J Natl Cancer Inst 1983;51:1527.
53. Sherman B, Wallace R, Bean J. Estrogen use and breast cancer: interaction with body mass. Cancer 1983;51:1527.
54. Volker W. Estrogen and estrogen-progestogen compounds: is there a risk for the

development of endometrial and breast cancer in the perimenopausal woman? In: Pasetto N, Paoletti R, Ambrus JL, eds. The menopause and postmenopause. Lancaster, England: MTP Press Ltd, 1980:273.

55. Wingo PA, Layde PM, Lee NC, et al. The risk of breast cancer in postmenopausal women who have used estrogen replacement therapy. JAMA 1987;257:209.
56. Wynder EL, MacCornack FA, Stellman SD. The epidemiology of breast cancer in 785 United States Caucasian women. Cancer 1978;41:2341.
56a. Armstrong BK. Oestrogen therapy after the menopause—boon or bane? Med J Austr 1988;148:213.
56b. Bates SK. Postmenopausal estrogen replacement therapy and breast cancer. J Soc Obstet Gynaecol Can 1990;12:9.
56c. Dupont WD, Page DL. Menopausal estrogen replacement therapy and breast cancer. Arch Intern Med 1991;151:67.
56d. Sillero-Arenas M, Delgado-Rodriguez M, Rodigues-Canteras R, et al. Menopausal hormone replacement therapy and breast cancer: a meta-analysis. Obstet Gynecol 1992;79:286.
56e. Steinberg KK, Thacker SB, Smith SJ, et al. A meta-analysis of the effect of estrogen replacement therapy on the risk of breast cancer. JAMA 1991;265:1985.
57. Bergkvist L, Adami H-O, Persson I, et al. Prognosis after breast cancer diagnosis in women exposed to estrogen and estrogen-progestogen replacement therapy. Am J Epidemiol 1989;130:221.
58. Gambrell RD Jr. Proposal to decrease the risk and improve the prognosis of breast cancer. Am J Obstet Gynecol 1984;150:119.
59. Cutler SJ, Young JL Jr. Third national cancer survey: incidence data. Monograph 41. Bethesda, MD: National Cancer Institute, 1975:110.
60. National Cancer Institute. Surveillance, epidemiology and end results (SEER). Bethesda, MD, Biometry Branch of the National Cancer Institute, 1980:47.
61. Cowan LD, Gordis L, Tonascia JA, et al. Breast cancer incidence in women with a history of progesterone deficiency. Am J Epidemiol 1981;114:209.
62. Coulan CB, Annegers JF. Chronic anovulation may increase postmenopausal breast cancer risk. JAMA 1983;249:445.
63. Hammond CB, Jelovsek FR, Lee KL, et al. Effects of long term estrogen replacement therapy. I - Metabolic. Am J Obstet Gynecol 1979;133:525.
64. Barrett-Conner E, Brown V, Turner J, et al. Heart disease risk factors and hormone use in postmenopausal women. JAMA 1978;241:2167.
65. Gambrell RD Jr, Maier RC, Sanders BI. Decreased incidence of breast cancer in postmenopausal estrogen-progestogen users. Obstet Gynecol 1983;62:435.
66. Wren BO, Routledge AD. The effect of type and dose of oestrogen on the blood pressure of post-menopausal women. Maturitas 1983;5:135.
67. Lind T, Cameron FC, Hunter FM, et al. A prospective controlled trial of six forms of hormone replacement therapy given to postmenopausal women. Br J Obstet Gynaecol 1979;86:1.
68. Notelovitz M. Effect of natural oestrogens on blood pressure and weight in postmenopausal women. S Afr Med J 1975;49:2251.
69. Utian WH. Effect of postmenopausal estrogen therapy on diastolic blood pressure and body weight. Maturitas 1978;1:3.
70. Punnonen R, Lammintausta R, Erkkda R, et al. Estradiol valerate therapy and the renin-aldosterone system in castrated women. Maturitas 1980;2:91.
71. Pallas KG, Holzwarth GJ, Stern MP, et al. The effect of conjugated estrogens on the renin-angiotensin system. J Clin Endocrinol Metab 1977;44:1061.

72. von Eiff AW. Blood pressure and estrogens. Front Horm Res 1975;3:177.
73. Notelovitz M. Exercise, nutrition, and the coagulation effects of estrogen replacement on cardiovascular health. Obstet Gynecol Clin North Am 1987;14:121.
74. Wilson PWF, Garrison RJ, Castelli WP. Postmenopausal estrogen use, cigarette smoking, and cardiovascular morbidity in women over 50. N Engl J Med 1985;313:1038.
75. Paganini-Hill A, Ross RK, Henderson BE. Postmenopausal oestrogen treatment and stroke: a prospective study. Br Med J 1988;297:519.
76. Sarles H, Gerolami A, Cros RC. Diet and cholesterol gallstones: a further study. Digestion 1978;17:128.
77. Honore LH. Increased incidence of symptomatic cholesterol cholelithiasis in perimenopausal women receiving estrogen replacement therapy. J Reprod Med 1980;25:187.
78. Kakar F, Weiss NS, Strite SA. Noncontraceptive estrogen use and the risk of gallstone disease in women. Am J Public Health 1988;78:564.
79. Gambrell RD Jr. The menopause: benefits and risks of estrogen-progestogen replacement therapy. IM—Int Med Specialists 1985;6:135.
79a. Gambrell RD Jr, Teran A-Z. Changes in lipids and lipoproteins with long-term estrogen deficiency and hormone replacement therapy. Am J Obstet Gynecol 1991;165:307.
80. Jensen J, Riis BJ, Strom V, et al. Long-term effects of percutaneous estrogen and oral progesterone on serum lipoproteins in postmenopausal women. Am J Obstet Gynecol 1987;156:66.
81. Jensen J, Nilas L, Christiansen C. Cyclic changes in serum cholesterol and lipoproteins following different doses of combined postmenopausal hormone replacement therapy. Br J Obstet Gynaecol 1986;93:613.
82. Creasman WT, Henderson D, Hinshaw W, et al. Estrogen replacement therapy in the patient treated for endometrial cancer. Obstet Gynecol 1986;67:326.
83. Gambrell RD Jr. Role of progestogens in the prevention of breast cancer. Maturitas 1986;8:169.

10

Estrogen-Androgen Hormone Replacement Therapy

Morrie M. Gelfand

The normal premenopausal ovary produces estrogen, progestin, and androgen. The postmenopausal ovary produces androgen. The total postmenopausal levels of androgens are slightly lower than the premenopausal levels, and data from Longcope (1) and Judd et al. (2) indicate that the postmenopausal ovary produces androstenedione, dehydroepiandrosterone, and testosterone. Testosterone is the most potent androgen, followed in order of decreasing activity by androstenedione and dehydroepiandrosterone; but testosterone must be converted to dihydrotestosterone by 5α-reductase to be effective at the cell's target level. The extent of stromal hyperplasia present in postmenopausal ovaries has been related to the amount of estradiol and androstenedione that are produced (3).

The ovaries and the adrenal glands are responsible for the secretion of androgen in the adult female. Conversion to androgen also takes place in the liver and peripheral tissue. Androstenedione is derived 50% from the ovaries and 50% from the adrenal cortex. Testosterone is derived 25% from the ovaries, 25% from the adrenal glands, and the remaining 50% from the conversion of androstenedione in the skin and liver. Testosterone in the circulation is bound to sex hormone–binding globulin (SHBG), and only 1 to 3% is present as free testosterone. This is the active form and can be measured in the blood. Serum free testosterone is the measurement we use in determining the patient's hormone profile. Noltz and Schwartz (4) summarized the situation involving circulating androgens by stating that none of the circulating androgens has an exclusive gonadal or adrenal source. Concentrations reflect the sum of entry into the circulation from glandular secretions and extraglandular production as well as their hepatic and extrahepatic clearance. The estimation of secretion rates is complicated by the complexities of ovarian and adrenal steroidogenesis. Multiple variables have to be taken into account, e.g., episodic, diurnal, cyclic, and age-related variations. Testosterone may in a very real sense be considered a weak estrogen. In the relative scarcity of endogenous estrogens, testosterone per se can bind to and activate the estrogen receptors, with subsequent regulation of the expression of a specific gene that is generally considered estrogen responsive (5).

Accepting the fact that androgens are produced in postmenopausal ovaries, it is therefore not surprising that one should consider the use of estrogen-androgen hormone replacement therapy (EA HRT) in women who have had ovariectomies or in postmenopausal women in whom the level of androgen hormones becomes negligible. The reasons for considering EA HRT are the findings that the androgen component has an important function in the maintenance of sexual functions and libido as well as psychological well-being. Oophorectomized women merit special attention in the field of hormone replacement therapy.

In North America, estrogen-androgen hormone replacement therapy was first employed in the early 1950s. Greenblatt et al. (6) in 1950 compared the use of estrogen, estrogen-androgen, androgen alone, and placebo in the treatment of symptoms of the menopause. The results were encouraging in terms of increased libido and sexual functioning, but the number of cases evaluated was very small and there was no extensive basic psychological evaluation or determination of the blood levels of the hormones. Furthermore, the androgen preparations used were oral androgen combined with oral estrogen. In 1953 Grody et al. (7) also reported the results of estrogen-androgen substitution therapy in menopausal females. The thrust of their investigation dealt with the effect on the endometrium. In Europe, Australia, and Canada, estrogen-androgen replacement therapy has been under study for a long period of time. Studd and coworkers (8) described a study of 76 women who received pellet implants of 50 mg of estradiol, a combination of 50 mg of estradiol and 100 mg of testosterone, or a placebo. They showed that only women on the combination therapy experienced a decided increase in sexual response and frequency of coitus. Brincat et al. (9) also showed in a study that sexual status was enhanced by the use of the combination estrogen-androgen subcutaneous pellets. In Canada, Sherwin and Gelfand have done extensive research in this field (10–14), and their specific findings are discussed in this chapter.

The objectives for this chapter are clinical considerations involving EA HRT in the treatment of patients. There are three basic categories of patients who should be considered for the use of EA HRT therapy. These are illustrated in Table 10.1, and are (*a*) the patient who has had a total

Table 10.1.
Pelvic Status of Patients Considered for EA HRT

Hysterectomy: bilateral salpingo-oophorectomy
Hysterectomy, ovaries intact
Uterus and ovaries intact

hysterectomy and bilateral salpingo-oophorectomy, (*b*) the patient who has had hysterectomy but who has her ovaries intact, and (*c*) the patient who has her uterus and ovaries intact.

It is estimated that approximately 30% of women in the United States and Canada over the age of 50 have had a total hysterectomy and bilateral salpingo-oophorectoy. Approximately 650,000 women each year undergo hysterectomy, making it the most common major operation performed in the United States (15). These patients, who have had hysterectomy and bilateral salpingo-oophorectomy, constitute the prime group for consideration of estrogen-androgen hormone replacement therapy. Patients who have had a hysterectomy but whose ovaries are still present and in whom the clinical symptoms of loss of sexuality and decreased libido have become evident, should also be considered for the EA hormone replacement regime. These patients do not require the addition of a progestin to their therapy, because the uterus has been removed. Patients who have their uterus and ovaries intact, but have the clinical symptoms of androgen deprivation, also require therapy. In these patients, one has to remember that with the uterus in place, the addition of the androgen to the estrogen has an effect on the endometrial response to the hormones.

It is known that the use of estrogen alone causes hyperplasia of the endometrium in a substantial number of patients. Using 0.625 mg Premarin daily for 25 of 30 days results in 30% hyperplasia at the end of 1 year (16). The addition of medroxyprogesterone acetate (MPA) (Provera) in a 5-mg dose for days 15 to 25 of the 30-day cycle eliminates the hyperplasia. Adding the androgen to the estrogen regime increases the number of cases with hyperplasia to 42%. Gelfand et al. (17) have shown that one has to add 10 mg of MPA for days 12 to 25 of each cycle to reduce the hyperplasia to 0 (Table 10.2).

The Sherwin-Gelfand research involved a study that evaluated premenopausal, hysterectomized, oophorectomized women who were studied prospectively in a blinded, randomized, crossover study. The drugs used for comparison were estrogen alone, androgen alone, an estrogen-androgen combination, and a placebo. In addition, there was a control group of patients who had undergone hysterectomy without bilateral oophorectomy. Figures

10.1, 10.2, and 10.3 indicate the results obtained in the areas of sexual desire (Fig. 10.1), sexual fantasies (Fig. 10.2) and sexual arousal (Fig. 10.3). It is evident from the representations that there was enhancement in all evaluated areas when the androgen hormone was part of the treatment regime. In addition to the above, the energy levels and well-being were monitored in the same fashion, and Figures 10.4 and 10.5 indicate the same kind of positive response. The data are quite convincing in terms of the effect of adding the androgen hormone to the estrogen hormone replacement therapy.

Table 10.2.
Incidence of Endometrial Hyperplasia at 6 Months and Type of Estrogen-Androgen[a] and Provera Therapy[b]

	Endometrial Hyperplasia	
Provera	No. of Cases	%
5 mg (days 12–25)	5/20	25
$P<0.01$		
10 mg (days 12–25)	0/26	0

[a]Climacteron 1 ml IM.
[b]From Gelfand MM, Ferenczy A, Bergeron C. Endometrial response to estrogen-androgen stimulation. In: Hammond CB, Haseltine FP (eds): Menopause: evaluation, treatment, and health concerns. New York: Alan R. Liss, 1989:29–40.

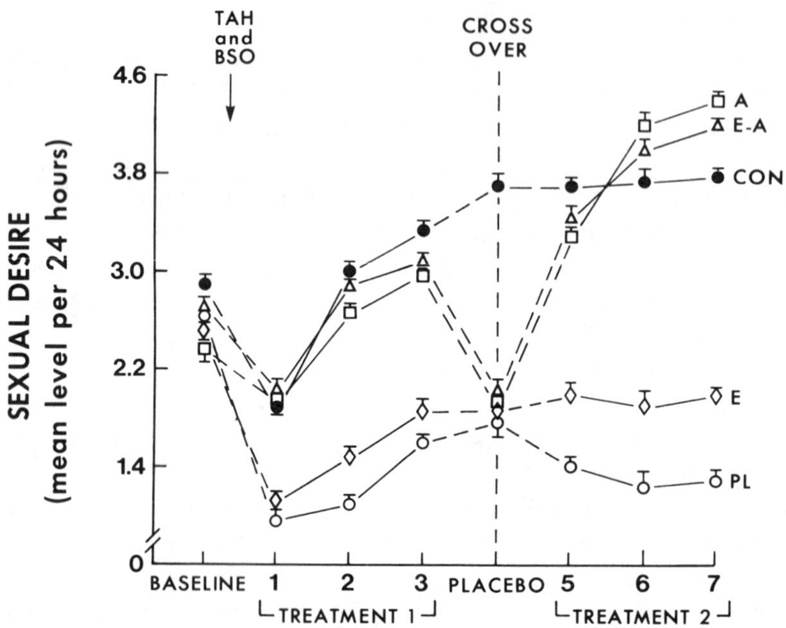

Figure 10.1.

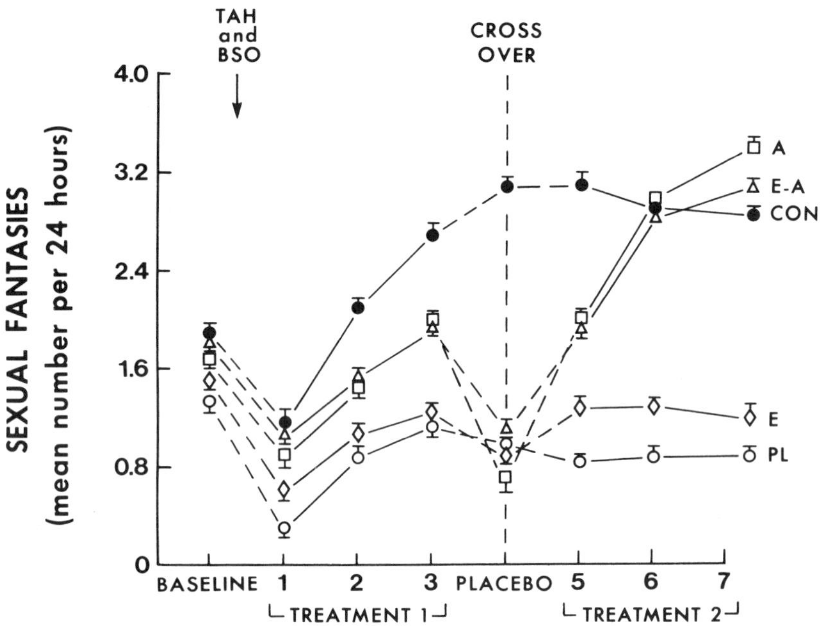

Figure 10.2.

Having accepted the positive response, are there risk factors to be considered in long-term estrogen-androgen hormone replacement therapy? The first area that comes to mind is the long-term effect on the lipid profile. Sherwin, Gelfand, et al. (18) evaluated patients who had been receiving estrogen-androgen replacement therapy for a minimum of 2 years and matched these subjects against patients who had been on estrogen alone, or patients who had received no hormones after their hysterectomy and bilateral salpingo-oophorectomy. Table 10.3 shows the LDL/HDL atherogenic risk ratio of the three groups. It is evident from these data that the addition of testosterone in long-term parenteral estrogen-androgen replacement regimens does not have a negative effect on the lipid profile compared to the parenteral administration of estrogen alone. These findings were corroborated in a study by Burger et al. (19) involving the implantation of pellets containing estradiol and testosterone. There were no significant lipid changes during the course of their study.

One of the major indications and benefits for using hormone replacement therapy has been the prevention of osteoporosis. It is agreed that estrogen is particularly effective in the inhibition of cortical bone loss as well as trabecular bone loss. In a review article, Dequeker and Geusens (20) discussed the treat-

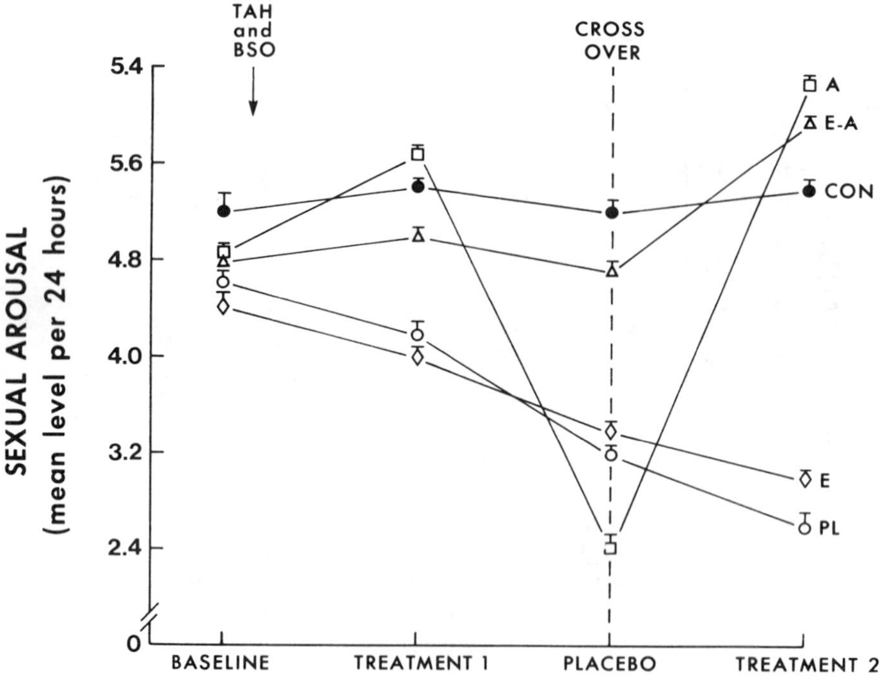

Figure 10.3.

ment of established osteoporosis and rehabilitation with reference to the current practice, and clearly show that the anabolic steroids are the only substances capable of inhibiting bone loss and stimulating bone formation. This has been our experience over the past 10 years, and there is at present ongoing research and evaluation of the effects of estrogen-androgen hormone replacement therapy on osteoporosis. Patients who have been receiving EA HRT for a minimum of 2 years are being compared to matched controls, and preliminary results indicate that we have not had a case of moderate to severe osteoporosis in the patients who have been receiving estrogen-androgen hormone replacement therapy.

In a recent publication, Myers et al. (21) studied the effects of estrogen, androgen, and progestin on sexual psychophysiology in postmenopausal women. They concluded that in physically sexually healthy women, gonadal steroids do not influence the major components of sexual function, including arousal and a wide variety of sexual experiences. These were patients who had their ovaries intact and had undergone a natural menopause. It must be stated that the androgen they used in their study was methyltestosterone, 5 mg orally. The possibility of a potentially different response to oral versus parenteral

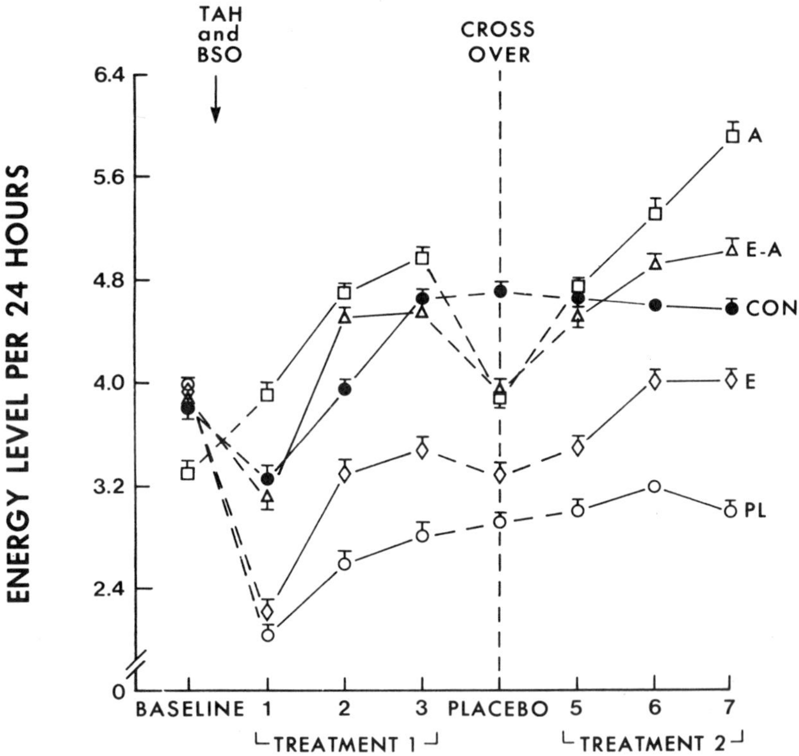

Figure 10.4.

testosterone should be considered. As with estrogen, the first liver bypass of the oral testosterone might also be of great significance. It is agreed that the total testosterone levels that were reported in Sherwin and Gelfand's studies were above the normal values for the adult female. In recent readjustments of dosages, it was found that, by decreasing the injectable androgen Climacteron from 150 mg to 75 mg (that is, 0.5 ml instead of 1 ml), the free testosterone blood levels were all within the normal range and there was still the positive enhancement of sexuality. It is clear that the free testosterone blood levels are dose related.

In all patients who are considered for the estrogen-androgen replacement regimen, there are certain baselines that have to be established before the initiation of hormone therapy. The blood levels of estradiol and free testosterone should be estimated. It has been our experience that the postmenopausal range of estradiol is less than 110 pmol/liter, and the free testosterone below the normal range of 3 to 13 pmol/liter. Patients who have their ovaries intact, are symptomatic, and still have a free testosterone level within the normal range can

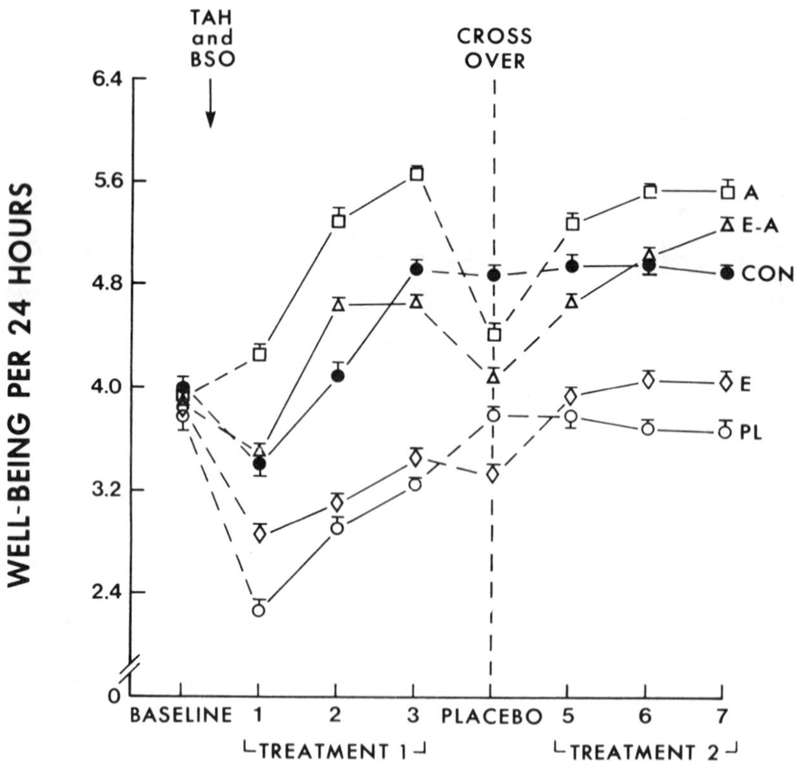

Figure 10.5.

Table 10.3.
LDL/HDL Ratios (Mean ± SD) for the Three Groups at Each Test Time[a]

Time	Group 1 (Estrogen-Androgen)	Group 2 (Estrogen Alone)	Group 3 (Control, Untreated)
Baseline	3.11 ± 1.2	3.08 ± 1.6	3.15 ± 0.6
Day 2	3.16 ± 1.4	2.78 ± 1.6	—
Day 4	3.04 ± 1.3	2.54 ± 1.3	—
Day 8	2.98 ± 1.3	2.63 ± 1.1	—
Day 15	4.15 ± 1.2	2.87 ± 1.4	—
Day 21	3.04 ± 1.3	2.90 ± 1.5	—
Day 28	2.92 ± 1.3	2.96 ± 1.6	3.22 ± 0.8

[a]From Sherwin BB, Gelfand MM, Schucher R, et al. Postmenopausal estrogen and androgen replacement and lipoprotein-lipid concentrations. Am J Obstet Gynecol 1987;4:414–419.

be given the opportunity to have EA HRT, but the testosterone levels have to be monitored regularly. It has been our experience that the clinical symptoms can be improved, and the free testosterone levels kept within normal limits, by using lower doses of the estrogen-androgen.

Hormone replacement therapy that incorporates the use of androgen with the estrogen-androgen or the estrogen-and-progestin hormone replacement regimen requires one to decide which androgen preparation to use and what dosage and to be aware of the potential positive and negative effects of the hormone use. Available estrogen-androgen preparations, both oral and parenteral, are noted in Table 10.4. Our experience indicates that the best regimen is 1 or 0.5 ml of Climacteron every 4 to 6 weeks. The clinical applications of the replacement therapy are noted in Figures 10.6 to 10.9, which outline the use of estrogen alone, estrogen-progestin, estrogen-

Table 10.4.
EA HRT—Parenteral Estrogen-Androgen Combinations

Product Name	Manufacturer	Generic Name	How Supplied
Injectable			(***per 1 ml solution***)
Climacteron (Canada)	Merck Sharp Dohme	Estradiol dienanthante	7.5 mg
		Estradiol benzoate	1.0 mg
		Testosterone enanthate	150 mg
Depo-Testadiol	Upjohn	Estradiol cypionate	2 mg
		Testosterone cypionate	50 mg
Oral			(***per tablet***)
Estratest	Reid-Rowell	Esterified estrogens	1.25 mg
		Methyltestosterone	2.5 mg
Estratest H.S.	Reid-Rowell	Esterified estrogens	0.625 mg
		Methyltestosterone	1.25 mg
Premarin with methyltestosterone	Wyeth-Ayerst	Conjugated estrogens	1.25 mg
		Methyltestosterone	10 mg
Premarin with methyltestosterone	Wyeth-Ayerst	Conjugated estrogens	0.625 mg
		Methyltestosterone	5 mg

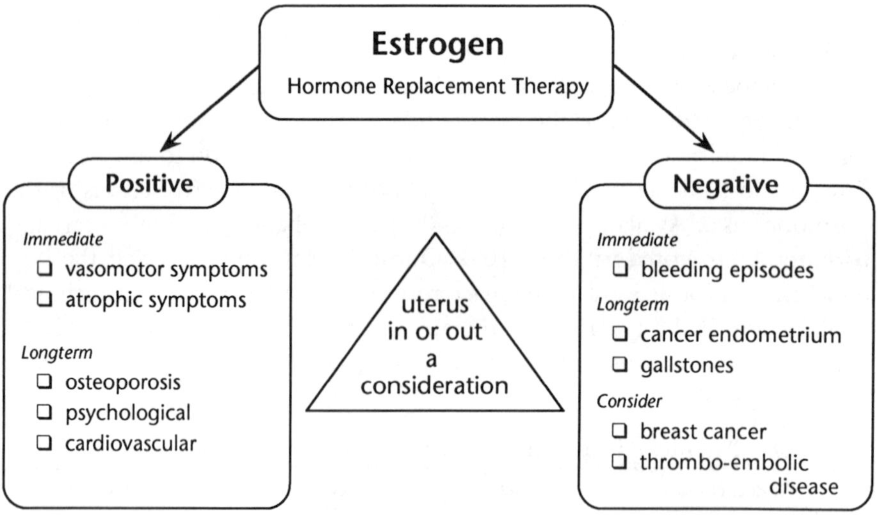

Figure 10.6.

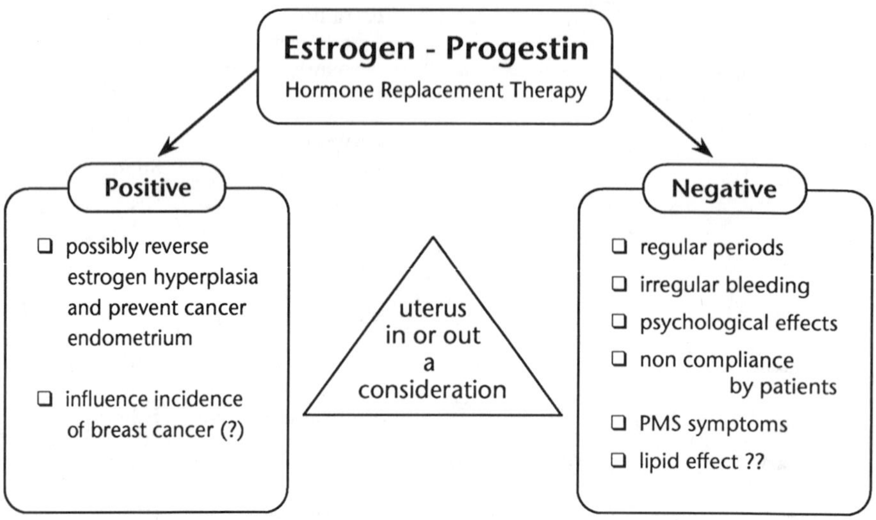

Figure 10.7.

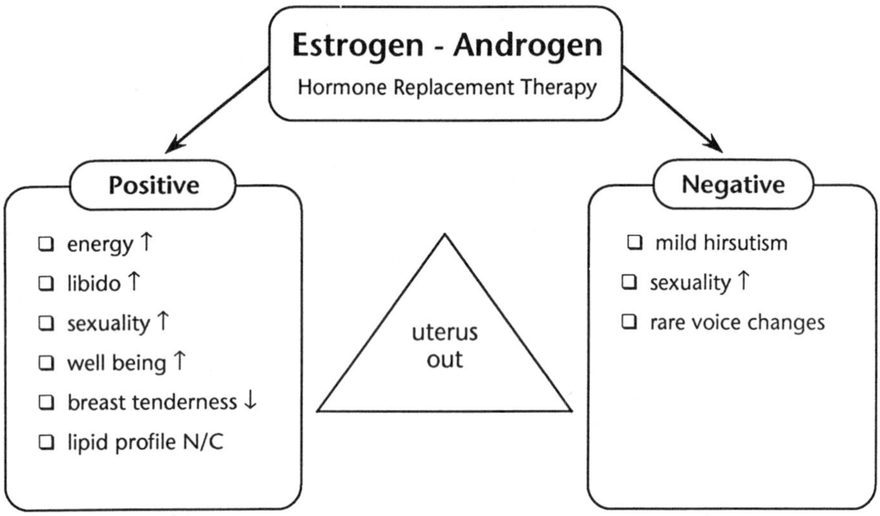

Figure 10.8.

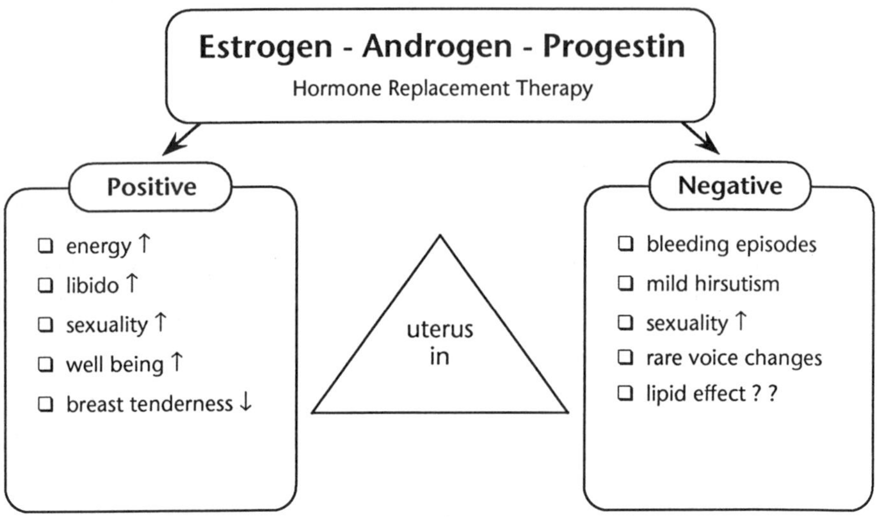

Figure 10.9.

androgen, and estrogen-androgen-progestin therapy. Figures 10.6 and 10.7 indicate today's accepted approach to estrogen and estrogen-progestin HRT. When one adds the androgen, one has to keep in mind the positive and negative effects as outlined in Figures 10.6 and 10.7. Figures 10.8 and 10.9 incorporate the androgen component into the system. In the column entitled Negative Effects in Figure 10.9, if the uterus is intact, one must remember that bleeding episodes can occur and that progestin should be added to prevent hyperplasia. In addition, there is a question of mild hirsutism, which was noted in 15 to 20% of our patients, and which was corrected when the androgen doses were lowered from 150 mg every 4 to 6 weeks to 75 mg every 4 to 6 weeks. This symptom is reversible, and the patient should be so informed. The question of increased sexuality as a negative side effect is mentioned in the context of patients who do not have relationships in which their sexuality is needed. These particular patients should be informed that they will have increased libido with their sexuality. The rare voice changes are uncommon but are mentioned as an isolated anecdotal finding.

CONCLUSION

Robert Greenblatt was a pioneer in the field of EA-HRT, and as a credit to his endeavors, we quote from one of his last publications (22):

> The post-menopausal woman lives in a catabolic milieu, and the addition of androgen to estrogen medication may serve to counteract this state. Androgens affect both the physiologic and psychologic components of sexuality. In physiologic doses, they are synergistic and complementary, and may be employed in combination with the estrogen to enhance the feelings of well-being, energy and sexuality. Patients who have had total hysterectomy, bilateral salpingo-oophorectomy, with the implied loss of the androgen production by the ovaries should be offered a trial of the estrogen-androgen combination to enhance the expected benefits of the estrogen replacement therapy. The ongoing research in the field of osteoporosis, breast cancer and psychologic behaviour which includes the sexuality component are areas to be considered for future management of the menopausal patient, whether it be surgical menopause or natural menopause.

Key Points

- The postmenopausal ovary produces androgen hormone.
- Serum free testosterone, the active form of testosterone, can be measured in the patient's blood.
- Patients who have had their ovaries removed have a particular need for estrogen-androgen hormone replacement therapy, but patients with intact

ovaries should also be considered as candidates for estrogen-androgen hormone replacement therapy after careful evaluation.

- Estrogen-androgen hormone replacement therapy in patients who have an intact uterus necessitates the addition of provera, 10 mg for days 12 to 25 of the cycle.
- Sexuality in terms of desire, fantasies, and arousal are enhanced by the addition of androgen to the estrogen hormone replacement regimen.
- Well-being and energy levels are improved with estrogen-androgen hormone replacement therapy.
- Long-term (more than 2 years) estrogen-androgen hormone replacement therapy has not been shown to affect the lipid profile adversely.
- Estrogen-androgen hormone replacement therapy can be an important adjunct in the treatment of osteoporosis.
- The action of parenteral estrogen-androgen hormone replacement therapy may have a different end result on sexuality than oral androgen therapy.
- Side effects such as mild hirsutism are dose related and can be monitored readily.
- Patients should be given the choice of receiving estrogen-androgen hormone replacement therapy when the need for it is evident clinically.

References

1. Longcope C. Adrenal and androgen secretions of normal females. Clin Endocrinol Metab 1986;15:213–228.
2. Judd HL, Judd GE, Lucas WE, et al. Endocrine function of the postmenopausal ovary—concentration of androgens and estrogens in ovarian and peripheral vein blood. J Clin Endocrinol Metab 1974;39:1020–1024.
3. Lucisano A, Russo N, Acampora MG, et al. Ovarian and peripheral androgen and estrogen levels in post-menopausal women. Correlations with ovarian histology. Maturitas 1986; 8:57–65.
4. Noltz L, Schwartz U. Gonadal and adrenal androgen secretion in hirsute females. Clin Endocrinol Metab 1986;15:229–245.
5. Watson GH, Korack KS, Muldoon TG. Obstruction of estrogen-receptor complex formation. Further analysis of the nature and steroidal specificity of the effect. Endocrinology 1977;101:1733.
6. Greenblatt RB, Williams E, Barfield, et al. Evaluation of an estrogen-androgen combination and a placebo in the treatment of the menopause. J Clin Endocrinol Metab 1950;10:15, 47–52.
7. Grody MH, Lampie EH. Masters WA. Estrogen-androgen substitution therapy in the aged female. Obstet Gynecol 1953;2:36–41.

8. Studd JWW, Collins WP. Estradiol and testosterone implants in the treatment of psychosexual problems in the postmenopausal woman. Br J Gynecol 1977;84:314–315.
9. Brincat, Studd JWW, O'Dowd T, et al. Subcutaneous implants for control of climacteric symptoms. Lancet 1984;1:16–18.
10. Sherwin BB, Gelfand MM. Effects of parenteral administration of estrogen and androgen on plasma hormone levels and hot flushes in the surgical menopause. Am J Obstet Gynecol 1984;148(5):552–557.
11. Sherwin BB, Gelfand MM. Differential symptom response to parenteral estrogen and/or androgen administration in the surgical menopause. Am J Obstet Gynecol 1985;151(2):153–160.
12. Sherwin BB, Gelfand MM, Brender W. Androgen enhances sexual motivation in females: a prospective cross-over study of sex steroid administration in the surgical menopause. Psychosom Med 1985;47(2):339–351.
13. Sherwin BB, Gelfand MM. Sex steroids and effect in the surgical menopause: a double-blind, cross-over study. Psychoneuroendocrinology 1985;10:325–335.
14. Sherwin BB, Gelfand MM. The role of androgen in the maintenance of sexual functioning in oophorectomized women. Psychosom Med 1987;49:397–409.
15. Dicker RC, Scalia MJ, Greenspan JR, et al. Hysterectomy among women of reproductive age trans-United States 1970–1978. JAMA 1982;248:323–327.
16. Gelfand MM, Ferenczy A. A prospective one-year study of estrogen and progestin in post-menopausal women: effects in the endometrium. Obstet Gynecol 1989;74:398–402.
17. Gelfand MM, Ferenczy A, Bergeron C. Endometrial response to estrogen-androgen stimulation. In: Hammond CB, Haseltine FP (eds): Menopause: evaluation, treatment and health concerns. New York: Alan R. Liss, 1989:29–40.
18. Sherwin BB, Gelfand MM, Schucher R, et al. Postmenopausal estrogen and androgen replacement and lipoprotein-lipid concentrations. Am J Obstet Gynecol 1987;4:414–419.
19. Burger HG, Hailes J, Menelaus M, et al. Management of persistent symptoms with estradiol-testosterone implants. Clinical, lipid and hormonal results. Maturitas 1984;6:351–358.
20. Dequeker J, Geusens P. Treatment of established osteoporosis in rehabilitation. Current practice and responsibilities. Maturitas 1990;112:1–36.
21. Myers LS, Dicksen J, Morrissette V, et al. Effects of estrogen, androgen and progestin on sexual psychophysiology and behaviour of postmenopausal women. J Clin Endocrinol Metab 1990;70:1124–1131.
22. Greenblatt RB. The use of androgens in the menopause and other gynecic disorders. Obstet Gynecol Clin North Am 1987;40:251–268.

11

Hormonal Replacement Therapy in the Cancer Patient

William T. Creasman

Today it is appreciated that estrogen replacement therapy (ERT) is the rational approach to the endocrinopathy of estrogen deprivation. Before the cancer scare of the 1970s, ERT was used mainly for the symptoms of the menopause with good results. Vasomotor symptoms were eliminated, but in general women receiving ERT also felt better and it was suggested that the fountain of youth was at hand.

In the early 1970s it became apparent that endometrial cancer was on the increase. This was reflected in several state and local cancer registries, although the National Cancer Institute (NCI) and their data base did not see an increased incidence of endometrial cancer. Other countries (Czechoslovakia and Norway) also noted similar increases as reported by some in the United States. The magic elixir balloon burst in the mid-1970s when two articles appearing back to back in the *New England Journal of Medicine* suggested that estrogen caused endometrial cancer. Ziel and Finkle compared 94 patients with endometrial cancer with two matched controls for each patient (1). The controls were pulled charts; therefore, some of these women could have had carcinoma. The investigators reported a risk ratio of 7.6, and this increased with the length of exposure to estrogen. In the same issue Smith and associates reported on 317 patients with matched controls (2). The controls were patients with other gynecological malignancies and over 200 had carcinoma of the cervix. Patients with carcinoma of the cervix are at a low risk for endometrial carcinoma. The investigators noted a 4.5 risk ratio. Again the risk increased with time and exposure to estrogen but also decreased with the age of the patient. Smith and associates were the first to report that the effect was greater in the so-called normal patient without other known predisposing factors of endometrial cancer. In 1976, Mack and associates reported similar findings from a retirement community in southern California (3). They reported a risk ratio of 8, with the risk increasing with the dose of estrogen, the period of exposure, and again in women without predisposing factor. Since then, many other articles have shown similar results. The use of ERT was therefore linked to endometrial cancer. Several authors suggested that the increased incidence of endometrial cancer was directly related to the amount of estrogen sold, even though the increased incidence in foreign countries could not be related to estrogen, because the hormones were not available or were not used for replacement therapy in those countries.

As a result of this cancer scare, the use of estrogen decreased tremendously. During the late 1970s and early 1980s, as a consequence of this new information, investigation in the field increased greatly and brought to light several important additional benefits of ERT. Nachtigall reported the long-term follow-up of a prospective randomized study of elderly women who received either estrogen plus progesterone (E + P) or placebo (4). She noted no increase in endometrial cancer, with the progestin apparently offering protection even when estrogen was used. Hammond (5), in reporting the Duke material, and Gambrell (6), evaluating a large data base at Wilford Hall Hospital, noted the same protection (Table 11.1). The recommendation at that time was to use estrogen for menopausal symptoms but to use it with progestins and only for a limited period of time.

Not only was it noted that endometrial cancer could be decreased by the use of E + P, but there also appeared to be an increased amount of data that suggested that the use of ERT was important in the prevention of osteoporosis, which is a major health problem for older patients (7, 8). Compression fractures of the vertebral column with its ensuing loss of stature, increased pulmonary restriction, and decreased ambulation are well appreciated as causes of major morbidity from this aging process. Osteoporosis, which

Table 11.1.
Estrogens-Progesterone Replacement Therapy and Endometrial Cancer

	Incidence/1000 Patient Years		
Study (Reference)	Untreated	E only[a]	E + P[b]
Nachtigall (4)	1.2	—	0.0
Hammond (5)	0.5	6.5	0.0
Gambrell (6)	2.5	3.9	0.5

[a]E, Estrogen.
[b]E + P, Estrogen + progesterone.

accounts for the majority of approximately 250,000 hip fractures per year, is a significant cause of mortality in the postmenopausal patient. Subsequent data have confirmed this protective effect, and ERT does prevent bone mass loss, which occurs naturally with the loss of estrogen.

In the 1970s several authors noted that patients receiving estrogen also seemed to have substantial protection from cardiovascular disease (9, 10). In the non-randomized study from Duke, patients who were estrogen deprived and never replaced had a much higher risk of many cardiovascular diseases compared with like patients who received ERT (8) (Table 11.2). During the last decade considerable research has been carried out in this field, and it is appreciated that this protection is probably due to the fact that women receiving estrogen have a decrease in total cholesterol and low-density lipoprotein with a concomitant increase in high-density lipoprotein, which is the reversal of what happens to these lipoproteins as the woman goes through the menopause. Authors who had reported an increase in endometrial cancer due to estrogen in the 1970s and recommended against its use suggested in the 1980s that its use could provide marked cardiac protection (9). Since the incidence of cardiovascular disease is so much greater than the effects of increased incidence of endometrial cancer (with essentially no increase in deaths), the risk-benefit ratio swung markedly in the direction of estrogen use (Table 11.3).

One area of controversy that has risen over the last decade or so has been the relationship of ERT to breast cancer. Gambrell has been a strong proponent of E + P, and his data suggest actual protection in breast cancer with the hormone combination (11). There are many who would argue with his data, stating that selection as well as other bias may have affected his

Table 11.2.
Cardiovascular Disease and Estrogen[a]

Disease	*p*
Stroke	<.05
CHD	<.05
CHF	<.001
ASCVD	<.001
Total diagnosis	<.001
Thrombus/embolus	NS
Arrhythmia	NS

[a]Data from Hammond CB, Jelovsek FR, Lee KL, et al. Effects of long-term estrogen replacement therapy. I. Metabolic effects. Am J Obstet Gynecol 1979;133:525–536.

Table 11.3.
Estimated Change in Mortality when Estrogen Is Used in Women Aged 50 to 75 Years

	Relative Risk	Cumulative Change in Mortality/100,000
Breast cancer	1.0	0
Endometrial cancer	4.0	0
Osteoporotic fracture	0.4	−563
Ischemic heart disease	0.5	−5,250

results. Nachtigall, in a prospective randomized study, noted that there may be a protection against breast cancer with E + P (4).

Even with its proven benefits in the prevention of vasomotor symptoms, osteoporosis, and cardiovascular disease, there still remain physicians and patients concerned over the possible role of ERT and cancer. The two cancers appreciated as hormonally related are endometrial and breast cancer. As noted previously, E + P appears to protect against endometrial cancer, possibly decreasing the risk by as much as 50%. As a result, it has become standard protocol in women with the uterus in situ to receive E + P when replacement therapy is given. The obvious side effect is withdrawal bleeding at the end of progestin. Several different E + P regimens have been suggested in an attempt to decrease or eliminate the bleeding; these are being evaluated further in regard to their effects on osteoporosis and cardiovascular disease.

In the late 1970s and early 1980s it also became apparent that estrogen-induced endometrial cancers had really very little if any impact on survival in these women. These cancers for the most part are well differentiated, tend to be limited to the endometrium, and are only superficially invasive. Data suggest that if a woman took estrogen and developed cancer, her survival was equal to or even better than her next door neighbor who never took estrogen or developed cancer (12, 13). This is presumed to be due to the protective effects of estrogen with regard to osteoporosis and cardiovascular disease. It has been estimated that the chance of a woman today taking estrogen, developing cancer, and dying from her cancer is one in 20,000. The real issue today is not that estrogen should not be taken because of endometrial cancer risk, but whether or not it can be given to the patient who has been successfully treated for endometrial cancer.

ENDOMETRIAL CANCER

For many years it was widely acknowledged that it was an absolute contraindication to use ERT in postendometrial cancer patients. The *Physicians' Desk Reference* (PDR) notes this contraindication, as do other publications (14). It is interesting to note that although this is listed as a contraindication in the PDR, there are no data or references provided to substantiate that admonition. In fact, as recently as 1992, the latest of 41 references listed in the PDR was dated 1976—certainly a considerable amount of data concerning ERT has been collected since then.

It became apparent that many endometrial cancer patients who were cured of adenocarcinoma of the endometrium were having frequent vasomotor symptoms secondary to bilateral oophorectomy. Many patients who are several years postmenopausal will develop vasomotor symptoms secondary to bilateral oophorectomy. This is probably due to the removal of the androgens produced by the ovarian stroma which are then being converted peripherally to estrogens. It has been well known for many years that progestins can eliminate vasomotor symptoms; however, if used for prolonged periods of time they will lead to vaginal atrophy and sexual dysfunction. Because of these disturbing symptoms, some patients successfully treated for their endometrial cancer were treated with estrogens. We initially treated our patients with local estrogen with the presumption that it would affect the vaginal mucosa but was not absorbed. Subsequent data indicated that local estrogen is readily absorbed by the vaginal mucosa. As a result, for the last several years we have used oral preparations in these patients. In 1985, an experience in a non-randomized study evaluating 221 stage I endometrial cancer patients treated between 1975 and 1980 was reported (15). Forty-seven patients (22%) received estrogen after cancer treatment for their endometrial malignancy. The main indication for estrogen treatment was vasomotor symptoms. Since this was not a prospective randomized study, the two groups of patients (estrogen treated versus non–estrogen treated) were evaluated for risk factors. None of the known prognostic factors (substage, grade, depth of invasion, node metastasis, peritoneal cytology, or hormone receptors) were statistically significantly different between the two groups. There were 26 (14.9%) recurrences among 174 estrogen untreated patients compared to only 1 (2.1%) recurrence in the estrogen-treated group ($P = 0.0147$). In the patients not receiving estrogen, 26 died compared to only one among those taking estrogen ($P = 0.0140$). Of the non–estrogen-treated patients, 16 died from cancer and 10 from intercurrent disease. In a multivariant analysis it was noted that the patients who had metastases to the pelvic nodes had poorly differentiated cancers and those who had malignant cells present in their peritoneal cytology were at risk for recurrence. The patients who had received estrogen appeared to be protected against recurrence ($P = 0.0336$). Since this initial report, there have been other publications suggesting that estrogen replacement therapy can be given to endometrial cancer patients after therapy (16). The American College of Obstetricians and Gynecologists has issued a committee opinion on this subject suggesting that in "women with a history of endometrial cancer, estrogens could be used for the same indications as for any other woman except that the selection of appropriate candidates should be based on prognostic indicators and the risk the patient is willing to assume." (17)

Although it has been said that estrogen replacement therapy is contraindicated in patients who had endometrial cancer, there are no data to substantiate that admonition. Many patients with endometrial cancers do have significant menopausal symptoms, and to restrict benefits of estrogen replacement therapy in these patients does not appear to be appropriate. The long-term benefits of estrogen replacement therapy, particularly as it relates to osteoporosis and cardiovascular disease, appear to be indication enough to treat these patients. Certainly many of the endometrial cancer patients would have more potential problems with these medical conditions—and the nature of the problems seems to outweigh the unknown increased risk of developing a recurrence.

BREAST CANCER

Although many physicians now feel relatively comfortable in treating endometrial cancer patients with estrogen replacement therapy, there still remains considerable hesitancy to do so in patients who have had breast cancer. The contraindications to estrogen replacement therapy as already noted in the PDR list a patient who has breast cancer unless she is specifically being treated with hormones for metastases or recurrence. Certainly the vast majority of surgical and medical oncologists appear to feel very strongly with regard to this dictum. Unfortunately, there are no data available in the literature today that would substantiate the rationale for not using ERT in breast cancer patients. Many of these patients have significant vasomotor symptomatology, particularly if they had their breast cancer premenopausally. Since there are no data that directly support the pros or cons of estrogen replacement therapy in these patients, are there any other related studies from which we can possibly draw some conclusions that might support the role of ERT in these individuals?

Over the last several years, there have been some reports in the literature that suggest oral contraceptives (OCs) might increase the risk for breast cancer. Pike was one of the first to suggest that there might be an increased risk for developing breast cancer in a subset of patients taking OCs (18). He noted an increased risk only in patients less than 37 years of age who had used high-progestin OCs before 25 years of age. A relative risk of 4.9 was noted if OCs had been used for longer than 6 years. This was a very small subset of his patients, as only 24 (7% of his total study population) fit this category. A study from Sweden and Norway noted an association between total duration of pill use and a risk of breast cancer before 45 years of age (19). The relative risk was 2.2 but it involved only 39 patients of 422 breast cancer patients evaluated. Recently the Royal College of General Practice suggested that there was a threefold increase in risk for young women aged 30 to 34 who had ever used OCs (20). There was a sixfold increase in risk for patients who were parous 1 but no increase in risk for nulliparous women or in women who had had more than one child (of 229 cancer patients only 27 were between 30 and 34 years of age). This study suggested that the absolute excess risk was 1 in 7000 ever-users per year. Researchers from the Centers for Disease Control (CDC) have evaluated the largest number of OC users with regard to breast cancer in the Cancer and Steroid Hormone (CASH) study (21). They evaluated 4711 cases of breast cancer and a similar number of controls in women 20 to 54 years of age. They noted an association between the risk of breast cancer before age 45, if the patient was nulliparous, had an early marriage, and used OCs for longer than 8 years—this represented only 39 cases, which was less than 1% of their total population. They noted no association with either pill use before first pregnancy or total duration of use in parous women. They suggested that there was no effect of OC use even long-term on aggregate risk of premenopausal breast cancer. Most studies in the literature suggest that there is no relationship between OCs and breast cancer; in fact, several organizations, including the U.S. Food and Drug Administration, the American College of Obstetricians and Gynecologists, and the World Health Organization, have recently suggested that there should be no change in OC labeling, no change in OC prescribing, and no change in OC use.

Although OCs do not have an influence on breast cancer, it should be remembered that there is a beneficial effect on both endometrial and ovarian cancer. A case control study from the CDC showed that the risks for endometrial cancer were 50% lower in the ever-users of combination OCs than in never-users (22). Other studies have confirmed the CDC's study. The aggregate data note that 7 or more years of use confers an approximately 60% reduction in risk. There was also a 40% decrease in ovarian cancer in users compared to never-users (23). Fourteen studies in the literature all show a decreased risk for ovarian cancer with 4 years' use. With 7 or more years of use there is a 60 to 80% reduction in ovarian cancer.

There have now been over 20 studies in the literature that have evaluated ERT in breast cancer. Most of these suggest that there is no effect one way or the other with regard to ERT and breast cancer. A recent study by Bergkvist from Sweden was published in the *New England Journal of Medicine* and received considerable publicity both within the medical community and in the public media (24). It was suggested that their study population involved over 23,000 women when in fact just over 700 patients had questionnaires sent to them in an attempt to enroll them into the study. Less than 90% of these women returned their questionnaires. Of the 253 cancer patients identified, only 77% had provided enough information to enter into the cancer data base. Several other problems were apparent from this study, including the mean duration of follow-up being only 5.7 years, while most breast cancers require 7 to 8 years to become clinically detectable. In the 208 estrogen users in the study, only 29 had been taking the estrogen for 9 or more years. The fact that women who never used estrogen had a risk of 1.6 times that of the overall population indicates that some other variable must have contributed to the high incidence of breast cancer in the study. The risk of 1.6 in non-users was very close to the risk of 1.7 in the estrogen users. Most of the patients in the study who had taken estrogen had used estradiol valerate, and only 22% had used conjugated estrogen. Very little, if any, estradiol valerate is used as replacement therapy in the United States. The authors intimated that the relative risk of breast cancer increased with the duration of estrogen use. Actually the data base showed a trend, but even after 9 years it was not statistically significant. More important, they noted no increase with conjugated estrogen. A considerable amount of emphasis in the lay literature was made on the fact that the authors reported the risk of breast cancer was highest among women who took E + P for an extended period. They noted that the relative risk was 4.4 for those who took E + P for longer than 6 years. This information was based on only 10 patients, and even with a relative risk of 4.4 it was not statistically significant. A significant finding of the study notes a suggestion that even with up to 6 years of ERT, there was no increased risk of breast cancer. This suggests that estrogen does not accelerate the subclinical growth that might be present during the period of estrogen use.

At the same time that the article mentioned above was receiving notoriety in the American press, the authors published an article in the *American Journal of Epidemiology* based on this same patient population (25). This article received essentially no media coverage. The second article noted that patients who were receiving estrogen prior to discovery of their breast cancer actually had a better prognosis than those patients not on ERT who also developed breast cancer. The difference between the two groups was greatest in the older patients. It also seemed to be related to the elapsed time from ERT commencement to the discovery of the breast cancer. The greatest increase in survival was noted in patients who were receiving ERT at the time of breast cancer diagnosis. If it was more than 12 months since ERT was used, the survival was equal to those who were not on ERT. This is not the first data base that has suggested that women on estrogen replacement therapy who develop breast cancer had a better survival than those not on estrogen who develop breast cancer. Gambrell noted that in women who were hormone users, 22% of these died from breast cancer whereas nonhormone users had a death rate of 45% ($P = 0.002$) (26). In this data base it was also noted that a larger number of the hormone users had negative axillary nodes compared with those not on hormones. Even when corrected for nodal status the patients on hormones appeared to have better survival in the node-negative category, one to three positive nodes, and four or more positive node groups.

In a recent meta-analysis of 23 studies on ERT and breast cancer, it is noted that in all studies the relative risk was 1.01 and in the postmenopausal women all studies noted a relative risk of 0.96 (27). Most in the field today would suggest that estrogen replacement therapy really has no effect one way or the other on whether or not a woman will subsequently develop a breast cancer. The role of E + P in the prevention of breast cancer still remains debatable.

In addition to the above OC and ERT data, there appear to be three "natural" experiences that might give us some important data to consider whether or not it is appropriate to use ERT in patients who have had breast cancer:

1. It used to be stated that if a woman had a breast cancer while she was pregnant, the prognosis was considerably worse than for women of the same age who were not pregnant. The data suggest that pregnant women tend to have more advanced disease because of the engorged breasts secondary to pregnancy. When corrected for age and stage, the survival of

the pregnant patient with cancer is similar to that of the non-pregnant patient (28). Termination of pregnancy, which at one time was suggested to remove the high levels of hormones secondary to the pregnancy, does not improve survival.

2. In the past, there was considerable reluctance to allow a woman with a history of breast cancer to have a subsequent pregnancy. This was believed desirable because of the very high level of estrogen that was present during the pregnancy. It is now suggested that subsequent pregnancies do not increase the recurrence rates in these women (29). When controlled for multiple factors, patients who have a subsequent pregnancy actually have a better survival than those not having a pregnancy. The time from breast cancer to subsequent pregnancy does not appear to be a factor (i.e. less than or more than 2 years). Even patients who receive chemotherapy did not have a survival status adversely affected by a subsequent pregnancy.
3. Several years ago, part of the primary treatment for breast cancer in the premenopausal patient was a bilateral oophorectomy or medically induced menopause. Prospective randomized studies have failed to show any benefits of prophylactic oophorectomy with regard to time of recurrence or survival in the premenopausal patient (30). It makes absolutely no sense to this observer that a woman at the age of 35 who has a cancer of the breast and has the benefits of 15 years of endogenous estrogen and then goes through a menopause cannot receive exogenous replacement. Presently patients with stage I cancer of the breast without axillary node involvement have greater than a 95% 5-year survival. It is appreciated that recurrences can occur many years later, yet in this patient it would appear that she would have substantially higher risks from the effects of osteoporosis and cardiovascular disease than she would have from a recurrence of her breast cancer. We all appreciate that quality of life is as important as, if not more important than, duration.

One more caveat: it is advocated today by many investigators that in the postmenopausal woman who has breast cancer, many should be placed on tamoxifen for prolonged periods of time. We know that tamoxifen not only is an antiestrogen but also is a weak estrogen. There are studies now reporting an increased incidence of endometrial cancer in women who have taken tamoxifen (31). Of interest is the fact that in premenopausal women taking tamoxifen the serum estradiol level is several times higher than those not on the drug. This may explain why the lipoprotein levels in these tamoxifen-treated patients are similar to those in postmenopausal women on ERT. Is the ERT story repeating itself with regard to tamoxifen?

Since there are no data to support the admonition that estrogen replacement therapy is absolutely contraindicated in women who have had breast cancer, circumstantial data suggest that hormones in and of themselves are probably not contraindicated. It appears reasonable at this point in time to discuss the risks and benefits with our patients who have had breast cancer and who are approaching menopause or are already postmenopausal. It also seems reasonable that in some of these women estrogen replacement therapy can be used without an adverse effect. Whether or not E + P has an advantage over estrogen by itself in this group of women is unknown.

Key Points

- There is an increased incidence of endometrial cancer when unopposed estrogen is used.
- Patients taking estrogen who develop endometrial cancer actually have a longer life than similarly aged women not on estrogen who do not develop endometrial cancer.
- Estrogen replacement therapy does not appear to be contraindicated in patients previously treated for endometrial cancer.
- There is no relationship between estrogen use and the development of breast cancer.
- Although ERT is said to be contraindicated in women who have had breast cancer, there are no data to confirm that dictum.
- ERT in individual post–breast cancer patients may not be contraindicated.

References

1. Ziel HK, Finkle WD. Increased risk of endometrial carcinoma among users of conjugated estrogens. N Engl J Med 1976:293:1167.
2. Smith DC, Prentice R, Thompson DJ, Herrmann WL. Association of exogenous estrogen and endometrial carcinoma. N Engl J Med 1975;293:1164.
3. Mack TM, Pike MC, Henderson BE, et al. Estrogen and endometrial cancer in a retirement community. N Engl J Med 1976;294:1262.
4. Nachtigall L, Nachtigall R, Nachtigall RD, Beckman EM. Estrogen replacement therapy. II. A prospective study in the relationship to carcinoma and cardiovascular and metabolic problems. Obstet Gynecol 1979;54:74–79.

5. Hammond CB, Jelovsek FR, Lee KL, et al. Effects of long term estrogen replacement therapy. II: Neoplasia. Am J Obstet Gynecol 1979;133:537–547.
6. Gambrell RD. Prevention of endometrial cancer with progestogens. Maturitas 1986;8:8159–8168.
7. Nachtigall L, Nachtigall R, Nachtigall RD, Beckman EM. Estrogen replacement therapy. I. A 10-year prospective study in the relationship of osteoporosis. Obstet Gynecol 1979;53:277–281.
8. Hammond CB, Jelovsek FR, Lee KL, et al. Effects of long-term estrogen replacement therapy. I. Metabolic effects. Am J Obstet Gynecol 1979;133:525–536.
9. Bush TL, Barrett-Conner E, Cowan DK, et al. Cardiovascular mortality and non-contraceptive use of estrogen in woman: results from the Lipid Research Clinics Program Followup Study. Circulation 1987;75:1102.
10. Henderson BE, Paganini-Hill A, Ross RK, et al. Estrogen replacement and protection from acute myocardial infarction. Am J Obstet Gynecol 1988;159:312.
11. Gambrell RD Jr. Role of progestogens in the prevention of breast cancer. Maturitas 1986;8:169.
12. Collins J, Allen LH, Donner A, et al. Oestrogen use and survival in endometrial cancer. Lancet 1980;2:961–963.
13. Chu J, Schweid AL, Weiss NS. Survival among women with endometrial cancer: a comparison of estrogen users and non-users. Am J Obstet Gynecol 1982;143:569.
14. Physicians' desk reference. Inc. Oradell, NJ: Medical Economics Company, 1990.
15. Creasman WT, Henderson D, Hinshaw W, Clarke-Pearson D. Estrogen replacement therapy in the patient treated for endometrial cancer. Obstet Gynecol 1986;67:326–330.
16. Baker DP. Estrogen replacement therapy in patients with previous endometrial carcinoma. Compr Ther 1990;16:28–35.
17. Committee opinion Number 80. Washington DC: American College of Obstetricians and Gynecologists, February 1990.
18. Pike MC, Henderson BE, Krailo MD, et al. Breast cancer in young women and use of oral contraceptives: possible modifying effect of formulation and age at risk. Lancet 1983;2:926–930.
19. Meirik O, Adami HO, Christoffersen T, et al. Oral contraceptive use and breast cancer in young women. Lancet 1986;2:650–653.
20. Kay CR, Hannaford PC. Breast cancer and the pill: a further report from the Royal College of General Practitioners' Oral Contraceptive Study. Br J Cancer 1988;58:675.
21. Centers for Disease Control and National Institutes of Child Health and Human Development Cancer and Steroid Hormone Study. Oral contraceptive use and the risk of breast cancer. N Engl J Med 1986;315:405.
22. Centers for Disease Control Cancer and Steroid Hormone Study. Oral contraceptive use and the risk of endometrial cancer. JAMA 1983;249:1600.
23. Centers for Disease Control Cancer and Steroid Hormone Study: Oral contraceptive use and the risk of ovarian cancer. JAMA 1983;249:1596.
24. Bergkvist L, Hans-Olov A, Persson I, et al. The risk of breast cancer after estrogen and estrogen-progestin replacement. N Engl J Med 1989;321:293.
25. Bergkvist L, Hans-Olov A, Persson I, et al. Prognosis after breast cancer diagnosis in women exposed to estrogen and progesterone replacement therapy. Am J Epidemiol 1989;130:221.
26. Gambrell RD Jr. Proposal to decrease the risk and improve the prognosis of breast cancer. Am J Obstet Gynecol 1984;150:119–132.
27. Armstrong BK. Estrogen therapy after the menopause—bone or bane? Med J of Aust 1988;148:213–214.

28. King RM, Welch JS, Martin JK Jr, et al. Carcinoma of the breast associated with pregnancy. Surg Gynecol Obstet 1985;160:228–232.
29. Ribeiro G, Jones DA, Jones M. Carcinoma of the breast associated with pregnancy. Br J Surg 1986;73:607–609.
30. Ravdin RG, Lewison EF, Slack NH, et al. Results of a clinical trial concerning the worth of prophylactic oophorectomy for breast carcinoma. Surg Gynecol Obstet 1970;121:1055–1064.
31. Mathew A, Clabon, AB, Kabakow B, et al. Endometrial carcinoma in five breast cancer patients receiving tamoxifen. Proc Am Soc Clin Oncol Annu Meet 1989;8:95.

12

The Future of Ovarian Hormonal Replacement

Donald P. Swartz

Almost a century has passed since Knauer reported that the changes that followed gonadectomy in experimental animals could be prevented by ovarian transplants (1). By 1935 the chemical structures of the estrogens and of progesterone had been identified, and A. Butenandt was awarded the Nobel prize in chemistry for his synthesis of progesterone (2). Testosterone and its chemical derivatives were understood sufficiently by 1937 that F. C. Koch was able to write an extensive review (3).

The discovery reported in 1938 that pregnant mares' urine contained water-soluble conjugated estrogens in large quantities was the impetus to make available for clinical use the orally active estrogen product known as Premarin (4). The availability of that product stimulated the widespread use of estrogen replacement in women.

During the succeeding 5 decades, the ability to localize the sites of hormonal action through understanding the hormone receptor binding concept has greatly broadened our understanding of the potential importance of the sex steroid hormones in general and of the estrogens in particular in helping to maintain many normal body functions.

No field of study exemplifies this more prominently than the area of greatest current interest, namely, the cardiovascular research area.

A number of reports point to estrogen effects directly upon arterial walls (5). Stumpf has summarized the extensive distribution of estradiol receptor activity in the myocardium and throughout the nervous system (6). Figure 12.1 is a reproduction of Stumpf's in which A-B-C circuitry refers to his concept of allocortex–brain stem–core circuitry of autonomic endocrine integration and regulation. Stumpf continues his review of the present evidence that the neuronal distribution of nuclear estradiol receptors "again indicates a direct involvement of estradiol in autonomic and cardiovascular regulations" (6).

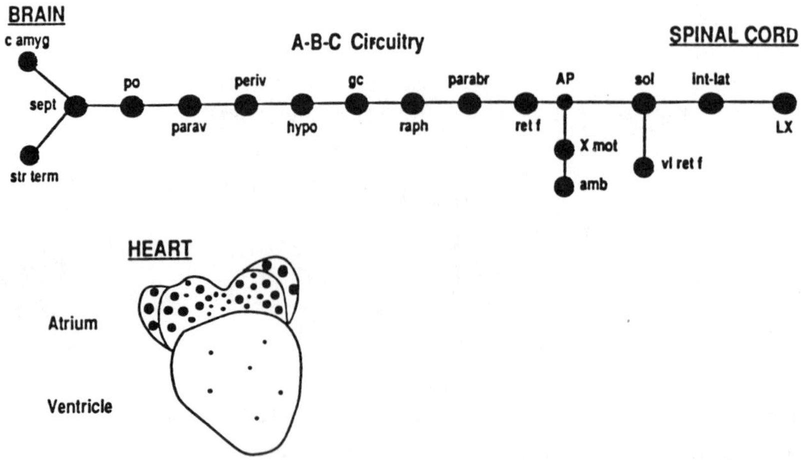

Figure 12.1. Estradiol sites of action in the heart and central neuronal regions involved in the control of cardiovascular functions. In brain and spinal cord, sites implicated in cardiovascular central regulation correspond to those that had been identified earlier as the estradiol-controlled A-B-C(allocortex-brainstem-core) circuitry of endocrine-autonomic integration and regulation. c amyg, nucleus (n.) centralis amygdalae; str term, bednucleus of the stria terminalis; sept, septum; po, preoptic area; parav, n. paraventricularis; peri, n. periventricularis; hypo, hypothalamus; cg, central gray; parabr, n. parabrachialis; ret f, reticular formation; sol, n. tractus solitarii; X mot, dorsal motor nucleus of vagus nerve; ambig, n. ambiguus; int-lat, n. intermediolateralis; LX, lamina X of spinal cord. (From Stumpf WE. Steroid hormones and the cardiovascular system. Direct actions of estradiol, progesterone, testosterone, gluco and mineralocorticoids and soltriol on central nervous regulatory and peripheral tissues. Experientia 1990;46:13.)

The direct vascular effect of normal endogenous estrogen production and of exogenously administered estrogen replacement has long been observed clinically by gynecologic surgeons. The increased vascularity during gynecologic surgery on estrogenized pelvic structures is quite apparent. Semmens et al. (7) and Sarrel (8) have reported confirming quantitative measurements in the vagina and the vulva, respectively. Bourne and his fellow workers claim the first proof in women that the administration of estradiol by the transdermal route reduced the pulsatility index in uterine arteries by 50%. Pulsatility index was measured by intravaginal ultrasound probe and pulsed Doppler and indicated that "estradiol reduces arterial impedance and decreases vascular tone in postmenopausal women" (9). Sarrel has also measured another aspect of the neural effects of estrogen deprivation; namely, decreased vibration

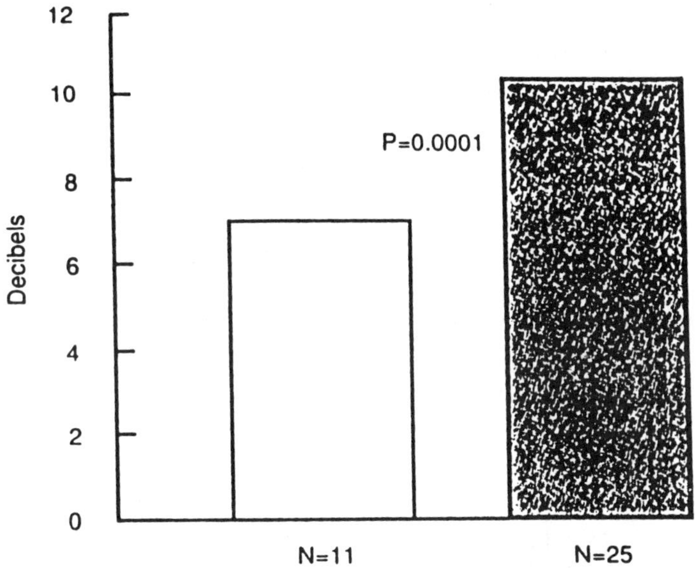

Figure 12.2. Comparison of right thenar vibration threshold in premenopausal (*white bar*) and postmenopausal (*shaded bar*) women, ages 47 to 51 years. (From Sarrel PM. Sexuality and menopause. Obstet Gynecol 1990;4(suppl):27S. Reprinted with permission from The American College of Obstetricians and Gynecologists.)

sense in the estrogen-deficient subject, which improved with estrogen replacement (8) (Figure 12.2).

As the many locations of estrogen receptors have become known, the hypothesis that estrogen may influence cardiovascular function and hence health in diverse ways has been strengthened. With the present large public health focus on the role of cholesterol, both quantitatively and qualitatively, in atherogenesis it was natural for a great deal of attention to be directed toward the effect of exogenous estrogen on cholesterol and its fractions. Current status indicates that, overall, when the dose administered is sufficient to produce a measurable effect on cholesterol, the effect is in the direction currently believed to be beneficial. However, as our knowledge evolves to point in the direction that estrogen can influence cardiovascular function through its effects on many neurovascular control mechanisms as well as possibly by its direct effect on vessels themselves, the effect of exogenous estrogen on cholesterol may be of somewhat less critical importance to the debate surrounding the question, "does exogenous estrogen significantly benefit cardiovascular health in the human female?"

An earlier focus of the benefit of estrogen replacement therapy was on the problem of osteoporosis and its complications, especially of hip and vertebral fracture. The extensive evidence supporting a preventive effect on the rate of loss of bone mineral content (BMC) from the central and appendicular skeleton is discussed in Chapter 3. Although efforts are ongoing to find an effective substitute for estrogen in this role, to date none of those proposed have proved satisfactory (e.g., fluoride, bisphosphonate etidronate, calcitonin) even for the desired effect on bone. The evidence for specific estrogen receptors in bone tissue adds support for the general principle of maintaining an adequate level of circulating estrogen for the maintenance of bone health and at least for the most important years of osteoporosis prevention.

Growing understanding of the multiple sites of estrogen nuclear receptors—especially in the neurovascular control centers and vascular structures—will likely argue strongly for the use of estrogen replacement therapy in clinical practice in the forseeable future, even if, for example, a new substance specifically effective in preventing osteoporosis might be developed. The same conclusion seems probable if biochemists succeed in synthesizing new drugs with specific serum cholesterol benefits without present disadvantages.

Current discussions regarding *which women* should receive estrogen replacement generally emphasize that *not all* women need replacement hormonal therapy. But the indicators of need are not defined clearly. Lindsay has provided data to support estrogen prescription according to BMC determinations insofar as the osteoporosis indication is concerned (see Chapter 3). But the neurological and cardiovascular aspects of our knowledge will most certainly undergo significant advances in the coming decade. Other aspects such as healthy sleep, energy, skin health, libido, depression, and that mysterious state of "well being" are all extremely difficult to study and quantitate. Will the dosage of hormone replacement currently in vogue require change? Current dosage is based very largely on the quantity of estrogen required to prevent the acceleration of loss of BMC at the time of withdrawal of exogenous gonadal estrogen production by oophorectomy. If one wishes to prescribe an estrogen dose that will both lower LDL cholesterol and elevate HDL cholesterol more effectively, the present popular dose of estrogen may need to be increased (9) (see Table 7.3). Product, mode of administration and dosage will continue to occupy research attention. It can be argued that the most "physiologic" replacement program currently available is the continuous transdermal administration of 17β-estradiol and sequential oral microcrystalline progesterone for 12 to 14 days monthly. Presumably, with the growing experience with subcutaneous implant progestin for contraception, a similar subcutaneous implant system for 17β-estradiol may become an option. With any route of estrogen administration (oral, transdermal, or implant) it may be possible to demonstrate that it is safe to administer sequential progesterone or progestins less frequently than monthly and possibly derive more constant and maximum estrogenic cardiovascular benefit. However, data available thus far suggests that oral progesterone may not diminish at least the cholesterol benefit effect of estrogen, as the weight of evidence indicates is the case with many synthetic oral progestins. Newer synthetic progestins may be marketed that may diminish or eliminate such benefit reductions.

In the ongoing discussion regarding indications and contraindications for hormone replacement therapy, the woman who has been treated for breast cancer presents a special dilemma. Because approximately one of nine women will develop this malignancy, they represent a very large population. Since many breast cancers are estrogen receptor positive and since all of the most common histologic types respond to some degree to hormonal manipulation, there exists an almost universal fear of prescribing a potent growth factor such as estrogen to the breast cancer positive patient. And yet many of these women are extremely symptomatic either from the vasomotor symptomatology or their vaginal atrophy. Considering the rapid evolution of our knowledge supporting a neurocardiovascular benefit of exogenous estrogen and the absence of proof that low-dose replacement estrogen therapy to the breast cancer patient is detrimental to long-term prognosis, one may look ahead to one of two possible resolutions of this dilemma:

1. Especially as the cardiovascular and possibly neurological benefits become clearer and more firmly established, it may be possible to structure a double-blind prospective study entering volunteer women with breast cancer who are presented in full the comfort, osteoporosis, neural, and cardiovascular benefits of estrogen replacement against the relatively unknown hypothesis of risk. It is highly plausible that well-informed women may choose to participate either in a double-blind prospective study or at least in a prospective evaluation of those who choose to use estrogen vs. those who choose on the basis of the same information not to use estrogen.
2. The alternative clinical development may be that if current directions of osteoporosis, neural, and cardiovascular benefits continue to be confirmed, more physicians will decide that it is appropriate and ethical clinical practice to present the data as objectively as possible to the newly

treated breast cancer woman and follow her personal wishes and direction with respect to prescription of hormonal replacement rather than declining to do so as is currently the majority philosophy.

The development of newer methodology for providing vaginal lubrication has assisted the breast cancer woman greatly, and nonhormonal agents that may be more effective in controlling vasomotor symptomatology could evolve and could also significantly alleviate that aspect of the breast cancer woman's symptoms.

The evolving philosophy with respect to the potential place of the addition of testosterone in hormonal replacement therapy is discussed in Chapter 10. The coming decade should add a great deal to the understanding of the role of testosterone and the possible selection of patients who may benefit most from its inclusion in a replacement program.

The current majority practice of prescribing estrogen-only replacement therapy to the ovarian-deficient woman whose uterus has been removed developed because of the demonstrated ability of the synthetic oral progestins to reduce the cholesterol benefit of an estrogen-only prescription (10). An early differing view promulgated by Gambrell (11) argued for the sequential prescription of estrogen and progestin to derive a reduction in breast cancer incidence. While the claimed reduction in breast cancer has not been substantiated, the expanding use of oral microcrystalline progesterone in lieu of synthetic progestins does not appear to reduce the cholesterol benefit of estrogen-only prescription. It may be anticipated that this decade of research will gather evidence to clarify whether continuous estrogen alone or continuous estrogen together with sequential microcrystalline progesterone is the more beneficial and physiologic replacement program for all women or whether women without a uterus should continue an estrogen-only replacement prescription.

The next decade will almost certainly witness an increased emphasis, especially from adolescence onward, on the aspects of personal health practice that can minimize future osteoporosis risks—such as appropriate nutrition (including adequate calcium intake) and weight-bearing exercise—and that can reduce atherosclerosis development and progression by following new dietary guidelines. Also, it seems reasonable to expect that the decade will witness significant expansion of knowledge regarding the proper place of exogenous steroid sex hormone replacement in women with decreased or absent ovarian function. The study of the balance between the risks and benefits of ovarian hormonal replacement therapy will continue to occupy major research attention. It is to be hoped that if the best replacement prescription that can be devised poses any significant risk—especially in the direction of increasing breast cancer—researchers may be able to quantify it accurately, and if not, that convincing evidence of its safety may be accumulated and disseminated widely.

References

1. Knauer R. Die Overientransplantation. Arch Gynaekol 1900;60:322.
2. Butenandt A. Progynon a crystalline female sexual hormone. Naturwissenschaften 1929; 17:879.
3. Koch FC. Male sex hormones. Physiol Rev 1937;17:153.
4. Schachter B, Marrian GF. Isolation of estrone sulfate from the urine of pregnant mares. J Biol Chem 1938;126:663–666.
5. Fischer GM, Bashey RI, Rosenbaum H, Lyttle CRA. A possible mechanism in arterial wall for mediation of sex difference in atherosclerosis. Exp Mol Pathol 1985;43:288.
6. Stumpf, WE. Steroid hormones and the cardiovascular system—direct actions of estradiol, progesterone, testosterone, glucocorticoids, mineral corticoids, and soltriol on central nervous regulatory and peripheral tissues. Experientia 1990;46:13.
7. Semmens JP, Wagner G. Estrogen deprivation and vaginal function in postmenopausal women. JAMA 1982;248:445.
8. Sarrel P. Effects of ovarian steroids on the cardiovascular system. In: Ginsberg J, ed. The circulation in the female from the cradle to the grave. U.K.: Carnforth, Parthenon Publishing, 1989:117–140.
9. Bourne T et al. Oestrogens, arterial status and postmenopausal women. Lancet 1990;335:1470.
10. Sherwin BB, Gelfand MM. A prospective one-year study of estrogen and progestin in postmenopausal women: effects on clinical symptoms and lipoprotein lipids. Obstet Gynecol 1989;73:759–766.
11. Gambrell RD, Maier RC, Sanders B. Decreased incidence of breast cancer in postmenopausal estrogen-progestogen users. Obstet Gynecol 1983;62:435.

Index

Page numbers followed by "f" denote figures; those followed by "t" denote tables.